EPIDERMAL WOUND HEALING

THIS BOOK IS BASED ON A CONFERENCE SPONSORED BY

THE DEPARTMENT OF DERMATOLOGY, UNIVERSITY OF CALIFORNIA

SCHOOL OF MEDICINE, SAN FRANCISCO,

THE DEPARTMENT OF CONTINUING EDUCATION, HEALTH SCIENCES,

UNIVERSITY OF CALIFORNIA, SAN FRANCISCO

and

JOHNSON & JOHNSON RESEARCH

held at

Pebble Beach, California

Epidermal
Wound Healing

Edited by

HOWARD I. MAIBACH, M.D.

*Associate Professor and Vice-Chairman, Department of Dermatology,
University of California School of Medicine, San Francisco, California*

and

DAVID T. ROVEE, Ph.D.

*Department of Skin Biology, Johnson & Johnson Research,
New Brunswick, New Jersey*

YEAR BOOK MEDICAL PUBLISHERS, INC.

35 EAST WACKER DRIVE • CHICAGO

Library of Congress Catalog Card Number: 73-183581

International Standard Book Number: 0-8151-5730-4

Contributors

ROBERT E. BAIER, PH.D., *Head, Chemical Sciences Section, Cornell Aeronautical Laboratory of Cornell University, Buffalo, New York; Research Assistant Professor of Biophysics, State University of New York at Buffalo, New York*

ALAN E. BEER, M.D., *Department of Cell Biology, The University of Texas Southwestern Medical School at Dallas, Dallas, Texas*

S. N. BHASKAR, D.D.S., M.S., PH.D., *Col. DC, Director, United States Army Institute of Dental Research, Walter Reed Army Medical Center, Washington, D.C.*

R. E. BILLINGHAM, D.SC., *Department of Cell Biology, The University of Texas Southwestern Medical School at Dallas, Dallas, Texas*

JAMES W. BOTHWELL, PH.D., *Department of Skin Biology, Johnson & Johnson Research, New Brunswick, New Jersey*

ENNO CHRISTOPHERS, M.D., *Department of Dermatology, University of Munich, München, Germany*

STANLEY COHEN, PH.D., *Department of Biochemistry, Vanderbilt University School of Medicine, Nashville, Tennessee*

ANNE MARIE DOWNES, B.A., *Department of Skin Biology, Johnson & Johnson Research, New Brunswick, New Jersey*

PETER M. ELIAS, M.D., *Dermatology Branch, National Cancer Institute, National Institutes of Health, Bethesda, Maryland*

LOUIS B. FISHER, PH.D., *Research Fellow, Division of Dermatology, Scripps Clinic and Research Foundation, La Jolla, California*

PATRICIA A. FLANAGAN, R.N., B.A., *Department of Skin Biology, Johnson & Johnson Research, New Brunswick, New Jersey*

JOSE GARCIA-VELASCO, M.D., *Department of Plastic and Reconstructive Surgery, Hospital General Centro Médico Nacional, Instituto Mexicano del Seguro Social, Mexico City, Mexico*

RICHARD J. GOSS, PH.D., *Division of Biological and Medical Sciences, Brown University, Providence, Rhode Island*

MAJOR DAVID R. HARRIS, M.D., M.C., U.S.A., *Division of Dermatology, Letterman Army Institute of Research, Presidio of San Francisco, California*

THOMAS K. HUNT, M.D., *Associate Professor of Surgery, University of California (San Francisco) School of Medicine, San Francisco, California*

ALBERT M. KLIGMAN, M.D., PH.D., *Professor of Dermatology, University of Pennsylvania School of Medicine, Philadelphia, Pennsylvania*

WALTER S. KRAWCZYK, D.D.S., *Department of Oral Histopathology and Periodontology, School of Dental Medicine, Harvard University, and Department of Dermatologic Genetics, New England Medical Center Hospitals, Boston, Massachusetts*

CAROLE A. KUROWSKY, R.N., *Department of Skin Biology, Johnson & Johnson Research, New Brunswick, New Jersey*

JOAN LABUN, *Department of Skin Biology, Johnson & Johnson Research, New Brunswick, New Jersey*

IAN C. MACKENZIE, PH.D., F.D.S., R.C.S., B.D.S., *Research Fellow, Department of Oral Pathology, London Hospital Medical College, London, England*

HOWARD I. MAIBACH, M.D., *Associate Professor, Department of Dermatology, University of California (San Francisco) School of Medicine, San Francisco, California*

RICHARD R. MARPLES, B.M., M.Sc., MRCPATH., *Assistant Professor of (Research) Dermatology, University of Pennsylvania School of Medicine, Philadelphia, Pennsylvania*

I. RICARDO MARTINEZ, JR., M.D., PH.D., *Department of Dermatology, Ochsner Clinic and Ochsner Foundation Hospital; Clinical Assistant Professor of Dermatology and Anatomy, Louisiana State University Medical Center, New Orleans, Louisiana*

WILLIAM MONTAGNA, PH.D., *Director, Oregon Regional Primate Research Center, Beaverton, Oregon; Professor and Head, Division of Experimental Biology, University of Oregon Medical School, Portland, Oregon*

GARY L. PECK, M.D., *Dermatology Branch, National Cancer Institute, National Institutes of Health, Bethesda, Maryland*

NINA TYLER POLLARD, PH.D., *Clinical Associate in Surgery, University of Louisville School of Medicine, Louisville, Kentucky*

DAVID T. ROVEE, PH.D., *Department of Skin Biology, Johnson & Johnson Research, New Brunswick, New Jersey*

I. A. SILVER, M.A., M.R.C.V.S., *Professor of Comparative Pathology, University of Bristol, Bristol, England*

HAROLD C. SLAVKIN, D.D.S., *Chairman and Associate Professor, Department of Biochemistry, School of Dentistry, and Associate Professor, Graduate Program in Cellular and Molecular Biology, University of Southern California, Los Angeles, California*

DAVID SPRUIT, PH.D., *Department of Dermatology, University of Nijmegen, The Netherlands*

JOHN M. TAYLOR, PH.D., *Department of Biochemistry, Vanderbilt University School of Medicine, Nashville, Tennessee*

NORTON G. WATERMAN, M.D., *Associate Clinical Professor of Surgery, University of Louisville School of Medicine, Health Sciences Center, Louisville, Kentucky*

GEORGE D. WINTER, PH.D., *Department of Biomedical Engineering, Institute of Orthopaedics (University of London), Royal National Orthopaedic Hospital, Brockley Hill, Stanmore, Middlesex, England*

LT. JERRY R. YOUKEY, M.S.C., U.S.A., *Division of Dermatology, Letterman Army Institute of Research, Presidio of San Francisco, California*

Preface

Interest in wound healing has increased tremendously during the last decade as is clearly evidenced by the voluminous literature on wound healing research. Many texts have focused on the dermal problems of surgical wound repair, but the status of research into the problems of epidermal healing has not been presented. To facilitate the collection and coordination of data in this important aspect of healing, a number of international investigators in this area was assembled for a conference at Pebble Beach, California in the fall of 1971. This volume includes contributions by each of the speakers at the conference—chapters which were specially prepared for publication and reflect the latest findings on this problem.

The contributions, although they do deal primarily with findings relative to the epidermis, do not ignore the dermal aspects. Important questions of dermal-epidermal interactions are reviewed and discussed. The scope of the volume includes topics such as maintenance and differentiation of intact skin, processes of repair following disruption of epidermal continuity, and clinical applications of some of the recent findings. The disciplines involved ranged from the basic sciences of biology, experimental embryology and surface chemistry to clinical fields of dermatology, surgery, plastic surgery and dentistry. The editors hope that this presentation of information from different fields with varying vocabularies and approaches will lead to cross-fertilization of ideas and mutual advances. The basic sciences have and are producing much information that is not being applied to clinical aspects of wound healing. Many basic scientists have failed to appreciate the value of relatively simple models of wound healing (such as the linear wound in the skin) for studying critical problems in biology such as differentiation and neoplasia.

This collection of papers from noted workers in the field of epidermal biology will provide a useful reference and guide to students of wound healing. It will be clear from reading the papers that there are controversies in the interpretations of data, and that many fruitful areas of research remain open. Some readers may be surprised at how little firm data is available to aid in making recommendations for the treatment of even minor epidermal wounds. These position papers provide the basis for experiments that should provide practical solutions in this area.

The editors wish to thank the Department of Continuing Medical Education of the University of California Medical Center in San Francisco and Johnson & Johnson in New Brunswick, New Jersey for co-sponsoring the meetings. We also acknowledge the help of Drs. Rupert Billingham, J. E. Dunphy, Seymour Farber, Thomas Hunt, and William Montagna in planning the program and at the scientific sessions, and Misses Sadie Kaye and Eleanor Hahn for administering the details of the Symposium.

HOWARD I. MAIBACH
DAVID T. ROVEE

Contents

Part V. Physical and Chemical Factors Affecting Repair

Part VI. Supplementary Reports

Part I

Cellular Facets of Wound Repair

Introduction

William Montagna, Ph.D. *

Somewhere in the world at least one conference a year is devoted to wound healing. Most of these meetings, with rare exceptions, deal with the healing of skin and usually disregard the other organs which perform this feat with greater dispatch than skin. Perhaps because of their very redundancy, these conferences divulge little that is new; most of the material, unfortunately, is a dull repetition of previous observations, much of it lacking even a new twist or slant. Surely we have looked at the same things in the same way for too long. In this era when ultrastructure and ultramicrochemistry have made such giant strides, it is unthinkable that we still lack knowledge about gross structural patterns in the epidermis. Mackenzie's description of precisely ordered structural units disproves our former beliefs that epidermal cells rise to the surface in a casual, first-come basis. He has elegantly and ingeniously shown that these ordered structural units involve not only the keratinocytes but also the still enigmatic Langerhans cells. This is an enormously important observation that will give a progressively better and different perspective of the epidermis under normal and abnormal conditions. Now, because of our awareness of these architectural patterns, the epidermis, particularly where it is very thick and the structural units are not clearly seen, should be vigorously reinvestigated.

Together with different approaches to the study of structure, new methods must be brought to bear on the study of the interaction of adjacent epithelial cells. If cells are to maintain their integrity, they must have chemical communication with their neighbors. The chemical entities that enable cells to express surface specificity in response to their environment are now being studied with fresh new approaches. Baier's painstaking assessment of cell surface specificity is only the beginning. The two articles that follow may well have launched us into a deeper understanding of the biology of the epidermis. Once we understand its normal behavior, what happens during its healing will no longer puzzle us.

*Director, Oregon Regional Primate Center, Beaverton, Oregon.

3

1

The Ordered Structure of Mammalian Epidermis

Ian C. MacKenzie, Ph.D. *

The stratum corneum of the epidermis consists of a number of layers of extremely flattened keratinized cells. Recently it has been shown that, in mammalian epidermis, these flattened keratinizing cells tend to be stacked, one above the other, to form columns of cells which run from the stratum spinosum to the surface [1, 2]. This ordered structure is seldom apparent from an examination of sections of wax imbedded specimens of skin but it can be demonstrated by treating frozen sections of unfixed specimens of skin with dilute alkali to expand the stratum corneum [3]. There appear to be two principal reasons for the inability to visualize this order in normal preparations. First, the insults of fixation, dehydration and imbedding produce varying degrees of shrinkage and distortion of structure. Second, the individual squames of the stratum corneum, in which the pattern is most clearly seen, are rarely visible with the light microscope because they are closely packed and usually less than 1 μm in thickness. The method originally described for expansion of the stratum corneum [3] results in the destruction of the deeper layers of the epidermis. Modifications of the technique to preserve the stratum Malpighii have allowed the ordered structure of the stratum corneum to be related to the position of cell division [4] and the position of cell migration [2, 5]. Examination of tissues by electron microscopy also provides some information about the spatial relationship between cells both in the stratum corneum [6] and the stratum Malpighii.

In this chapter we will present a general description of the ordered structure of mammalian skin, mention briefly techniques which have been used in its study and speculate about the mechanisms by which ordered structure is established and maintained.

THE ORDERED STRUCTURE OF THE STRATUM CORNEUM

Treatment of cryostat sections of frozen, unfixed skin with an aqueous 0.1 M sodium hydroxide solution destroys most of the epidermis except for the cell boundaries of the keratinized cells of the stratum corneum. The alkali also

*Department of Oral Pathology, London Hospital Medical College, London, England.

causes the stratum corneum to swell to several times its original width and, as it swells, the outlines of the individual horny cells become visible to the light microscope (Fig. 1-1). A similar expansion of the stratum corneum is also produced by dilute acids. The cell boundaries which are seen after expansion appear to correspond chemically to the acid and alkali resistant cell envelope described by Matoltsy [7] and morphologically to the marginal band seen with the electron microscope [8]. A tendency for squames to be arranged into columns, appears to

Fig. 1–1 (top).—Hamster ear epidermis expanded in sodium hydroxide. Phase contrast, scale = 30 μm. The deeper epidermal strata have been destroyed by the alkali but the outlines of the individual squames of the expanded stratum corneum are visible. These squames are aligned to form columns of cells running from the stratum granulosum (below) to the surface. *Arrows* point to the regular step-like interdigitation of squames at the lateral junctions of columns.

Fig. 1–2 (bottom).—**A**, hamster ear epidermis prepared as for Figure 1–1. Part way through the stratum corneum a sudden break in the alignment of the lateral junctions of columns (*arrows*) is seen. The stratum corneum has fractured along the lateral boundary of the column above and to the left. Scale = 30 μm. **B**, stratum corneum of human plantar epidermis prepared as for Figure 1–1. Squames are not aligned and show a greater degree of expansion. Scale = 60 μm.

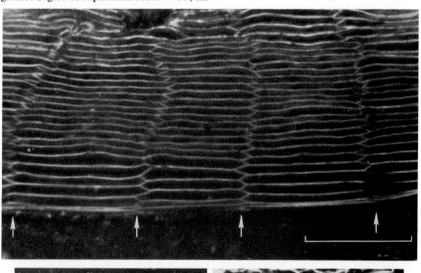

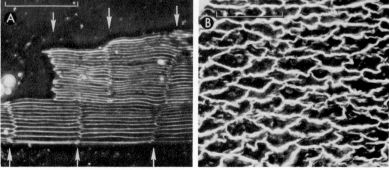

be typical of most mammalian epidermis except for specialized areas such as palmar and plantar surfaces.

The most precisely ordered stacking of squames is seen in a thin epidermis such as that covering the pinnae of rodents. After expansion with alkali, the stratum corneum of such tissues appears as a closely united assembly of squames in which individual squames lie one above the other to form columns of cells running from the stratum granulosum to the surface (Fig. 1-1). Within each column squames are in contact, for the greater part of their width, only with the squames immediately above and that below. Laterally, where squames of adjacent columns meet, there is a slight overlap and each squame interdigitates with its neighbors to produce a regular step like pattern. Usually these regions of lateral interdigitation maintain a vertical alignment throughout the thickness of the stratum corneum but occasionally a sudden break in the alignment of a group of squames may occur (Fig. 1-2A).

There is some variation with respect to both species and site in the regularity of positioning of individual squames and in the degree of their lateral interdigitation. Primate epidermis, whether from man or monkey, seldom demonstrates an order as precise as that seen in rodents; usually squames show a greater and more variable degree of overlap (Fig. 1-3). The stratum corneum of plantar and palmar surfaces and of the foot pads of rodents is thicker than that of other body regions, expands more readily in dilute acidic or alkaline solutions, and does not show an ordered arrangement of squames (Fig. 1-2B). Oral mucosa shows marked regional variations of keratinization [9] and fully keratinized regions such as the rodent palate and hamster cheek pouch are difficult to expand with sodium hydroxide. On the other hand the keratinized buccal mucosa of rodents, which has features in common with nonkeratinized human buccal mucosa [9], expands very readily. An ordered arrangement of squames has not so far been demonstrated in oral mucosa.

The lateral junctions of the squames of the stratum corneum may be studied in greater detail by electron microscopy. The methods of preparation of specimens for electron microscopy usually result in some separation of squames and perhaps loss of the most superficial cell layers but, if sections are cut at right angles to the epithelial surface and if a sufficiently large area of tissue is examined, a columnar arrangement of squames can be demonstrated (Fig. 1-4). When mouse ear epidermis is examined in this way, the junctional region of interdigitation between squames of adjacent columns is more complicated than the appearance of expanded sections suggests. For the greater part of their width squames show a simple, relatively flat profile but laterally, where they contact the squames of neighboring columns, a number of projections and depressions are found which complement those of the abutting squames and appear to lock the assembly together in a jigsaw like fashion (Fig. 1-5A). A step like depression of the superficial margin of cells is often seen [6] but occasionally cells abut end to end with very little overlap or bifurcate to join with two adjacent squames. Specimens prepared for electron microscopy also show that the flattened cells of the stratum granulosum and upper stratum spinosum are aligned beneath the columns in the stratum corneum (Fig. 1-5A).

Sections of skin provide only a two-dimensional picture of the structure of the stratum corneum. A three-dimensional concept can be obtained by relating

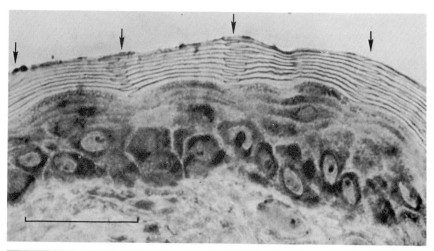

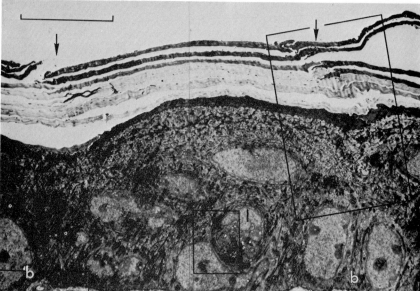

Fig. 1–3 (top).—Epidermis of thorax of monkey. Scale = 30 μm. The cells of the granular and spinous layers are aligned beneath columns of squames in the stratum corneum (lateral junctions are *arrowed*). There is a deeper and less regular interdigitation between the squames of adjacent columns than is found in rodent epidermis (Fig. 1–6).

Fig. 1–4 (bottom).—Electromicrograph of mouse ear epidermis. Scale = 10 μm. The junctions of the squames of the stratum corneum are aligned (*arrows*) and the basement membrane is indented beneath the junctional region (*b*). A Langerhans cell (*l*) lies beneath the center of the column.

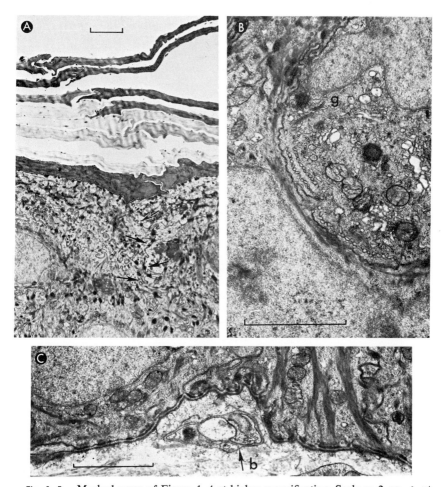

Fig. 1–5.—Marked areas of Figure 1–4 at higher magnification. Scale = 2 μm. **A,** at their lateral junctions the interdigitating squames show a number of small projections which appear to lock them together in a jigsaw-like fashion. The lateral borders of the cells of the spinous and granular layers (*arrows*) are aligned with the junctions of squames. **B,** the Langerhans cell contains a Langerhans granule (*g*) and shows considerable vesicular activity at the cell margins. **C,** beneath a lateral junction of the overlying column a small nerve, surrounded by a basal lamina (*b*), lies close to the epidermis within a dermal projection.

the appearance of sections of skin to the surface morphology of squames studied either after stripping with adhesive tape or after staining intact unsectioned sheets of epidermis. It has been shown [10] that squames are flattened discs with an irregularly polygonal, frequently hexagonal, outline. The junctions between squames are well demonstrated by staining sheets of epidermis, separated from the dermis by the action of EDTA, with suitable silver impregnation techniques [11]. This method has the advantage that the regularity of the alignment of

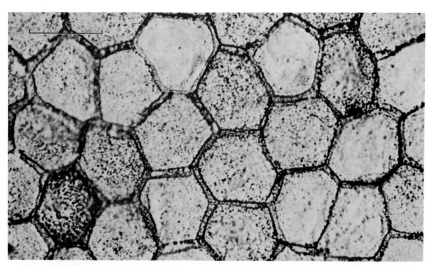

Fig. 1–6.—Squames of a sheet of mouse ear epidermis stained by silver impregnation. Scale = 30 μm. The polygonal, typically hexagonal, outlines of the columns of squames are seen. The region of interdigitation between columns appears as a band lying parallel to the boundaries of the columns.

squames into columns and their degree of overlap may be observed throughout the full thickness of the stratum corneum by changing the plane of focus of the microscope. In mouse ear epidermis, although there is some variation of polygonal outline from column to column (Fig. 1-6), all the squames of a particular column are found to have a very similar outline shape. The junctions between adjacent columns are remarkably straight and the regions of overlap appear as parallel bands running around each column. Scanning electron microscopy of squames [6] has shown that this area of overlap may form a steplike depression.

ORDERED STRUCTURE BELOW THE STRATUM CORNEUM

The existence of a regular columnar arrangement of the fully keratinized squames of the stratum corneum raises the question of how this pattern is established and at which level in the stratum Malpighii alignment first occurs. It was not until after the ordered structure of the stratum corneum had been observed in frozen sections, that a regular pattern in the contour of the stratum corneum and an alignment of the nuclei of the granular and spinous layers, both of which are apparent in many specimens, was detected in normal histological preparations of mouse ear epidermis even though this tissue had been examined previously on many occasions. To permit a study of cell position within the stratum Malpighii, the original alkali expansion technique was modified. A brief fixation of frozen sections slightly reduces expansion of the stratum corneum in acidic or alkaline solutions but has the advantage that it greatly reduces damage to the stratum Malpighii and allows sections to be stained prior to expansion. Cryostat sections were cut at approximately 4μm, collected on coverslips and fixed for 5

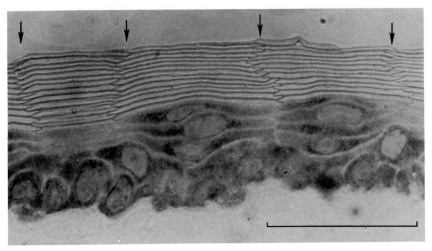

Fig. 1–7.—Hamster ear epidermis following staining in methylene blue and expansion. Scale = 30 μm. Suprabasal cells are aligned beneath columns of squames in the stratum corneum (lateral junctions are *arrowed*). To the left the plane of section passes through the periphery of a column.

minutes in 70% ethanol. Sections were then either stained for 2 minutes in 0.5% aqueous methylene blue prior to expansion in 0.1 M NaOH, or expanded in 0.5% methylene blue acidified to pH 3.5 with HCl.

In a thin epidermis, such as that of the rodent ear, almost all suprabasal cells are found to be flattened and aligned beneath overlying columns of squames (Fig. 1-7). The basal cells, which are considerably smaller than the overlying squames, showed no precise positioning. In a thicker epidermis, flattening and alignment beneath columns is found only in the 4 or 5 cell layers forming the stratum granulosum and upper stratum spinosum. No order is apparent in the spinous cells beneath this level or in the basal cells (Fig. 1-3).

THE ESTABLISHMENT OF ORDERED STRUCTURE

The mechanisms which produce a polygonal outline and regular stacking of squames within the stratum corneum are, at present, uncertain. It is clear that when an ordered epidermal structure is found, alignment is first seen in the flattening cells of the stratum spinosum some three to five cell layers beneath the stratum corneum but it is not clear whether alignment is first established at this level by mutual cell pressures developed during keratinization or by cell contact phenomena or whether cell alignment is the first morphological evidence of ordered activity at a deeper level.

An alignment of the flattened cells of the stratum corneum does not appear to be explained by any current concept of the behavior of epidermal cells and an attempt to explain its establishment serves principally to emphasize how little information is available to serve as a basis for speculation. A complete explanation of the mechanism by which ordered structure is established should presumably be able to account not only for its presence at most epidermal sites, but also for its absence from plantar and palmar epidermis and from other sites after damage.

Briefly, the events which occur during the establishment of a columnar structure may be described as follows: cells are formed by division in the basal layer and ascend into the stratum spinosum where, at a level which varies with epidermal thickness, by flattening and moving laterally in relation to the cells below, they become vertically aligned and form columns of flattened cells which have, within a particular column, a closely similar polygonal outline form.

Hexagonal close packing of cells is often found in both plant and animal tissues. Examples of its occurrence and a discussion of the principles governing its establishment were given, over fifty years ago, by D'Arcy Thompson [12]. When uniformly sized, circular discs are packed closely together in the same plane the six points of contact of each disc flatten and each disc tends to assume a hexagonal outline. Hexagonal packing can be demonstrated quite simply by blowing uniformly sized bubbles into the surface of soapy water. The polygonal outlines which are formed (Fig. 1-8A) have a similar appearance, to the stained outline of squames of sheets of stratum corneum (Fig. 1-6). However, the same model also demonstrates that simple physical packing does not produce a vertical alignment similar to that of the stratum corneum because, when a second layer of bubbles is blown beneath the first, a fairly regular overlap of half the diameter of a bubble is formed (Fig. 1-8B). Even apart from this inability to account for vertical alignment, an analogy between the formation of polygonal columns of squames and the mechanical packing together of circular bodies [6] is inaccurate in other ways. Squames are not originally flat circular bodies which only subsequently become compressed into a polygonal shape. Rather they should be considered as bodies, initially of relatively small area, which expand laterally to

Fig. 1–8.—**A**, bubbles packed together on the surface of water. A hexagonal outline similar to that of columns of squames (Fig. 1–6) is produced. **B**, unlike squames, which become vertically aligned, a second layer of bubbles blown beneath the first has a regular overlap of half the diameter of a bubble (see text).

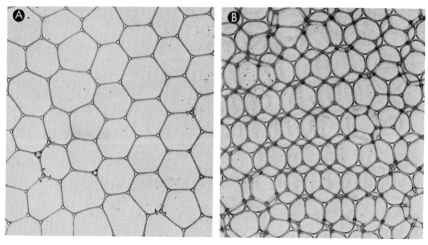

acquire a polygonal shape as the result of an inhibition of lateral expansion in certain directions by a lack of space or by some other factors. It is perhaps in the factors producing and controlling the lateral expansion which results in flattening that a mechanism for the establishment of alignment should be sought.

It is not clear how a relationship between cell population pressure and cell movement is affected by the presence of desmosomes at the cell interfaces. In order that lateral expansion of cells may take place it is necessary that desmosomal contact should be broken and reestablished but the presence of an alignment of cells into columns does not, in this respect, set any more problems about the nature of the desmosome than arise from the occurrence of lateral expansion in nonordered epithelial tissues, from a differential rate of movement of epithelial cells toward the surface [13] or from the rapid passage of inflammatory cells across epithelia [14]. It has been shown that desmosomes act as areas of attachment between epithelial cells [15] but it is clear that a suggestion of desmosomal stability based on their ultrastructural appearance would be at variance with the observed movement of epidermal cells [16]. Disruption and reformation of desmosomes within 72 hours has been observed after epidermal damage [17] but the way in which cell attachments are lost and reestablished during the normal turnover of epidermal cells is not known. However, some idea of the rate at which membrane changes normally occur in the flattening cells of an undamaged epithelium can be obtained from estimates of the increase in cell area and the rate of cell turnover. In mouse ear epidermis, cells flatten immediately after leaving the basal layer to cover an area equivalent to that occupied by 10 basal cells [4] and in so doing increase their surface area threefold. Since the turnover time of the basal layer is about 20 days [18], a new cell is added to each column every two days. Therefore, it appears that in less than 48 hours cells completely readjust their surface relationship to other cells and synthesize over double their original complement of plasma membrane and desmosomes.

The mechanism by which cell flattening and an increase in cell area occur during keratinization is unclear. Cells show a great increase in volume and in dry weight during their passage from the basal to the granular layers but their volume, and to a lesser extent their dry weight, decreases on entering the stratum corneum [19]. Dehydration is probably a factor associated with some of the reduction in cell volume which occurs during keratinization but it appears unlikely that dehydration can account for the lateral movement between adjacent cells which is necessarily associated with cell flattening if an increase in cell area is to occur. Furthermore, in a thin epidermis, lateral expansion of cells and the establishment of cell columns occur immediately after cells leave the basal layer (Fig. 1-7) and apparently while cells are still increasing in volume. It has been suggested [20] that an enhancement of intercellular adhesion may, during hair formation, play an active role in molding the shape of cells and that an area of contact between two epidermal cells, by spreading in a zipper like fashion, could produce relative movement and cell flattening [21]. Branson [22] described orthogonal arrays of microtubules in flattening cells of the granular layer of newborn rat epidermis and suggested that their presence was associated with the changes in cell shape occurring at this level. Although the mechanism is uncertain, the finding that flattening occurs during the keratinization of cells of small cultured outgrowths of epidermis [23] suggests that the ability to flatten is an active property of individual epithelial cells rather than the result of cell population pressure.

Christophers [5] has suggested that maintenance of alignment of cells into columns may depend upon the effects on cell flattening of the rate or sequence of addition of cells to adjoining columns. A cell which has flattened into line beneath a particular column lies below cells previously added to the adjacent columns and therefore interdigitates beneath them forming a step like boundary at its lateral margins (Fig. 1-9). When the next cell which is to flatten moves up from below, the presence of this step may tend to guide it away or limit its bilateral expansion into, the territory of the first column. This cell therefore flattens into line beneath an adjacent column and, since after flattening it lies slightly below the first column, it reestablishes a step which determines the position of further cell addition. Although a repetition of this sequence can be sustained with a two-dimensional model, when the third dimension is considered it is apparent that each column has not two, but five or six boundaries; it would require a regular and rather complex sequential addition of squames to a group of columns to result in each column being bounded in turn. The problem of explaining such a sequence in terms of a deflection of ascending cells by the presence of differing numbers of flattened cells in overlying columns, makes it difficult to interpret the establishment of columnar structure solely in terms of physical interference between flattening cells. The establishment of columnar structure may be explained, without involving

Fig. 1–9.—Diagram of cell flattening and alignment. **Top,** in vertical section, the relative age of cells can be determined by the sequence of their addition to columns which is indicated numerically. The cells last added to columns lie slightly below previously flattened cells (*3*) and at their lateral borders, form a step which may tend to limit the lateral expansion of subsequently flattening cells (*5*). During flattening cell 5 must break the junctions between cell *3* and cells *X*. **Bottom,** a surface view of cell flattening: for cell alignment to occur the lateral expansion of cell *5* is arrested at the borders of six previously flattened cells (*4*). For further explanation see text.

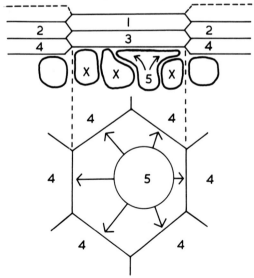

cell pressures or a sequential addition of cells, as the result of an inhibition of lateral expansion of flattening cells by the junctions between previously aligned cells [(Fig. 1-9). However, while there is a considerable body of evidence for a contact inhibition of movement between sheets of cultured epidermal cells and between epidermal cells during wound healing [24], a selective contact inhibition of movement between cells of an intact epithelium does not appear to have been considered and no experimental evidence can be cited to support this suggestion. If contact inhibition is to account for cell alignment, the lateral movement of flattening cells between junctions involving nonflattened cells (Fig. 1-9) makes it necessary to postulate that inhibition of lateral expansion occurs only at the junctions of cells which are more mature than those which are in the process of flattening.

The maintenance of columnar structure appears to depend on a slow rate of formation and maturation of epidermal cells. In this context, maturation is taken to imply the changes occurring in a cell as it passes toward the fully keratinized state. An increased mitotic rate is associated with an increase in the rate of cell maturation and entry into the stratum corneum [25, 26]. The most precisely ordered stacking of squames is found in epidermis from regions such as the rodent ear in which the mitotic rate is normally relatively low [18]. In tissues with a somewhat higher mitotic rate, such as the general body epidermis, the pattern tends to be less regular. Plantar and palmar epidermis have a high turnover [27] and show no evidence of column formation. A relationship between a low mitotic rate and the formation of columns is suggested by the finding that stacking of squames is lost from guinea pig ear epidermis during the period of increased mitotic activity which follows Scotch tape stripping but that it is reestablished after about 10 days when the rate of cell regeneration has returned to a low level [28]. The thickening of the stratum corneum which is produced by chronic frictional stimuli is associated with an increase in the mitotic rate and the rate of maturation of keratinocytes [26] and also with a less regular columnar structure. Christophers [28] has suggested that loss of columnar structure under conditions of rapid epidermal regeneration results from the lack of time which is available for maturation of flattened cells before further cells start to flatten beneath them. If the formation of lateral steps or some other property of the lateral junctions of the more mature flattened cells is responsible for inhibiting lateral expansion of younger cells, an increased rate of cell formation possibly might not allow this degree of maturation to become established in time to control the flattening of the next layer of cells.

ORDERED STRUCTURE AND THE FUNCTIONS OF THE STRATUM CORNEUM

The stratum corneum has two principal functions: one to protect the underlying tissues from physical or chemical damage, the other to act as a barrier to water loss [29]. The columnar arrangement of cells within the epidermis raises the question of how the functions of the stratum corneum may be affected by a spatially ordered cellular structure. At present, however, no clear functional advantage of an ordered structure has been demonstrated and it is necessary to bear in mind that a columnar arrangement of squames could be related to some deeper pattern of epidermal organization rather than to a function of the stratum corneum.

A columnar arrangement of squames might affect the resistance of the stratum corneum to minor mechanical trauma. This may be illustrated by considering, as a model, a heap of randomly scattered slates or tiles. If one slate in such a heap is lifted by the edge, the slates which overlap it are also lifted and these in turn lift others and in this way a cleavage plane is formed which runs deeply into the heap. If, however, the slates are neatly stacked one upon the other, individual slates may be removed from the top of each stack without dislodging the adjacent slates. The regular stacking of the squames of the stratum corneum may likewise tend to prevent minor surface trauma from producing cleavage planes which run deeply into the stratum corneum. A similar effect may also be important during desquamation. Where there is a columnar arrangement, the greatest area of attachment appears to be between squames of the same column and the passive shedding of individual squames from each column can thus be largely independent of the shedding of squames from adjacent columns. A loss of columnar arrangement might affect desquamation by producing cleavage planes which might result in the formation of scales. It is of interest in this connection that the stratum corneum often breaks along the lateral junctions of columns during the sectioning of frozen specimens of skin (Fig. 1-2A).

In opposition to the suggestion that a columnar structure may tend to limit mechanical damage to the stratum corneum is the absence of a columnar structure from epidermis, such as that covering plantar and palmar surfaces, which is adapted to withstand considerable mechanical damage. Possibly the maintenance of the integrity of an epidermis with a thin stratum corneum and a low rate of turnover is more dependent upon factors assisting shedding and increasing resistance to minor trauma than is palmar or plantar epidermis which is adapted to resist mechanical trauma by having a higher rate of turnover [27], a greater bulk of stratum corneum and thicker individual squames [29].

The permeability of the stratum corneum to substances passing through material in the extracellular space [30], is perhaps affected by the vertical alignment of the lateral junctions of columns of squames, which establishes a more direct channel across this layer. Alignment of squames would not affect substances which pass through the cells themselves. Palmar and plantar epidermis from which columns are absent is a poorer barrier to the passage of water than the general body epidermis [29] which has an ordered structure. On the other hand the skin of rodents is more permeable than human skin [31] but has a more precise ordered stacking of squames. Permeability may thus be more related to differences in the chemical composition of the stratum corneum than to the spatial arrangement of its squames. From the information which is available there appears to be little correlation between the presence of ordered stacking and permeability.

OTHER PATTERNS OF CELL DISTRIBUTION AND ACTIVITY RELATED TO ORDERED STRUCTURE

It is clear from a number of reports of tissue culture experiments that the initial establishment of epidermal structure depends on a complex interplay between the dermis and the epidermis but the nature of the inductive process remains to be elucidated [32, 33]. Grafting experiments using the epidermis of adult animals [34] and studies of epidermal changes during wound healing [35] suggest that epidermal cells exist in a modulated [36] rather than a fully differentiated state and that the maintenance of epidermal structure is thus continually dependent on factors extrinsic to the epidermis. The interfollicular surface epidermis of mammalian skin has not generally been considered to display a directional growth other than that imposed by the presence of a basement membrane [37] nor to show a spatial distribution of cells such as that found in hair or claw which have a more or less precise cellular architecture. However, Komnick [38] using amphibia has demonstrated a series of epidermal structures ranging from a stratified squamous epithelium showing little cellular order, to more complex epidermal structures such as claws. There is an ordered columnar structure in this series which is, in its spatial organization, similar to a thin columnar mammalian epidermis. This led Komnick to suggest that the more complex structures arise as the result of directional growth pressure produced by focal mitotic activity. Dermal influences may be as important to the establishment of these structures, however, as they appear to be to formation of hair which also involves localized mitotic activity and a differential rate of movement of post mitotic cells [39] and to the formation of less complex keratinized epithelial structures such as lingual papillae in which fine localized regional differences of differentiation are found [40]. The presence of a columnar structure in the stratum corneum raises the question of whether the establishment of this limited degree of spatial organization is in any way similar to the establishment of more complex epidermal structures. More particularly, are there patterns of mitosis or cell emigration in the deeper epithelial strata, or patterns in the structure of the dermis, that are related to the overlying epidermal columns? Some preliminary results of investigations of these points using the thin epidermis of the mouse ear, give hints of organization in the deeper epithelial strata which is related to the overlying columns.

The Relationship between Ordered Structure and the Position of Cell Division

Although mitosis has previously been described to occur randomly among basal cells [41], an examination of sections of wax imbedded specimens of mouse ear epidermis suggested that there was a tendency for mitotic figures to occur more frequently beneath regions corresponding to the junctions of overlying columns than beneath the central regions. To investigate this relationship in more detail, adult male mice were injected with Colcemid (Ciba) at a dose rate of 0.2 mg. per 100 Gm. body weight and six hours later specimens of ear epidermis were frozen in liquid nitrogen for sectioning on the cryostat [4]. Sections, cut at 5 μm, were fixed and expanded by the methods described above for preservation of the stratum Malpighii and areas of epidermis containing blocked metaphase figures were identified and photographed. From the lowermost squamous junctions of each column that lay above a metaphase figure, lines were drawn perpendicular to the plane of the epithelium to define a length of basal region which corresponded to the overlying column (Fig. 1-10). The distance of the center of each metaphase figure from the edge of the region so defined together with the

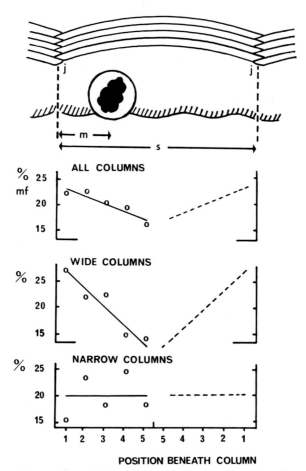

Fig. 1–10.—The position of mitosis in relation to the columns of squames in the stratum corneum. The width of a column (*s*) and the distance of a metaphase figure from its boundary (*m*) were measured using lines dropped perpendicular to the plane of the epithelium from the lowermost squamous junctions. The distribution of metaphase figures (*mf*), derived from the ratio of m/s for each column, is plotted as the number of metaphase figures in each of five equal divisions from the edge to the center of columns. There is a tendency for fewer metaphase figures to be found in relation to the central regions of columns (*All Columns*). This tendency is greater for columns sectioned through the central region (*Wide Columns*) and is absent from columns sectioned through the periphery (*Narrow Columns*). See text.

overall width of its related column was measured, and from measurements of 346 mitotic figures the frequency of occurrence of mitosis beneath various regions of columns from the edge to the center was calculated.

If mitosis were to occur randomly among basal cells, equal lengths of the basal region would have an equal probability of containing mitotic figures. The results of the measurements that were made (Fig. 1-10) showed that a greater number of mitotic figures were situated beneath the edges of columns of squames than beneath the central region ($p < 0.05$). Relating this pattern to the polygonal outline of unsectioned columns suggested that cells with a low mitotic potential lie beneath the center of each column and are surrounded by rings of more mitotically active cells lying beneath the periphery. With such an arrangement of cells, an increased probability of the position of mitosis being toward the edge of an overlying sectioned column would only be expected when the plane of section passed through the central area of low mitotic potential. As columns sectioned through this central region are more likely to show a wider cut surface than those sectioned through the periphery, the columns lying above metaphase figures were allocated to one of two approximately numerically equal groups according to their width. After grouping columns in this way it was found that the group composed of the wider columns showed a more marked tendency for metaphase figures to be situated beneath the junctional region ($p < 0.01$) than was shown by ungrouped columns, whereas the group composed of the narrower columns showed an essentially random distribution of mitosis (Fig. 1-10). A distribution of this type lends support to the hypothesis that mitotic activity occurs more frequently beneath the periphery of overlying columns.

On the basis of these findings and of the finding that cell emigration from the basal layer is restricted to the oldest post mitotic cells [42] it was suggested [4] that rings of mitotically active cells lying beneath the periphery of overlying columns might produce cells which move centrally to become aligned beneath the overlying columns before emigrating from the basal layer. Recently, however, Christophers [5] has reported a fluorescence staining technique with which it appears possible to distinguish between undifferentiated cells and cells which have started to differentiate toward the formation of keratin, and he has described cells having a pedunculated shape which appear to be emigrating from the basal layer beneath the junctional region of the overlying columns. Further investigations of the migration and emigration of basal cells by labelling with tritiated thymidine have been delayed by the difficulty of accurately identifying columns of squames after autoradiography but recently a method for selectively staining the junctions of squames in intact sheets of epidermis has been found [11] and may enable the sequence of basal cell proliferation and emigration to be more accurately determined.

The Relationship between Ordered Epidermal Structure and the Dermis

Except for a slight scalloping of the dermo-epidermal junction, no dermal pattern corresponding to the columnar pattern of overlying epidermis has been detected with the light microscope. Epidermal columns are only of the order of 30 μm wide and are, in general, too small to be related to regularly spaced dermal structures such as the larger dermal papillae and blood vessels. No pattern has been seen in the distribution of the cellular component of the dermis. After staining with silver methods [43, 44] fine nerve fibers are seen close to the dermo-epidermal junction but, by these methods of demonstration, they appear too few in number to be regularly related to the overlying columns.

Scalloping of the dermo-epidermal junction of a thin, well ordered epidermis is a fairly common feature of specimens processed for electron microscopy. The basement membrane bulges into the dermis beneath the center of overlying columns and rises again on either side (Fig. 1-4). Beneath the junctions of overlying columns the basement membrane often rises more sharply and in these regions small dermal papillae project upwards between the basal cells. Within these papillae small subepithelial nerve fibers are often found lying close to the basement membrane (Fig. 1-5C).

As the aligned cells of the stratum spinosum and stratum granulosum are usually spindle shaped in section (Fig. 1-7), the downward bulging of the dermoepidermal junction may reflect the greater volume occupied by those cells beneath the center of each column. Alternatively, scalloping of the dermoepidermal junction might be due to a difference in degree of shrinkage between the stratum corneum and the underlying tissue during dehydration and embedding. The siting of small dermal nerve fibers close to the epidermis beneath the junction region cannot be explained in these terms but, as yet, insufficient material has been examined to show that there is in fact a significant correlation between these structures.

The Relationship between Ordered Epidermal Structure and Langerhans Cells

Despite numerous experimental, histological, histochemical and ultrastructural studies the function of the Langerhans cell remains uncertain [45–50]. However, Wolff and Winklemann [45, 46] have shown that in guinea pig epidermis Langerhans cells form a regularly spaced and numerically constant population and, by analogy with the epidermal melanin unit, have speculated that a functional association might exist between a Langerhans cell and its surrounding clone of keratinocytes [45]. From their figures of 920 Langerhans cells per mm.^{2} it can be seen that such a clone would have an area of about 1000 μm^2 and a diameter of approximately 36 μm; that is, it would form a unit of similar size to an epidermal column. The position of Langerhans cells in relation to epidermal columns was therefore investigated.

Sheets of ear epidermis from adult albino Balb/C mice were separated from the dermis by the action of sodium bromide and processed and incubated for the demonstration of Langerhans cells by the ATPase method of Wolff and Winklemann [45]. After sulphiding, the epidermal sheets were refixed in Formol calcium and stained in a solution of Sudan Black B in propylene glycol for 24 hours at 37°C. The sheets were then mounted flat in glycerin jelly on microscope slides.

Prolonged staining with Sudan Black B appears to stain selectively the intercellular material of the stratum corneum and, after staining the ATPase preparations in this way, the outlines of columns of squames were identified by the denser blue staining of the regions of lateral interdigitation between columns (Fig. 1-11B). These preparations also demonstrated a numerous and evenly distributed population of ATPase-positive dendritic Langerhans cells (Fig. 1-11A). Focusing through the thickness of the epidermal sheets showed that the number of Langerhans cells per area of epidermis was similar to the number of columns of squames and, furthermore, that Langerhans cells appeared to have a tendency to lie beneath the center of the overlying columns: in some fields of vision this positioning was more premise than in others (Fig. 1-11).

Measurements of the position of 450 Langerhans cells in relation to columns were made using tracings of random fields of vision. These were projected onto

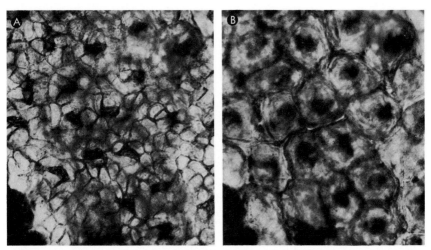

Fig. 1–11.—Sheet of mouse ear epidermis after incubation for ATPase and staining with Sudan Black. **A**, a number of ATPase-positive dendritic Langerhans cells are regularly distributed in the basal region of the epidermis. **B**, on changing the plane of focus, outlines of columns of squames in the stratum corneum are seen. Beneath these columns the position of ATPase-positive cells can still be defined. They appear to occupy a central position.

paper and the center of a column of squames was found by superimposing on the tracing a transparent template on which a number of concentric circles were scored. The position of each Langerhans cell was then derived from the ratio of the distance of the Langerhans cell from the center of the column to the distance from the center to the periphery of the column along a line drawn through the center of the Langerhans cell. When the region beneath each column was divided into central and peripheral zones of equal area it was found that 60 per cent of the Langerhans cells examined lay within the central zone. This nonrandom distribution of Langerhans cells suggests that Langerhans cells may have a function related to some aspect of the activity of keratinocytes during the establishment of columnar structure.

At present, evidence is lacking that the ATPase method of Wolff and Winklemann [45] specifically demonstrates Langerhans cells: cytochemical evidence for its specificity has been presented [51] but these results have been challenged [52]. During the present study an increasing deposition of a nonspecific reaction product at the plasma membrane of basal cells was found with increasing incubation times but, with all incubation times investigated, a number of dendritic cells, more strongly ATPase positive than the basal cells, was identifiable. An ultrastructural investigation has shown the presence of Langerhans cells beneath the columns of the ear epidermis of Balb/C mice (Fig. 1-5B); melanocytes were not identified in any of the sections examined. It is therefore highly probable that the strongly ATPase-positive dendritic cells found in relation to the epidermal columns correspond to the Langerhans cells which were identified ultrastructurally.

Recent investigations [46–48, 50] have provided new information about the morphology and behavior of the Langerhans cell and, although its function is still undecided, present opinion tends to the view that the Langerhans cell is of mesenchymal origin and corresponds to the dermal histiocyte [47, 48, 53, 54]. Two postulated functions of the Langerhans cell appear to be of interest in any discussion of the formation of columns: that of its role in assisting the movement of keratinocytes [47] and its relationship to the control of cell proliferation [48, 54, 55]. A nonrandom position of Langerhans cells might be expected to arise from either of these functions as the alignment of cells into columns is established by a lateral movement of cells during cell flattening and as the position of mitosis has been found to be related to the columnar structure. However, the role of the Langerhans cells as a more active organizer of epidermal structure should perhaps not be excluded at this stage.

DISCUSSION AND SUMMARY

One of the principal problems raised by the findings mentioned in this chapter is that of deciding at which level the factors controlling the establishment of a columnar structure are situated; that is, whether the patterns of cell distribution and activity which have been detected below the level at which cells become aligned are partly responsible for the alignment or whether they are a result of a feedback from alignment established at a higher level by some local factor. Ways in which a columnar structure could be established by factors operating during the cell flattening associated with keratinization have been discussed and if stacks of cells were established in the upper epidermal strata by such mechanisms their presence might affect the underlying cells. For example the diffusion toward the basal cells of a mitosis depressing chalone produced by differentiating cells [25] might be affected by their alignment and produce regions of high and low mitotic activity related to the columns; the contour of the dermoepidermal junction may reflect the greater cell volume beneath in the center of each column. At present, only a tendency can be shown for certain cell activities and cell positions in the deeper epidermal to be related to the columns and this is more in keeping with these patterns being a result rather than a cause of cell alignment. However, the importance of dermo-epidermal interactions to the maintenance of normal epidermal structure [56, 57] and to the differentiation of more complex spatially organized epidermal structures such as hair [57] or feathers [33], to which the limited spatial organization of epidermal columns may be analogous, suggests a possibility that the establishment of epidermal columns results from mechanisms situated at a deeper level than that at which cell alignment occurs.

Irrespective of the level at which the mechanism responsible for column formation is situated, the presence of an ordered alignment of cells in the upper epidermal strata indicates that the maintenance of normal epidermal structure involves more than a control of the type of cellular synthetic activity and a balance between the rates of cell formation and maturation [25]; a further mechanism controlling the spatial organizations of cells has also to be considered.

The apparent relationship of epidermal columns to the position of Langerhans cells and to the position of cell division and emigration, together with the segmented appearance of the epidermis produced by the contour of the basement membrane suggests that the full thickness of a thin epidermis may be divided into a series of functional units. However, further work is required to define the degree of autonomy exercised by the clone of epidermal cells lying beneath each column and to examine the activity of the cells of the deeper strata of thicker epidermis in which columnar patterns are less precise. Furthermore, investigation of the problems concerned with the establishment of the ordered columnar structure of the epidermis may, by focusing attention on the poorly understood interrelationship between the various activities of keratinocytes and their association with Langerhans cells and the underlying dermis, help to resolve some of the enigmas of the maintenance of epidermal structure.

ACKNOWLEDGMENTS

I express my gratitude to Professor A. E. W. Miles, Dr. C. A. Squier and Mr. J. E. Linder for their advice and assistance during the course of this work and in the preparation of the manuscript. This work was supported by a grant from the Medical Research Council.

REFERENCES

1. Mackenzie, I. C.: Ordered structure of the stratum corneum of mammalian skin, Nature 222: 881, 1969.
2. Christophers, E.: Cellular architecture of the stratum corneum, J. Invest. Dermat. 56:165, 1971.
3. Christophers, E., and Kligman, A. M.: Visualization of the cell layers of the stratum corneum, J. Invest. Dermat. 42:407, 1964.
4. Mackenzie, I. C.: Relationship between mitosis and the ordered structure of the stratum corneum in mouse epidermis, Nature 226:653, 1970.
5. Christophers, E.: Die epidermale columnärstruktur, Ztschr. Zellforsch. u. mikr. Anat. 114:441, 1971.
6. Menton, D. N., and Eisen, A. Z.: Structure and organisation of mammalian stratum corneum, J. Ultrastruct. Res. 35:247, 1971.
7. Matoltsy, A. G., and Parakkal, P. F.: Keratinization, in Zelickson, A. S. (ed.): *Ultrastructure of Normal and Abnormal Skin* (London: Henry Kimpton, 1967).
8. Hashimoto, K.: Cellular envelopes of keratinized cells of the human epidermis, Arch. klin. exper. Dermat. 235:374, 1969.
9. Meyer, J., and Medak, H.: Keratinization of the Oral Mucosa, in Butcher, E. O., and Sognnaes, R. F. (eds.): *Fundamentals of Keratinization* (Washington, D.C.: American Association for the Advancement of Science, 1962).
10. Goldschmidt, H., and Kligman, A. M.: Exfoliative cytology of human horny layer, Arch. Dermat. 96:572, 1967.
11. Mackenzie, I. C., and Linder, J. E.: In preparation.
12. Thompson, D'Arcy: in Bonner, J. T. (ed.): *On Growth and Form,* Abridged Edition (Cambridge: Cambridge University Press, 1961).
13. Epstein, W. L., Conant, M. A., and Krasnobrod, H.: Molluscum contagiosum: normal and virus infected epidermal cell kinetics, J. Invest. Dermat. 46:91, 1966.
14. Schroeder, H. E.: Quantitative parameters of early gingival inflammation, Arch. oral Biol. 15:383, 1970.
15. Chambers, R., and Renyi, G. S.: The structure of the cells in tissues as revealed by microdissection I. The physical relationships of the cells in epithelia, Am. J. Anat. 35:385, 1925.
16. Braun-Falco, O., and Vogell, W.: Elektronenmikvoskopische Untersuchungen zur Dyanamik der Acantholyse bei Pemphigus vulgaris, Arch. klin. exper. Dermat. 223:328, 1965.

17. Mishima, Y., and Pinkus, H.: Electron microscopy of keratin layer stripped human epidermis, J. Invest. Dermat. 50:89, 1968.
18. Sherman, F. G., Quastler, H., and Wimber, D. R.: Cell population kinetics in the ear epidermis of mice, Exper. Cell Res. 25:114, 1961.
19. Meyer, J., Alvares, O. F., and Barrington, E. P.: Volume and dry weight of cells in the epithelium of rat cheek and palate, Growth 34:57, 1970.
20. Birbeck, M. S. C., and Mercer, E. H.: Electron microscopy of the human hair follicle II. The hair cuticle, J. Biophys. & Biochem. Cytol. 3:215, 1957.
21. Mercer, E. H.: *Keratin and Keratinization,* International Series of Monographs in Pure and Applied Biology (New York: Pergamon Press, 1961).
22. Branson, R. J.: Orthogonal arrays of microtubules in flattening cells of the epidermis, Anat. Rec. 160:109, 1968.
23. Friedman, Kien, A. E., Morrill, S., Prose, P. H., and Liebhaber, H.: Culture of adult human skin: *in vitro* growth and keratinization of epidermal cells, Nature 212:1583, 1966.
24. Abercrombie, M.: Behaviour of cells toward one another, Advances Biol. Skin 5:95, 1964.
25. Bullough, W. S.: *The Evolution of Differentiation* (New York and London: Academic Press, Inc., 1967).
26. Mackenzie, I. C.: An experimental study of the effects of mechanical stimulation on keratinizing epithelia of rodents, Ph.D. Thesis, University of London, 1970.
27. Goldschmidt, H., and Kligman, A. M.: Quantitative estimation of keratin production by the epidermis, Arch. Dermat. 88:709, 1964.
28. Christophers, E., and Braun-Falco, O.: The architecture of the stratum corneum after wounding (Abst.), J. Invest. Dermat. 54:437, 1970.
29. Kligman, A. M.: The Biology of the Stratum Corneum, in Montagna, W., and Lobitz, W. C. (eds.): *The Epidermis* (New York and London: Academic Press, Inc., 1964).
30. Middleton, J. D.: Pathways of penetration of electrolytes through stratum corneum, Brit. J. Dermat. 81:56, 1969.
31. Tregear, R. T.: Permeability of Skin to Molecules of Widely Differing Properties, in Rook, A., and Champion, R. H. (eds.): *Progress in the Biological Sciences in Relation to Dermatology,* Vol. 2 (Cambridge: Cambridge University Press, 1964).
32. McLoughlin, C. B.: Mesenchymal influences on epithelial differentiation, Symp. Soc. Exptl. Biol. 17:359, 1963.
33. Sengel, P.: The Determinism of the Differentiation of the Skin and Cutaneous Appendages of the Chick Embryo, in Montagna, W., and Lobitz, W. C. (eds.): *The Epidermis* (New York and London: Academic Press, Inc., 1964).
34. Billingham, R. E., and Silvers, W. K.: Studies of the conservation of epithelial specificities of skin and certain mucosas in adult mammals, J. Exper. Med. 125:429, 1967.
35. Winter, G. D.: Regeneration of Epidermis, in Rook, A., and Champion, R. H. (eds.): *Progress in the Biological Sciences in Relation to Dermatology* (Cambridge: Cambridge University Press, 1964).
36. Montagna, W.: *The Structure and Function of Skin,* 2d ed. (New York and London: Academic Press, Inc., 1962).
37. Van Scott, E. J.: Definition of epidermal cancer, in Montagna, W., and Lobitz, W. C. (eds.): *The Epidermis* (New York and London: Academic Press, Inc., 1964).
38. Komnick, H., and Stockem, W.: Die Feinstruktur der Epidermisoberfläche an der Extremitäten des Krallenfrosches, Arch. histol. jap. 32:17, 1970.
39. Epstein, W. L., and Maibach, H. I.: Cell proliferation and movement in human hair bulbs, Adv. Biol. Skin 9:83, 1967.
40. Farbman, A. I.: The dual pattern of keratinization in filiform papillae on rat tongue, J. Anat. 106:233, 1970.
41. Leblond, C. P., Greulich, R. C., and Pereira, J. P. M.: Relationship of cell formation and cell migration in the renewal of stratified squamous epithelia, Adv. Biol. Skin 5:39, 1964.

42. Iversen, O. H., Bjerknes, R., and Devik, F.: Kinetics of cell renewal, cell migration and cell loss in the hairless mouse dorsal epidermis, Cell Tis. Kinet. 1:351, 1968.
43. Rowles, S. L., and Brain, E. B.: An improved silver method for staining nerve fibres, Arch. Oral Biol. 2:64, 1959.
44. Roman, N. A., Ford, D., and Montagna, W.: Demonstration of cutaneous nerves, J. Invest. Dermat. 53:328, 1969.
45. Wolff, K., and Winklemann, R. K.: Quantitative studies on the Langerhans cell population of guinea pig epidermis, J. Invest. Dermat. 48:504, 1967.
46. Wolff, K., and Winklemann, R. K.: The influence of ultraviolet light on the Langerhans cell population and its hydrolytic enzymes in guinea pigs, J. Invest. Dermat. 48:531, 1967.
47. Breathnach, A. S., and Wyllie, L. M. A.: The problem of the Langerhans cell, Adv. Biol. Skin 8:97, 1966.
48. Prunieras, M.: Interactions between keratinocytes and dendritic cells, J. Invest. Dermat. 52:1, 1969.
49. Zelickson, A. S.: The Langerhans cell, J. Invest. Dermat. 44:201, 1965.
50. Kiistala, V., and Mustakallio, K. K.: Electron microscopic evidence of synthetic activity in Langerhans cells of human epidermis, Ztschr. Zellforsch. u. mikr. Anat. 78:427, 1967.
51. Wolff, K., and Winklemann, R. K.: Ultrastructural localization of nucleoside triphosphatase in Langerhans cells, J. Invest. Dermat. 48:50, 1967.
52. Zelickson, A. S., and Mottaz, B. S.: Localization of gold chloride and adenosine triphosphatase in human Langerhans cells, J. Invest. Dermat. 51:365, 1968.
53. Hashimoto, K., and Tarnowski, W. M.: Some new aspects of the Langerhans cell, Arch. Dermat. 97:450, 1968.
54. Wong, Y. C., and Buck, R. C.: Langerhans cells in epidermoid metaplasia, J. Invest. Dermat. 56:10, 1971.
55. Giacometti, L.: The healing of skin wounds in primates III. Behaviour of the cells of Langerhans, J. Invest. Dermat. 53:151, 1969.
56. Gillman, T.: Possible Importance of Dermal-epidermal Interactions in the Pathogenesis of Human and Experimental Wound Healing and Skin Cancers, in Rook, A., and Champion, R. H. (eds.): *Progress in the Biological Sciences in Relation to Dermatology* (Cambridge: Cambridge University Press, 1964).
57. Cohen, J.: Dermis, epidermis and dermal papillae interacting, Adv. Biol. Skin 9:1, 1969.

2

Surface Chemistry in Epidermal Repair

Robert E. Baier, Ph.D. *

All higher organisms, including man, are well integrated assemblages of trillions of separate cells which, though stemming from a single progenitor, are marvelously differentiated to perform specific functions. Thus, everything that occurs in a living biological organism must take place through the agency of cells or of cell products. The cell types most specialized for participation in closure of any breach in the environmental seal of the higher organisms are the epidermal cells. Therefore, a central issue in wound repair is epidermal cell behavior at the wound edges. This behavior can be modified when exposed to various environmental conditions, including self-modification by cellular exudates, and by intercession of either adventitious contaminants or deliberately applied medical products.

It is also crucial to observe that epidermal cells (and many other cell types in nature) normally live, expand and grow at various interfaces between solids and liquids, between immiscible solids and liquids of different types, or between solids and gases and liquids and gases. In a very real sense, it is already "nature's way" that living cells organize into thin (often monolayer) films and spread at these various interfaces. In a lecture summarizing nearly three decades of sustained study of this problem, Paul Weiss [1] reviewed "The Biological Foundations of Wound Repair." His pioneering work sets the theme for future studies of cell spreading and organization at interfaces. Although sustained research into cell spreading and cell adhesion has been reported, proper insight into the mechanisms of wound healing has not yet been achieved because appropriate methods are either not available or well known for assessing the proper level of surface specificity which cells actually demonstrate in their response to their environment. Rather, the best Weiss was able to do was to present a profusion of examples to convey an impression of the enormous multiplicity, diversity and complexity of the processes involved in this most vital mechanism, wound closure.

The goal of the present writer is to summarize some of the currently recognized surface chemical interferences and aids to cell adhesion which must be

*Head, Chemical Sciences Section, Cornell Aeronautical Laboratory of Cornell University, Buffalo, N. Y.

considered in any characterization of biological joints. The interferences must be overcome in some way by the living cells during their migration, and making and breaking of contacts, over one another and over foreign materials. It is certain that their behavior is complicated during such contact reactions by the presence of cell exudates themselves, of wound fluids or of other organic secretions. These behave as "conditioning" layers between adjacent cell surfaces, or between cell surfaces and foreign substrates, before any true adhesive bonds are made. Throughout the following discussion, we also review some of the methods and equipment which will prove useful for surface chemical characterizations of cells and substrates which participate in normal wound closure or are under consideration as deliberately applied prosthetics (wound covers, for example).

The following sections take up, in order, the influence of blood clotting and of wound fluids in the wound environment and present some surface chemical methods for study of these factors. Next, cell-to-cell contact is considered, especially with respect to mechanisms which can favor more rapid wound closure. Then we discuss cell-to-foreign surface contact at some length because this represents the area where we have the greatest freedom to interfere with the wound closure process, hopefully beneficially. This interference might include use of additives to the wound itself, provision of wound covers of various types or other modifications in the wound environment. Surface chemical factors which influence cell adhesion are considered in detail. The penultimate section deals with proteins and other adsorbed films and suggests the enormous influence that these materials must have in modifying all of the previously discussed situations. Finally, we provide a brief indication of other important areas for further research along these lines.

BLOOD CLOTTING AND WOUND FLUIDS

An up-to-date understanding of the problems of blood clotting, which are— in more careful terms—described as problems of platelet adhesion, thrombus formation and blood protein coagulation, must precede consideration of the mechanisms of epidermal cellular movement and participation in wound healing. Two symposia presented during 1971 on the various aspects of these problems are already in the process of publication, so additional discussion of these details need not be given here [2, 3].

Almost every conceivable definition of a wound includes attention to the damaged tissue which is produced. Similar damage, although to a variable extent, is done to the vascular system at the capillary level. In any case of sufficient damage to be considered more than a casual abrasion, blood and tissue fluids rapidly find their way into the wounded area. As the first "seal" to the environment, the blood clot is especially important to all wounds. It prevents contamination by foreign materials, prevents the continued loss of body fluids, including additional blood, and provides substrate materials on, in and through which epidermal and dermal cell growth may occur. Definitive healing can neither begin nor carry on to completion without continued favorable conditions for cell propagation and movement throughout the resolution of the originally-formed blood clot.

The blood clot can unfortunately act as a nutrient source for bacteria and as an additional energy source for cells that could then propagate excessively to form an unseemly amount of scar. Therefore, it is important to prevent large accumulations of blood in any open wound or to remove such accumulations before final covering with a foreign surface. Any factor, whether in the wound cleft itself, accompanying an antiseptic additive or deliberately applied as a wound cover, which delays cell growth and motion, causes perturbations in cell adhesiveness which will delay the healing process. Once the universally recognized detrimental influence of infection is contravened, other responses by the attending physician may be ill advised because of their possible interference with the basic natural responses normally attending wound closure. After wounding, endothelial capillary buds proliferate and grow into the wound site under the protective stabilizing scab. This endothelial development follows closely the white cell phagocytosis of debris and of the exudate from the inflammatory stage [4]. About seven days after initial damage, granulation tissue and the epithelial layer have both grown in under the scab to close the initial wound completely. There is some evidence that maintenance of a high relative humidity external to the wound can shorten this period [5]. During the formation of the blood clot in the gap between the cleaved wound edges, the phenomenon of clot retraction (mediated by changes in platelets, called viscous metamorphosis, and their subsequent contraction) leads to an orientation of the fibrin net to produce an abundance of fibers oriented from wound edge to wound edge, as will be discussed in a subsequent section. Such fibers can impart a measure of cell guidance to the epidermal cells as they migrate into the gap. If the blood clot forms improperly, or is interfered with unduly, the fibrin net may set at random (or cross-wise) such that clot retraction cannot preferentially orient it normal to the wound edges. These unorganized or wrongly organized fibers will, rather than assisting cell guidance, constitute an effective barrier to the transit of the migrating cells. A large amount of disoriented cell motion will occur to delay the process of healing and to produce a less cosmetic closure.

Although blood is the first fluid to enter the damaged area, a primary colloidal wound exudate also collects in that region. Not much is known about this early exudate. Unfortunately, it seems to be difficult to study effectively. It is usually present in tiny quantities and appears to be changing its composition regularly during the healing process. It can be presumed, however, that the exudate contains components from damaged tissue, cytoplasm, blood and actual "formed" debris (e.g., organelles) from the disturbed cells, in addition to cell discharges elaborated in response to the physical trauma. The presence of blood fibrin and any other fibrous materials in this wound exudate is important because such fibers can act as favorable guiding "rails" for the moving cells. Now that there are simple, elegant and directly applicable surface chemical techniques available for study of the very early events in blood clotting [6] and for analysis of the elaborated wound fluids, it is expected that rapid advances in our state of knowledge of these initial events in wound healing will be achieved.

Figure 2-1 presents a composite diagram indicating four essentially nondestructive surface chemical measurements that can be made simultaneously, or in sequence, on as little as a microgram of fluid produced in a damaged epidermal mass. The diagram indicates that the actual molecular structure of the material, that is, its basic chemical "fingerprint," can be deduced by a technique called surface spectroscopy or internal reflection spectroscopy [7]. This method

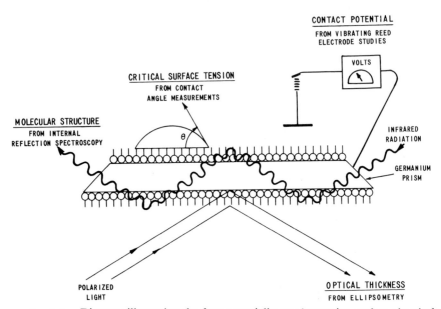

Fig. 2–1.—Diagram illustrating the four essentially nondestructive surface chemical measurements that can be made on as little as one microgram of the fluid produced in a damaged epidermal mass.

allows the recording of the diagnostic infrared spectra for the most important first few molecular layers of a material without interfering signals from the adjacent bulk, assuming that a bulk quantity of the material is available.

The absence of a large amount of material from wound sites requires that the technique be sensitive enough to detect and identify organic materials in extremely thin films. Films as thin as 10 Angström units have been studied by this method, and it has been possible to follow changes in the configuration and bonding within these films [8]. Since the method is nondestructive, it is admirably supplemented by other techniques which also judge the qualities of the material without removing it at all from the substrate to which it had originally been applied for surface spectroscopy.

A major supporting technique is that of ellipsometry [9], which allows a nondestructive assessment of the refractive index and thickness of the material. Similarly, a nondestructive estimate of the abundance and orientation of polar groups (which have associated dipole moments) can be made from a contact potential measurement on the same thin film arrayed in a layer even as thin as a single monomolecular film. We have reported elsewhere the simultaneous use of these methods to provide this multiple parametric description of monomolecular layers of protein analogs having various chain configurations [8]. Since the methods mentioned do not in any way modify the film or the organic specimen under analysis, it remains suitable for subsequent inspection by electron microscopy or electron diffraction, by autoradiography or any other ancillary technique.

Surface chemical characterization of even minute quantities of wound exudate can be carried out to discover the actual physical characteristics of the liquid itself including, for example, its liquid/vapor surface tension. A test as simple as that of placing a single droplet of the wound fluid on a piece of cleaned, smooth Teflon and recording the contact angle which that drop makes on the solid surface allows one to immediately infer the operational surface tension of that liquid. The basic concept behind this simple test is that the drop profile reflects its equilibrium contact with a surface of known relative surface energy. For Teflon, standard plots have been produced of the contact angles of a large variety of liquids (of various structural types and having various liquid/vapor surface tensions). Thus, once one has recorded the apparent contact angle for the tiny quantity of biological fluid of interest, one goes immediately to a standard Teflon plot [10] and reads out the surface tension which corresponds to the observed contact angle. This simple test works because Teflon has a markedly lower surface energy than any of the organic liquids which would be placed upon it. As defined in a later section, all solids, including Teflon, have a specific "critical surface tension" (a parameter of the solid surface only) independent of the nature of the liquids used originally to obtain that parameter.

Another most useful surface chemical method involves positioning the tiny quantities of biological fluids available immediately after wounding and at various stages during wound healing, at various gas/liquid interfaces. A versatile research instrument which allows the formation and characterization of extraordinarily tiny amounts of such organic materials and thin films is a Langmuir-Adam trough [11]. Such an apparatus is the two-dimensional analog to a piston and cylinder arrangement. It allows the determination of surface pressure versus surface area isotherms for interfacial films in much the same manner that pressure versus volume relationships are established for gases in piston and cylinder devices. Use of this research instrument, in addition to allowing characterization of the organic materials according to their molecular architecture, allows film samples to be taken at pressures, areas and temperatures known in advance. Such samples are appropriate for immediate analysis by the methods depicted in Figure 2-1 (internal reflection spectroscopy, ellipsometry, contact angle measurements and contact potential measurements) as well as for direct inspection in the electron microscope.

There has long been a need for careful definition of the surface properties of living cells, of their substrates and, in particular, of the fluids which make up their special microenvironment directly after the wounding event. Based upon the availability of surface chemical knowledge, experimental methodology and equipment as noted above, it is certain that surface chemical characterization of components in the wound healing cycle will be an important factor in advancing our state of understanding of this subject in the near future.

CELL MOTION AND CELL-TO-CELL CONTACT

The surface chemical phenomena of coagulation of dispersed colloids [12] and the coalescence of immiscible liquid droplets [13] in model systems show definite similarities to the behavior of living cells in contact in aqueous media. It was recognized many years ago [14] that general surface forces contributed most directly to the mutual adhesion of blood cells and to their aggregation, as opposed to the more common biological notion of a specific "stickiness" between adjacent cell surfaces. Microscopic inspection of cell aggregation processes generally supports the assumption of a simple physical/chemical mechanism tending to minimize the cell/fluid interface, as opposed to the presence of special adhesive factors at the individual cell surfaces. Individual cells do have the capability to join with other cells in their vicinity after they have made contact and similarly have the capability to break that association. Epidermal cells in normal tissue are quite firmly bound by what are now recognized as desmosomes and earlier characterized [15] as "lipid-rich bobbins" which were "veritable hold fast mechanisms." At the site of an injury, these apparently quite special and elaborate joints between epidermal cells are degraded. The individual cells, deprived of these anchors, become free of their tissue plate and begin to migrate and exhibit an almost ameboid motion. In tissue culture studies, it has become apparent that unlike cells from a variety of origins do not actively avoid mutual contact; but once such contact has been made, they preferentially exert activity at their furthest borders from their plane of meeting and thus actively separate. Neither do like cells seek one another out, actively, but instead ultimately aggregate with one another more because of a slightly stronger contact interaction among "like" neighbors. Like-to-like cell adhesion includes a slightly longer lifetime of the adhesive joint than is manifested in contacts between unlike cells. This apparently discriminatory reaction has been discovered with all of the following cell types in various combinations: embryonic chick liver, epidermis, lung, heart, kidney; embryonic mouse liver and lung, and neonatal rat liver; cultured strains of human conjunctiva; human liver and rabbit kidney. Certain of these cells like human conjunctiva and human liver do not coalesce with any other fresh tissues but do sometimes associate well with one another [15, 16].

Epithelial cells initially make random contacts with one another. There is no actual attraction or repulsion among individual cells but when two isolated epithelial cells meet at random, if they are of the same type, they cease their vigorous activity at the interfaces where they make contact with one another and only the free parts remain active and mobile. As time passes, the inactivity along the joint border spreads and becomes permanent. Repeated manifestations of this interaction cause the building up, in tissue culture, of small islands of identical cells and in this way it seems that epithelial tissue recruits like cells from a mixed tissue culture conglomerate of cells. When the epithelial cells are of different kinds, they also make indiscriminate physical contact with one another at first. However, their contact is tenuous and broken very soon with each one of the dissimilar cells going its own way. This reflects the poor quality of the cell-to-cell adhesion along their mutual border and the continued activity along the free parts. The apparent contact affinity among similar epithelial cells and lack of affinity among dissimilar cells readily leads to sorting out of mixed cell populations into groups of homogeneous clusters [17]. Such selection of similar-to-similar cell joints, as opposed to all unlike cell joints, leads eventually to the smooth repair of even a ragged wound edge. The presence of abundant cellular components from blood or damaged nonepidermal tissues does not seem to hinder eventual restoration of considerable tissue order and a cosmetically acceptable closure of most wounds. In tests directly bearing on wound healing [18], various epithelia were grafted into a surface wound in the skin. When the graft was likewise skin, or tissue normally found appended to adjoining skin, such as cornea, the two advancing cellular margins merged quite smoothly. When, on the other hand, the epithelial graft was foreign tissue (esophagus, gallbladder, lung), the wound edges did not join but the epidermis kept on migrating without apparent impediment either over or under the graft and did not cease its quest until confronted with another epidermal mass. When cartilages were used from a common source, either mesoderm or neural crest, they fused. When cartilage was used from either of these sources, they would not join with cartilage from the other [19].

To summarize, surface interactions seem to dominate the initial stage of contact among all types of cells and especially epidermal cells. Initial contact between cells has been recorded as essentially random and nonspecific, with any cell potentially adherent to any other cell or foreign surface [20]. Numerous experiments on cell aggregation [21, 22] demonstrated regularly this randomization of initial contacts. Since the ultimate results in all these studies were usually a sorting out of cells into specific tissue like collections, it is presumed that the quality of adhesion between the different cell types must be variable. The adhesion at the border between like cells must be of slightly greater tenacity than that between unlike cells.

Attention has been given to the possibilities that cell-to-cell interactions can be modified substantially by surface changes which would promote or inhibit cell proliferation into tumor masses. Such an achievement would be especially significant in cancer research. Phenomena called "contact inhibition" and "contact promotion" have been reviewed by Curtis [23]. Experiments designed and performed to test the possible relation of variation in cell surface properties to the spread of cancer, particularly with respect to the observed decreased adhesiveness and increased invasiveness of malignant cells, have been reported by Weiss [24, 25]. There have been continued difficulties, however, in applying experimental data in the tests of these concepts [26, 27].

It is cellular migration, as opposed to cellular growth, that establishes the primary closure of the skin wound. The cells at the edge of a wound, once detached from their nearest neighbors by either the trauma of the wounding action itself or the secondary effect of disintegration of the holdfast desmosomes, resume their ameboid type motion for no reason other than that their surface has been deprived of its former contact with neighboring cells [28]. It is equally clear, however, that this motile cell front at the border of a wound edge does not passively drag the remainder of the cohesive epithelial sheet along with it. Rather, in their migratory passage through the wound space, the epidermal cells move individually and without apparent influence from their neighbors. The orientation of cellular advance seems to depend critically upon the presence of "tactile" clues provided by their contact interactions with fibers, cellular debris, or deliberately applied materials of a variety of surface energies. Hence, the topic of cell interactions with "foreign" surfaces seems most pertinent to a better understanding of wound healing mechanisms.

CELL GUIDANCE AND CELL-TO-FOREIGN MATERIAL RELATIONS

At a freshly formed wound edge, the outwandering epidermal cells have the capability, as discussed previously, to move essentially at random. The locomotive apparatus of each free cell seems to reside in numerous pseudopods thrown from its surface in all directions. It is the attachment to and subsequent contraction of these blunt or pointed protrusions from the cell surface which physically drag the remainder of the cell in the various directions. Without a favorable substrate for these attachments to occur, the numbers and directions of cellular motions are as much a matter of chance as that expected from particles dancing in free Brownian motion in solution. How then, in most natural circumstances, is such potential randomness turned into the rigorous orientation associated with the efficient and cosmetic closure of epidermal wounds? How, also, can a medical practitioner assist such cell organization and speed the progress of advance of the epidermal cells by eliminating the wasteful energy expenditure in cell motions in directions and for distances not properly aligned toward the opposite wound edge? The orientation and tracking of cells across simple incised wounds seem to depend, in the natural instance, upon both the presence and orientation of fibers. In the simple incision, the immediately formed blood clot in the gap connects the two wound edges and during the subsequent clot retraction, the tension orients the fibrin in the clot longitudinally. Cells then seem to track most regularly over these fibrous strands to mend the break. In an open skin wound, where in addition to the blood clot one has a wound fluid exuded, the subsequent progress of the epidermal cells depends markedly upon the degree of drying and maintenance of aseptic conditions that will influence the formation of fibers from coagulating proteins in the exudates. A certain degree of drying will impart structure to the proteinaceous network of the exudate, as it does to the fibrin clot, and effect a ready alignment of the cells. If a more liquid state in the exudate persists, as would be the case if infection had set in, fibril organization would be inhibited. Rather than the wound healing, an open sore will develop and remain. Thus, we develop the picture that certain tensions (and absence from degradative interactions) are necessary to organize the fibers which provide the anchoring tracks for the pseudopods of the actively moving cells. It is, then, immediately hypothesized that the better oriented the medium, the more rigorously the cells can be aligned and the more efficiently can they make progress toward their neighbors from the opposite wound edge. Weiss [29, 30] showed that the tips of nerve fibers follow contact guidance according to this scheme and that by proper attention to this factor, the direction of nerve growth can be readily controlled. Instead of forcing the nerve ends together by suturing, he joined them by an elastic tube of some material which had an apparent low adherence toward the blood which filled the wound gap. Arterial segments were used, either fresh or after freezing, or cuffs from the metal tantalum were applied. The general point in the experiment was to force the blood clot to adhere preferentially to the nerve ends and not to the protecting sleeve so that during drying and clot retraction, no tensions could act except in one direction, namely, along the line connecting the two stumps of the original nerve axis. These experiments resulted in a well-oriented fibrous pathway system within the blood clot between the two nerve stumps which guided the outwandering cells and new nerve sprouts straight across the gap toward their most desirable destinations. Thus, by orienting fibers lengthwise between the faces of wounds, there is a strong probability that outgrowing epidermal cells will propagate preferentially along those pathways. Without such fibrous orientation or "tactile" clues, they would dissipate in random directions. The structure of the fibrillar matrix, and the organization of any essentially solid materials imbedded in the wounds, can even by minute changes in their organization drastically alter the microenvironment of the cells and turn successful healing into a gross failure to heal or cause healing with the presence of excess scar tissue.

Cartilage powders and other materials containing collagenous fibers have been employed to help close large incisions after many operations. If the fibrous components of these powders are providing tactile clues or specific points of surface attachment for the migrating epidermal cells, it should be cautioned strongly that the proper application of these materials is required to insure the correct organization of the fibers longitudinally along the wound axis.

The contact guidance achieved by the presence of fibrin, wound exudate fibrils or cartilage derived structures within the wound gap is perhaps explainable on the basis of a cell-to-foreign surface attachment according to increasingly well understood surface chemical mechanisms. Evidence is accumulating that the surface properties of materials, especially their relative surface energies and wettabilities by different organic phases, can be correlated with initial cell spreading and adhesion to these surfaces. Weiss [15] noted, for instance, that the most important of cell activities—cell motion—in wound healing could be viewed as fundamentally similar to phagocytosis where the spreading of cells on a foreign surface is likened to a vain attempt of the cell to encompass a giant substrate. Contact angle and surface tension changes also apparently contribute to the interaction of blood elements with normal blood vessel walls and with the walls in a wound environment. Copley [31] recorded observations of the modification of these surface properties caused by adsorbed films of fibrin which were reflected in changes in the wall adherence and the viscosity of blood flowing through tubes. There also exists reasonable evidence that blood coagulation times and platelet adhesion to various foreign surfaces can be correlated with the relative surface free energies of the various materials [32, 33].

The influence of surface properties of polymers on the adhesion and spreading of cells in tissue culture has been studied most carefully by Weiss [34] and Taylor [35, 36]. In these investigations, the speed with which initial cell attachment occurred and the lack of observed specificity among a variety of cells and foreign surfaces seemed to indicate that physiological or metabolic processes of the living cells are not major factors in the initial cell contact phenomenon. In Taylor's studies [35], for example, living and dead cells showed similar contact behavior at both clean and protein coated surfaces. Other studies of Weiss [20] produced results which could be interpreted as discounting the role of electrical properties in initial cell contact phenomena, since living and dead cells did exhibit different contact relations although the cell surface charge did not vary significantly after cell death.

Thus we contend that the initial adhesion and spreading of cells can be dictated by the peculiar surface properties of the cell/substrate interface. From the experiments previously discussed, it should not be surprising that surface modifications, even by adsorbed films of the same type of protein, can have variable effects on cell spreading [36]. Yet, we do not support the common generalization from many observations that cells adhere better to hydrophilic than hydrophobic surfaces, since the words hydrophilic and hydrophobic imply too narrow a measurement of a substrate surface property involving only an observation of its degree of wettability by water. Biological environments can so dramatically modify any form of substrate that a simple a priori hydrophobic or hydrophilic designation for a surface has little meaning. The accumulation of proteins, which can impart cell contact guidance to a variety of substrates is an important event. Water contact angles on proteinaceous coatings are notoriously unreliable, both because of hydrogen bonding interactions and penetration of the films. A more proper determination of surface wettability, still based on contact angle measurements, holds the promise of providing a more meaningful surface energy parameter which may correlate cell adhesion and cell/substrate interactions. Still, we remain cautious of extrapolating laboratory approaches to the complex environment in and surrounding a wound. Weiss and Blumenson [37] make special mention of the fact that relations of cell adhesion to the wettability of unmodified substrates, in their laboratory state, suffer from lack of knowledge of the actual surface character of that same substrate in the presence of the copious, adsorbable components found in vivo. Yet, contact angle relationships of various liquids and solid substrates are useful in predicting the tenacity and character of nonbiological joints, which, when the bond is properly made, always fail in one of the bulk phases and never at the interfacial plane where the two materials are mated. Therefore, a factor encouraging comparison of biological adhesion to adhesion in nonliving systems is the observation that cell adhesion also generally fails in cohesion. Weiss [24] has shown that the separation of cells from the foreign substrata to which they have adhered is usually a cohesive failure. Other experiments have shown that the attachment of mollusk ligaments to their calcareous shells is so firm that these joints also fail in either the organic or mineral phase but not at the interface [38].

Contact Angle Measurements

The most important requirement in current and future studies of wound fluids, the wound microenvironment, and especially the foreign substrates adventitiously or deliberately present in or adjacent to a wound, is for an extremely sensitive and reliable method of monitoring adhesive properties of the liquids and solids. A quite reliable technique for rapidly identifying changes in surface constitution of any material is based on contact angle measurement; one simply measures, generally with the aid of a goniometer stage and a telescope with a calibrated eyepiece, the angle (through the liquid phase) which a sessile drop makes when placed upon the surface of interest. When contact angles of zero degrees (or near zero) are obtained, this indicates that spontaneous spreading of the liquid can take place. When larger equilibrium contact angles are obtained, most often between 0 and 90 degrees, but occasionally greater than 90° as well, poorer or incomplete surface wetting of the solid by the liquid phase is indicated. This latter case would indicate the absence of strong adhesive interactions. Contact angle methods have been developed extensively over the past three decades by Zisman and co-workers at the Naval Research Laboratory [39]. A large body of reliable data is now available and a considerable literature exists on the subject. Contact angle data have been correlated best with the surface properties of liquids and solids by selecting an empirical parameter called the "critical surface tension" which is related to (some argue, identical to) the surface free energy of a material. The critical surface tension is determined by extrapolation from a graphical treatment of contact angle data. In this graphical treatment, one simply plots the cosines of the contact angles for a variety of test liquids versus the liquid/vapor surface tensions of the liquids, and empirically selects the best rectilinear fit to the data points. The intercept of this line through the data points, at the cos $\theta = 1$ (contact angle $= 0°$) axis is different for surfaces of different chemical quality. The intercept surface tension value is thus recorded as the critical surface tension for the solid in question. This value can be precisely defined only by the use of a series of homologous liquids, but it has been shown that liquids of all types generally fall along the same straight line, or cluster closely around it in a narrow rectilinear band. The critical surface tension inferred from a variety of liquids of different structural types is thus an even more valuable parameter than that inferred from a series of homologous liquids, since the former value is characteristic of the solid surface only and may be taken as independent of the liquids used in its determination. As mentioned earlier, the knowledge of the critical surface tension of a block of pure, smooth Teflon allows the interpolation of this plot in reverse, in what we have called "the Teflon test." Only a single droplet of biological fluid is sufficient to reliably infer its liquid/vapor surface tension from measurement of its contact angle on the precalibrated Teflon surface.

Another important consideration for research purposes is that the critical surface tension values have been intimately related to the actual outermost atomic layer, that is, to the true surface constitution of most solids. Simple hydrocarbon surfaces (for example, that of polyethylene) exhibit contact angle values leading to extrapolated critical surface tensions of between 30 and 40 dynes/cm. If the hydrogen atoms in a polyethylene surface were replaced by fluorine atoms, the critical surface tension zone would drop substantially to an intercept of only 18 dynes/cm. (as is typical with polytetrafluoroethylene). On the other hand, gradual replacement of the hydrogen atoms in polyethylene with chlorine atoms, causes an increase in critical surface tension of the material to above 40 dynes/cm. as is obtained with polyvinylidene chloride. It is, therefore, clear that contact angle methods, when applied with care and interpreted by experienced workers, can provide rapid and inexpensive answers to those questions of surface constitution and surface chemistry which must be answered during our search for a better understanding of wound healing mechanisms.

Potential Correlation of Biological Interactions with Critical Surface Tension

The rate of cell spreading and the ultimate degree of spreading achieved by a variety of cells on surfaces with different water affinities were observed by Taylor [35, 36]. The water affinity was ranked according to the measured water contact angle of each surface. Since no immediate and obvious correlation was shown, Taylor discounted the suggestion that there might exist some strong relationship between the intrinsic surface wettability and the cell contact behavior. We have discussed this situation in detail elsewhere [40] and highlighted two deficiencies in Taylor's thesis. First, the water contact angle is not a reliable indicator—by itself—of relative surface energies of materials and especially for materials of biological origin. Second, the water contact angles obtained by Taylor were not consistent with the contact angles obtained on cleaned surfaces of these substrates by numerous other investigators in recent years. Thus, some unknown type and quantity of contamination must have existed on his surfaces or, alternatively, they may have had strikingly different surface textures which anomalously influenced the contact angle results [41]. When the published cell spreading results on the various materials [35, 36] were reviewed in the context of the critical surface tension concept [40], they provided an encouraging correlation of the surface behavior of cells with the substrate surface properties of the foreign materials to which they became attached. The higher energy surfaces, including glass and cellulose derivatives, had strong liquid/solid interactions as indicated both by their high critical surface tensions and shallow slopes in their Zisman plots. These surfaces seemed to induce the greatest and most rapid cell spreading. The lower energy surfaces, down to a critical surface tension of about 22 dynes/cm., seemed to induce only minimal cell spreading. In recent scanning electron microscopic investigations of the behavior of blood platelets settling on solids of various surface characteristics, it has also been shown that the platelets tend to interact the least, that is, maintain the highest and most spherical (or native) cell profile, on surfaces whose critical surface tensions were in the 20 to 30 dynes/cm. range [42]. In Taylor's cell spreading studies [35, 36], increased cell spreading was noted on Teflon. This also reflects a departure of the substrate surface energy out of the zone for least interaction with cells (that is, minimum disturbance from their native shape and minimum adhesiveness) but on the lower energy side. Although it is admittedly speculative at this time, the probable zone of minimal cell spreading, and therefore minimal cell adhesion and minimal potential for contact guidance by such a substrate, lies in the critical surface tension range from 20 to 30 dynes/cm. This zone includes surfaces such as those of paraffin and medical grade silicones. It also may include the critical surface tension value for vascular endothelium [43, 44] and have some influence on the lack of initiation of thrombus formation and blood clotting at the walls of normal, healthy blood vessels. Since so little data are available on surfaces with critical surface tensions lower than 20 dynes/cm., Teflon being the only reported example, this zone of minimal cell adhesion might extend downward to all critical surface tensions less than about 30 dynes/cm. if the cell spreading studies on Teflon cannot be independently confirmed. For the time being, it should be considered that foreign surfaces emplaced in the wound environment will not provide effective contact guidance for migrating epidermal cells unless their critical surface tensions are above 30 dynes/cm.

It is interesting that films of fibrinogen, which Taylor reported to show a high degree of cell spreading [35, 36], do exhibit a critical surface tension of above 30 dynes/cm. (36 dynes/cm.) [6]. Thus, we have a ready example of a high degree of cell spreading, exhibited in tissue culture, correlating with a high critical surface tension for the substrate. Such cell spreading—and presumably cell migration—is definitely relevant to the wound environment. In the course of studies on the nature of platelet adhesion to various materials [45] it was determined that collagen, a protein with a critical surface tension of about 39 dynes/cm. [46, 47], caused platelets to adhere most strongly.

A possible objection to the use of the critical surface tension parameter, inferred from contact angle measurements, is that it is an average property of the surface and is insensitive to the microheterogeneities on the various substrates which are perhaps the most important determinants of cell adhesive phenomena. After all, the initial cell adhesions are made with pseudopodial probes sometimes of extremely small radius. The observation of cell behavior at isotropic liquid surfaces seems to validate the critical surface tension approach, however. Rosenberg [48] investigated cell cultures at various liquid-liquid interfaces formed between balanced salt solutions and liquids of silicone or halogenated hydrocarbon structure. The cell spreading behavior turned out to be quite sensitive to the chemical composition of the nonaqueous phase. In some cases, uniform cell spreading and aggregation occurred while in others the cells remained quite separate and assumed elongated shapes. Since these results were achieved at liquid-liquid interfaces with no apparent heterogeneities, and none of the steps or stresses which exist in the case of solids, the observation of differing cell behavior at these interfaces must reflect differences in the actual chemical composition of the surfaces which can be empirically correlated with surface energy parameters.

Autophobicity

The word "autophobicity" means literally, self hating. It has been adopted as the general term for the case when certain liquids will not spontaneously spread on clean, foreign surfaces nor on adsorbed monolayers created by diffusion of components from their own liquid mass or by adsorption of portions of the liquid constituents at the solid/liquid interface. The lack of spreading of these liquids, and the similar anomalous lack of spreading of living cells at foreign surfaces, could definitely impede adhesion. Autophobic behavior is noted particularly in hydrated systems where hydrolysis of certain liquid components (a pure organic ester, for example) exuded from living cells, could lead to fragmentation of the molecules and subsequent autophobic events. It will be important to learn how epidermal cells eliminate the potential difficulties from this problem.

Involvement of Water

The microstructure of a living cell surface almost certainly consists of a highly hydrated zone of material at the cell/solution interface. It is these hydrated zones which must mediate the first interaction of a cell with a foreign surface [20, 25]. Over forty years ago [14] it was proposed that adhesion among cells or between cells and other surfaces could be promoted by the increase of surface energy associated with desolvation of the cell surfaces. Schmitt, in particular [49], corroborated this thesis with evidence that the strong interaction between the basic hydrophilic protein, histone, and the phospholipid, cephalin, could cause the expulsion of water from between the faces of adjacent layers and produce an insoluble complex. This finding explained why monolayer amounts of histone, when added to red cell suspensions, caused strong cell-to-cell adhesion to be manifested [49]. All cell contacts are influenced by the state of solvation of the cell surface. Any factors that can play a role in desolvating proteinaceous interfaces, including divalent ions such as calcium and magnesium, can cause a marked increase in the strength of cell adhesion. Steinberg [50] disagreed with the suggestion that dehydration of cell surfaces by calcium was sufficient to explain its known adhesion promoting properties in some systems, but the general proposition that divalent ions may interact specifically with the hydration layers at cell surfaces (or with the hydrated layers separating cells from foreign solids or "guiding" protein fibers) to alter molecular conformation, hydrophilic-hydrophobic balances, and tenacity of the adhesive bonds merits increased attention.

In the course of forming strong adhesions, even of a temporary nature, between cell pseudopods and foreign surfaces in the wound environment, it might be possible that some of the cell exudates or cell surface coatings behave like the natural biological adhesives extruded by barnacles and mussels [51]. Such marine adhesives apparently displace the water, or react with or absorb the water during the course of their setting at the various interfaces. There are definite surface chemical principles which apply here, and which have been used recently in the design of finishes for glass fibers to enhance the resin-to-glass adhesion in fiberglass reinforced resin structures. These finishes also work by reacting with or dissolving the surface adsorbed water to some extent [52].

The Role of Adsorbed Water

Shifting our view from the wound's internal environment itself to a location immediately above the wound, where we might like to provide a specially designed wound cover, a consideration of the role of adsorbed water on various solid materials which might be considered as components of such wound covers is in order. When a polymolecular film of water is adsorbed on many common surfaces (which include glass, silica, alumina, metals, metal oxides, many organic solids and salts) the most firmly adsorbed portion cannot be removed by physical process such as heating, vacuum drying, or even the use of a water displacing agent. When residual water remains, the critical surface tension is generally markedly lower than that which would be found for the dry solid substrate. As the water layer increases in thickness, the critical surface tension of the bulk water surface (about 22 dynes/cm. at 20°C) is approached [53]. Therefore, if epidermal cells propagating across a wound gap make contact with such a moist surface, they might have a lower probability for spreading and forming strong adhesive bonds. This supposition assumes that the analogy we have made between the wetting and spreading in initial cell contact relations and wetting and spreading of pure liquid droplets is a useful one. In both cases, appreciable contact angles would be exhibited and neither cell nor test liquid could form a strong adhesive bond to that substrate. On the other hand, if the cell surfaces are dominated by active, hydrophilic groups a hydrated wound cover surface could present the disadvantage of causing these hydrophilic groups to spread more readily upon the moist surfaces. Substantial further research is required to discover whether cell surfaces themselves, cell surface secretions or natural bioadhesives do actively scavenge water from substrate surfaces or incorporate this water into their own structures. If so, they should persist in demonstrating good "tack" and strong initial bonding.

Environmental Contaminants

Exposure of any clean surface to any real environmental atmosphere most certainly results in rapid contamination of these surfaces by materials spontaneously adsorbed from the environment. Such films will in most instances induce varying degrees of adhesion and associated poor spreading. Wound closure might be inhibited by environmental contaminants. An adequate knowledge of the surface properties of the components in the wound system can explain this poor adhesion, which could be related to delayed wound healing and perhaps the maintenance of open sores, as well as good adhesion as discussed in previous sections.

Environmental contaminants in, on, or adjacent to open wounds can convert the substrates present there, which might originally be favorable for cell contact guidance, into substantially lower energy surfaces. These will cause large equilibrium contact angles between the various fluids and the substrates or between the cells and the substrates and result in diminished cell-to-substrate adhesion. Associated entrapment of voids, either of particulates or gases, cause potentially strong adhesive bonds to "unzip" when even gentle stress is applied. Therefore, effective separation of the joint could occur in situations when the bonds would not have failed in the absence of gaseous or particulate contaminants at the substrate surface. Earlier discussions of adhesion in the case of biological contact reactions [40] make it evident that, to maintain optimal cell adhesion, solid surfaces or other foreign surfaces in the wound microenvironment must remain as free as possible from contaminating organic layers of low surface energy. An apparently subtle change in the surface composition of these foreign materials can greatly increase, but more likely will greatly decrease, the potential adhesiveness. Outermost substituents which increase the critical surface tension, such as hydroxyl, sulfhydryl, carbonyl or amino groups would increase spreading of extruded organic droplets and enhance the formation of strong adhesive bonds between cell and substrate. Conversely, outermost substituents which decrease the critical surface tension, such as terminal methyl groups or hydrocarbon (CH_2) groups, would decrease that adhesion.

THE NEED FOR ATTENTION TO THE SURFACE CHEMISTRY OF PROTEINS

In even the simplest tissue culture systems, when cells are studied in pure salt solutions or in salt solutions containing supplemental protein, vast differences are noted in the adhesion of the living cells to various substrata depending upon both the presence of added protein and of the protein type. In the absence of protein, in most instances, cells adhere less firmly to the substratum, exhibit fewer advancing points on their margins, and similarly exhibit more retraction of the unbonded marginal zones. The identical cells take up strikingly different morphologies in solutions of identical makeup except for the addition of trace quantities of protein, as has been shown time and time again by time lapse cinemicrography of tissue cultures [15]. As an example of a situation where proteins can give the opposite effects, it has been noted by Weiss [1] that when cells were put into pure Eagle's medium (balanced salt solution) cell spreading was essentially complete in two hours; when that same medium was supplemented with 10% calf serum, the same degree of cell spreading was not achieved until 10 hours had elapsed. The extreme localization of surface forces, and the case which has been made for their importance in bioadhesion here and elsewhere [40], should be taken as a strong indication of the author's belief that the specific surface chemistry of protein fibers and of protein films must be elucidated for advances in all aspects of cell contact phenomena, including that of cell contact guidance and cell growth in wounds. Differences in the behavior of cells which were allowed to adhere to glass beads in columns were striking [37] when culture media with and without serum were used to suspend the cells. A major change occurred for adhesion to the glass surfaces which suggested a substantial lowering of the glasses' surface energy by adsorption of protein from the serum. It was also observed that the presence of protein in a cell suspending medium roughly equalized cell adhesion and spreading on surfaces as intrinsically different as Teflon and glass. Earlier work had shown that the culturing of cells in contact with nominally high critical surface tension glass surfaces was quite sensitive to the pretreatment given to these surfaces and to their various cleaning procedures [54, 55]. It was hypothesized [56] that serum additives in cell culture media functioned primarily by their modification of the surface properties of the substrates (usually glass) by their spontaneous adsorption to the solid/ liquid interface. As described earlier, blood proteins are among the first that are expected to be present in a fresh wound. Adsorption of blood proteins onto various solid surfaces is now known to proceed essentially instantaneously [6, 57–59]. The investigations of Lyman's group [32, 33] are particularly important because they were able to demonstrate that even though proteins were the first species to coat foreign solid surfaces, the initial adhesion of blood platelets could also be correlated with the critical surface tension of the underlying material. Thus, these substrate surface properties were able to influence initial cell adhesion through the influence they had on the adsorbed protein films. In Taylor's studies [36], gamma-globulin coatings retarded cell adhesion quite dramatically whereas fibrinogen seemed to favor it. It is therefore significant that the blood protein which has been most convincingly implicated in the formation of the initial "conditioning" layer on foreign substrates is fibrinogen [6, 58], and that the fibrin formed from polymerization of fibrinogen apparently makes up the bulk of the coating immediately and spontaneously formed on any foreign surface in the presence of fresh blood (as would be expected to occur with any rapidly applied wound dressing). It is now taken as a demonstrated fact [60–63] that an adsorbed proteinaceous "conditioning" film is a necessary precursor to cell adhesion to any foreign surface. It has been known for some time that, in addition to modifying the adhesive interactions of cells with one another and with substrates, proteins also provide a definite growth factor for certain cell lines in tissue culture [64]. Other evidence for the involvement of extracellular layers in biological adhesion has been reviewed by Curtis [23].

Quickly following the flooding of a fresh wound with blood proteins, and maybe simultaneous with that event, the accumulation of a wound fluid regularly occurs. This wound fluid, although of unknown composition, probably contains components actively extruded by the adjacent cells themselves, either damaged or undamaged. Rosenberg [65] demonstrated that cells could produce a proteinaceous microexudate which would coat clean foreign surfaces, and Taylor [36] showed that cells in culture, by means of these liberated products, could inhibit the spreading and adhesion of their own pseudopodial probes or those of adjacent cells. Paul Weiss [15] provided a review of the involvement of other extracellular factors in cases of cell contact interactions, and Rinaldini [66] suggested that the exudates play a major role as intercellular layers in all animal tissues. Finally, it has been noted [36] and should be repeated here that all body fluids contain a considerable quantity of adsorbable components, and that cells have the additional ability to contribute organic materials to any surface they contact. These observations should provide strong inducements for continued study of cell interactions with substrates of known properties, especially if medical practitioners are to have beneficial wound covers, dressings or healing rate accelerators available to them in the not too distant future. Such biomedical aids could be developed on the basis of deliberately produced structural modifications of certain fibrous proteins, including collagen, which has already been widely used. Collagen does have a conformation dependent wettability [46, 47]. In the course of future work, care will have to be taken that the modifications produced do not appear to the proliferating epidermal cells, or to their neighbors from subjacent layers, as strikingly foreign substances. For example, if normally nonantigenic proteins in the wound fluid have their surface properties so strikingly changed that—in addition to their being favorable to cell adhesion—they also activate antibody and rejection systems, they could be responsible for biological incompatibility of the healed tissue, or of the wound healing accelerator. This phenomenon might also lead to formation of excessive scar or even sloughing of the initial epidermal cover. Many advantages will accrue from developing new knowledge in how to exert controls over such surface interactions in vivo, either to promote or inhibit cell adhesion. We would like to promote cell adhesion to wound healing accelerating materials which could be added to the wound gap whereas we would—on the other hand—like to impede the adhesion of bandages to wound surfaces. In the latter case, the epidermal cells would not remain firmly attached and be inadvertently stripped as the cover is finally removed. The concept of tailor making surface active modifiers for a variety of surfaces holds considerable promise for eventually meeting these disparate requirements [67–69].

SPECIFIC FUTURE RESEARCH NEEDS

The Role of Metabolic Processes

Throughout the preceding discussion of cell adhesiveness, we have presumed that wetting power and critical surface tension relationships are definitely involved in the initial cell contact phenomena. The subsequent relationship between the observed initial events and the various assessable surface properties may not turn out to be as simple. In the longer term, the active role of each individual cell in the expansion of its surface that accompanies adhesion must be considered, even though such spreading initially might appear similar to that of an oil drop (or any organic droplet) at that same interface [70]. It is a gross oversimplification to suppose that the continued expansion of cell surfaces in contact with foreign substrates is a process dictated only by the surface tensions prevailing. Adhesional forces and interfacial tensions at the cell/substratum margin can be very highly influenced, and are almost certainly so influenced, by the cell's expenditure of metabolic energy. The net expansion of cells must be controlled by competition between the cell cohesional forces, adhesional forces, and the metabolic phenomena [70, 71]. There is some evidence that cell adhesion and cell contact phenomena, in general, are temperature dependent [72]. This reflects the state of development of the cells and the probable intervention of specifically exuded products dependent upon metabolic activity [73]. Low temperature studies, and support work with chemical inhibitors of cell aggregation [74], led to suggestions that a metabolically produced adhesive substance could underly all cell adhesion, as discussed in the previous section. Curtis [75], on the other hand, demonstrated reaggregation of certain cells in culture at temperatures as low as 1°C (where metabolic activity should not be significant) when extraneous proteinaceous components were excluded from the culture medium. Curtis and Greaves [76] subsequently isolated a pure serum protein which could inhibit cell aggregation unless destroyed metabolically by the cells. These few examples illustrate the opposite viewpoints on the role of cell metabolism which must be resolved by careful experimental work.

Wound Healing and Cellular Microenvironment

There is work now in progress to investigate the tissue microenvironment in wounds by using advanced microelectric and spectrometric techniques. Such work must be continued and expanded to determine all those physical conditions which now prevail during and which, by modification, might beneficially affect the healing process. Factors affecting capillary blood flow and permeability have been studied along with measurements of gradients of oxygen tension from the blood vessels to the cell suborganelles such as mitochondria [77]. It was demonstrated in this work that very steep oxygen gradients do exist in the rapidly proliferating cellular zone and that this gradient may be part of a stimulus for new cell growth. Many of the cells in this zone of most rapid growth appear to be oxygen deprived; the supply of oxygen may be a rate limiting factor in cell growth. This is an important observation to keep in mind when one is interested in determining the gas permeability characteristics of candidate wound covers. Other factors, such as shock, the release of vaso-active substances, or even stress, which reduce blood flow to wounds, could worsen conditions in the growing zone in any case.

Effects of Electrical Phenomena and Interfacial Potentials on Wound Healing

Since bioelectric phenomena are often important manifestations of the action and properties of living cells, the interfacial potential existing between rapidly proliferating epidermal cells and any other materials in the wound microenvironment should influence the rate of healing. Information on bioelectrical phenomena in wound healing is most limited. Interesting preliminary experiments were conducted on a small scale by allowing an electrical current to produce a potential difference across healing abdominal muscle incisions, using metal sutures as the active electrodes [78]. It was found in that study that wounds sutured with platinum wire were weaker, for unknown reasons, than those sutured with stainless steel wire whether or not an electrical current was passed through the metal/tissue interface. Neither polarity nor varying intensity of the electric current supplied, nor significant modifications of the interfacial potential, resulted in any measurable effect on wound tensile strength or histology of the healed zone. Studies of this type carried out in the future must definitely be supported by other characterizations of the substrate materials (for example, the platinum and stainless steel sutures) to discover what their true prevailing surface energy and surface textural properties were which might have overwhelmed the influence of the bioelectric phenomena.

Other Important Considerations

The availability of multiple attenuated internal reflection spectroscopy as described briefly here and in detail elsewhere [7], both in the infrared and ultraviolet visible ranges, should allow immediate new research on dissected skin and wound specimens to identify the true chemistry of these materials at various stages in their history. Experiments should also be undertaken on the culturing of fibroblasts and epithelial cells on well characterized substrates. The measures of surface properties and the "critical surface tension" concepts presented here should aid in selecting wound covering materials or wound additives which could accelerate cell growth, minimize adhesion of covers and maximize cell guidance along certain deliberately added substances. Experiments should also be designed to consider the tracking of cells along paths of different critical surface tensions to demonstrate that the contact guidance principle can have practical manifestations. One should also investigate the influence on wound closure and cell growth of various nonsolid or nonfibrous additives, including Vitamin C. Analysis of wound exudates can proceed immediately by both the Teflon test described herein and by internal reflection spectroscopy. Proposed proteinaceous or polymeric supplements to the wound environment can also be examined by these methods. Much of our hoped for advance in this field will depend upon the development of a reliable analytical technique for demonstrating both the presence and the role of ointments, salves and other medical applications on human skin in situ, eliminating the need for biopsies and the confusion from histological changes which do occur in all excised tissues. Attempts should also be made immediately for identification of all elaborated extracellular components in model wounds. Finally, the development of "artificial skin", already in progress [79], should be encouraged.

Recognition of areas where an interdisciplinary approach can relate fundamental knowledge of adhesive phenomena to bioadhesional problems is most important [80].

REFERENCES

1. Weiss, P.: The biological foundations of wound repair, Harvey Lect. 55:13, 1959-1960.
2. Mechanical surface and gas layer effects on moving blood, Fed. Proc. 30:1523, 1971.
3. Problems in evaluating the blood compatibility of biomaterials, Bull. New York Acad. Med. (In press).
4. Needham, A. E.: *Regeneration and Wound Healing* (London: Methuen, 1952).
5. Winter, G. D.: Movement of Epidermal Cells Over the Wound Surface, in Montagna, W., and Billingham, R. E. (eds.): *Advances in Biology of Skin Wound Healing*, Vol. 5 (Oxford: Pergamon Press, 1964).
6. Baier, R. E., and Dutton, R. C.: Initial events in interactions of blood with a foreign surface, J. Biomed. Mater. Res. 3:191, 1969.
7. Harrick, N. J.: *Internal Reflection Spectroscopy* (New York: Interscience Publishers, Inc., 1967).
8. Baier, R. E., and Loeb, G. I.: Multiple parameters characterizing interfacial films of a protein analogue, polymethylglutamate, Polymer Preprints 11:1137, 1970.

9. McCrackin, F. L., *et al.*: Measurement of the thickness and refractive index of very thin films and the optical properties of surfaces by ellipsometry, J. Res. Nat. Bur. Stds. 67A:363, 1963.

10. Baier, R. E., *et al.*: Surface chemical evaluation of thromboresistant materials before and after venous implantation, Tr. Am. Soc. Artif. Int. Organs 16:50, 1970.

11. Adamson, A.: *Physical Chemistry of Surfaces* (New York: Interscience Publishers, Inc., 1960).

12. Hogg, R., *et al.*: Mutual coagulation of colloidal dispersions, Tr. Faraday Soc. 62: 1638, 1966.

13. Torza, S., and Mason, S. G.: Coalescence of two immiscible liquid drops, Science 163:813, 1969.

14. Fahraeus, R.: The suspension stability of the blood, Physiol. Rev. 9:241, 1929.

15. Weiss, P.: Cell contact, Internat. Rev. Cytol. 7:391, 1958.

16. Abercrombie, M., and Heaysman, J. E. M.: Observations on the social behavior of cells in tissue culture. II. "Monolayering" of fibroblasts, Exper. Cell Research 6:293, 1954.

17. Moscona, A.: Development of heterotypic combinations of dissociated embryonic chick cells, Proc. Soc. Exper. Biol. & Med. 92:410, 1956.

18. Chiakulas, J. J.: The role of tissue specificity in the healing of epithelial wounds, J. Exper. Zool. 121:383, 1952.

19. Chiakulas, J. J.: The specificity and differential fusion of cartilage derived from mesendoderm and mesectoderm, J. Exper. Zool. 136:287, 1957.

20. Weiss, L.: Cellular locomotive pressure in relation to initial cell contacts, J. Theoret. Biol. 6:275, 1964.

21. Holtfreter, J.: Observations on the migration, aggregation and phagocytosis of embryonic cells, J. Morphol. 80:25, 1947.

22. Lucey, E. C. A., and Curtis, A. S. G.: Time-lapse film study of cell reaggregation, Med. & Biol. Illus. 9:86, 1959.

23. Curtis, A. S. G.: Cell contact and adhesion, Biol. Rev. 37:82, 1962.

24. Weiss, L.: Cell movement and cell surfaces: A working hypothesis, J. Theoret. Biol. 2:236, 1962.

25. Weiss, L.: *The Cell Periphery, Metastasis, and Other Contact Phenomena* (Amsterdam: North-Holland Publishing Company, 1967).

26. Weiss, L.: Studies on cellular adhesion in tissue culture: IX. Electrophoretic mobility and contact phenomena, Exper. Cell Res. 51:609, 1968.

27. Weiss, L.: Studies on cellular adhesion in tissue-culture: X. An experimental and theoretical approach to interaction forces between cells and glass, Exper. Cell Res. 53:603, 1968.

28. Weiss, P.: Perspectives in the field of morphogenesis, Quart. Rev. Biol. 25:177, 1950.

29. Weiss, P.: In vitro experiments on the factors determining the course of the outgrowing nerve fiber, J. Exper. Zool. 68:393, 1934.

30. Weiss, P.: Experiments in cell and axon orientation in vitro; the role of colleidal excudates in tissue reorganization, J. Exper. Zool. 100:353, 1945.

31. Copley, A. L.: Apparent Viscosity and Wall Adherence of Blood Systems, in Copley, A. L. and Stainsby, G. (eds.): *Flow Properties of Blood and Other Biological Systems* (Oxford: Pergamon Press, 1960).

32. Lyman, D. J., *et al.*: The effect of chemical structure and surface properties of polymers on the coagulation of blood. I. Surface free energy effects, Tr. Am. Soc. Artif. Int. Organs 11:301, 1965.

33. Lyman, D. J., *et al.*: The effect of chemical structure and surface properties of synthetic polymers on the coagulation of blood. II. Protein and platelet interaction with polymer surfaces, Tr. Am. Soc. Artif. Int. Organs 14:250, 1968.

34. Weiss, L.: The adhesion of cells, Internat. Rev. Cytol. 9:187, 1960.

35. Taylor, A. C.: Attachment and spreading of cells in culture, Exper. Cell Res. Suppl. 8:154, 1961.

36. Taylor, A. C.: Cell adhesiveness and the Adaptation of Cells to Surfaces, in Bren-

nan, M. J., and Simpson, W. L. (eds.): *Biological Interactions in Normal and Neoplastic Growth* (Boston: Little Brown & Company, 1962).

37. Weiss, L., and Blumenson, L. E.: Dynamic adhesion and separation of cells in vitro. 2. Interactions of cells with hydrophilic and hydrophobic surfaces, J. Cell. Physiol. 70:23, 1967.
38. Wakefield, H. F.: Adhesives, technology and marine organisms, Proc. Symp. Exper. Marine Ecol. 2:51, 1964.
39. Zisman, W. A.: Relation of the equilibrium contact angle to liquid and solid constitution, Adv. Chem. Ser. 43:1, 1964.
40. Baier, R. E.: Surface Properties Influencing Biological Adhesion, in Manly, R. S. (ed.): *Adhesion in Biological Systems* (New York: Academic Press, Inc., 1970).
41. Johnson, R. E., and Dettre, R. H.: Contact angle hysteresis. I. Study of an idealized rough surface, Adv. Chem. Series 43:112, 1964.
42. Schoen, F. J.: Gulf General Atomic Report, GA-10483, 1971.
43. Baier, R. E., *et al.*: Surface Chemical Features of Blood Vessel Walls and of Synthetic Materials Exhibiting Thromboresistance, in Blank, M. (ed.): *Surface Chemistry of Biological Systems* (New York: Plenum Press, 1970).
44. Baier, R. E., and DePalma, V. A.: The Relation of the Internal Surface of Grafts to Thrombosis, in Dale, W. A. (ed.): *Management of Arterial Occlusive Disease* (Chicago: Year Book Medical Publishers, Inc., 1971).
45. Mustard, J. F., *et al.*: Platelet-surface interactions: Relationship to thrombosis and hemostasis, Fed. Proc. 26:106, 1967.
46. Baier, R. E., and Zisman, W. A.: Critical surface tension of wetting for protein analogues, 153rd Nat'l Meeting, Am. Chem. Soc., p. 47 (Abstracts), 1967.
47. Baier, R. E., and Zisman, W. A.: In preparation.
48. Rosenberg, M. D.: Cell Surface Interactions and Interfacial Dynamics, in Emmelot, P., and Muhlebock, O. (eds.): *Cellular Control Mechanisms and Cancer* (Amsterdam: Elsevier Press, Inc., 1963).
49. Schmitt, F. O.: Some protein patterns in cells, Growth Supplement 5:1, 1941.
50. Steinberg, M. S.: Calcium Complexing by Embryonic Cell Surfaces: Relation to Intercellular Adhesiveness, in Brennan, M. J., and Simpson, W. L. (eds.): *Biological Interactions in Normal and Neoplastic Growth* (Boston: Little Brown & Company, 1962).
51. Manly, R. S.: *Adhesion in Biological Systems* (New York: Academic Press, Inc., 1970).
52. Shafrin, E. G., and Zisman, W. A.: Preparation and wettability of terminally chlorophenyl-substituted carboxylic acid films, Adv. Chem. 87:20, 1968.
53. Shafrin, E. G., and Zisman, W. A.: Effect of adsorbed water in the spreading of organic liquids on soda-lime glass, J. Am. Ceram. Soc. 50:478, 1967.
54. Nordling, S., *et al.*: The effects of different methods of washing, drying and sterilizing glass surfaces on cell attachment and growth behavior, Exper. Cell Res. 37:161, 1965.
55. Myllya, G., *et al.*: Serum lipoproteins in primary cell attachment and growth behavior of cells on glass, Ann. Med. & Exper. Biol. Fenniae (Helsinke) 44:171, 1966.
56. Rappaport, C., *et al.*: Studies on properties of surfaces required for growth of mammalian cells in synthetic medium, Exper. Cell Res. 20:465, 1960.
57. Brash, J. L., and Lyman, D. J.: Adsorption of plasma proteins in solution to uncharged, hydrophobic polymer surfaces, J. Biomed. Mater. Res. 3:175, 1969.
58. Vroman, L., and Adams, A. L.: Identification of rapid changes at plasma-solid interfaces, J. Biomed. Mater. Res. 3:43, 1969.
59. Scarborough, D. S., *et al.*: Morphologic manifestations of blood-solid interfacial reactions, Lab. Invest. 20:164, 1969.
60. Dutton, R. C., *et al.*: Microstructure of initial thrombus formation on foreign materials, J. Biomed. Mater. Res. 3:13, 1969.
61. Taylor, A. C.: Adhesion of Cells to Surfaces, in Manly, R. S. (ed.): *Adhesion in Biological Systems* (New York: Academic Press, Inc., 1970).

62. Baier, R. E., *et al.*: Role of an artificial boundary in modifying blood proteins, Fed. Proc. 30:1523, 1971.
63. Petschek, H. E., *et al.*: An experimental preparation for the study of thrombosis on artificial surfaces under controlled flow conditions, Avco Everett Res. Lab. Rept. No. 314, 1968.
64. Lieberman, I., and Ove, P.: A protein growth factor for mammalian cells in culture, J. Biol. Chem. 233:637, 1958.
65. Rosenberg, M. D.: Microexudates from cells grown in tissue culture, Biophys. J. 1:131, 1960.
66. Rinaldini, L. M. J.: The isolation of living cells from animal tissues, Internat. Rev. Cytol. 7:587, 1958.
67. Zisman, W. A.: Improving the performance of reinforced plastics, Ind. Eng. Chem. 57, No. 1:26, 1965.
68. O'Rear, J. G., *et al.*: Chlorophenyl-alkyl-substituted carboxylic acids and silanes designed as adhesion promoters, Adv. Chem. 87:10, 1968.
69. Bascom, W. D.: The wettability of ethyl- and vinyltriethoxysilane films formed at organic liquid silica interfaces, Adv. Chem. 87:38, 1968.
70. Weiss, P.: Guiding principles in cell locomotion and cell aggregation, Exper. Cell Res. Suppl. 8:260, 1961.
71. Weiss, P., and Garber, B.: Shape and movement of mesenchyme cells as functions of the physical structure of the medium. Contributions to a quantitative morphology, Proc. Nat. Acad. Sc. (U.S.) 38:264, 1952.
72. Moscona, A. A.: Effect of temperature on adhesion to glass and histogenetic cohesion of dissociated cells, Nature 190:408, 1961.
73. Moscona, A. A.: Synthesis of Tissues In Vitro from Cells in Suspension: Cellular and Environmental Factors, in Brennan, M. J., and Simpson, W. L. (eds.): *Biological Interactions in Normal and Neoplastic Growth* (Boston: Little Brown & Company, 1962).
74. Moscona, A. A.: Analysis of cell recombinations in experimental synthesis of tissues, J. Cell. & Comp. Physiol. 60, Suppl. 1:65, 1962.
75. Curtis, A. S. G.: Effect of pH and temperature on cell re-aggregation, Nature 200: 1235, 1963.
76. Curtis, A. S. G., and Greaves, M. S. F.: The inhibition of cell aggregation by a pure serum protein, J. Embry. Morph. 13:309, 1965.
77. Silver, I. A.: The measurement of oxygen tension in healing tissue, Prog. Resp. Res. 3:124, 1969.
78. Wu, K. T., *et al.*: Effects of electric currents and interfacial potentials on wound healing, J. Surg. Res. 1:122, 1967.
79. Hall, C. W., *et al.*: Evaluation of artificial skin models: Presentation of three clinical cases, Tr. Am. Soc. Artif. Int. Organs 16:12, 1970.
80. Baier, R. E., *et al.*: Adhesion: Mechanisms that assist or impede it, Science 162: 1360, 1968.

Part II

Cell Kinetics

Introduction

William Montagna, Ph.D. *

Because skin suffers so many different kinds of accidental or deliberate damage and because the different types of wounds apparently heal differently, the healing process seems to assume different modes under different conditions. Despite apparent differences, however, skin is probably endowed with a single complex mechanism of repair which must adjust to the various conditions inflicted by the wound and to the environment in which repair is effected. Too many aimless arguments have worried the question whether only the basal cells divide under normal and wounded conditions. When a wound breaks the continuity of the epidermis, the cells at the edge of the wound tumble out into the space in an attempt to bridge the gap; the cells heaped up at the cut edge probably come mostly from the basal layer. Therefore, cells dividing high up in the wound edge are not necessarily those that normally belong at that level of the epidermis. Christophers has shown that when the epidermis is damaged by stripping and the cells can only move linearly upwards, only the basal cells synthesize DNA. When considering cell division, one must remember that epidermal cells begin to synthesize keratinous substances even as they rest against the basal lamina. For that matter, basal cells in division normally possess some tonofilaments. However, those cells that have moved up from the lamina are no doubt already so committed to differentiation that they can no longer divide. Such cells, full of inert proteinous material, cannot dedifferentiate, and dedifferentiation is a prerequisite to mitosis.

Probably, the most important consideration in arriving at a better understanding of epidermal healing is the unfolding of the full spectrum of biological properties of normal epidermal cells and the physical and chemical environments in which they perform their task. Despite the attention given to these considerations in the following papers, we are still far from having arrived at an understanding of these phenomena. One of the major obstacles in these and other studies of wound healing is the limitations of the investigator's own techniques. Why, for example, have those who have studied cell kinetics with H^3-labeled substances usually injected the label *after* wounding and not before? Furthermore these studies require enormous technical skill, and much of the work published thus far has been unsatisfactory. Finally, although wound healing reveals much about

*Director, Oregon Regional Primate Center, Beaverton, Oregon.

the patrimony of epidermal cells, most scientists have chosen to focus upon the results of the process rather than upon the unfolding of the biological details of the cells themselves.

3

Kinetic Aspects of Epidermal Healing

E. Christophers, M.D. *

There is hardly any subject which has attracted more students in biology than the fascinating chain of events in wound repair and there is hardly any system which works with more precision than wound healing. In an attempt to understand better the response of epidermal cells to various degrees of injury and some of the underlying aspects of epidermal cell movement after wounding, two experimental models of epidermal wounding were analyzed:

1. *Partial epidermal defects* made by the removal of the stratum corneum by adhesive tape stripping.

2. *Deep epidermal defects* made by cutting.

The differences between the two systems are based upon the amount of tissue (either dead or living) removed.

Although both types of injury will show the general pattern of epidermal wound response, various aspects, especially cell migration and cornification, shall be shown to differ considerably. The parameters assessed in this study were:

1. Cell proliferation (using ^{3}H-TdR as a label)

2. Cell migration

3. Cornification

The term "kinetics" in recent years has increasingly been applied in the study of the cell cycle. However, tracing it back the term stems from "kinein", the Greek word for "to move." It therefore should be applicable also to such cellular activities as locomotion and transition.

MATERIALS AND METHODS

All experiments were carried out on the ears of male albino guinea pigs (200–250 Gm. body weight). Removal of the stratum corneum ("stripping") was performed as previously described. Open wounds were made by scratching the ears transversely using one arm of a surgical forceps, which was kept under constant pressure. This produced wounds of nearly 2 mm. width. By this method the stratum corneum remained in close proximity to the wound and the extent of

---

*Department of Dermatology, University of Munich, Munich, Germany.

subcorneal cell damage was easy to assess. The techniques of tissue preparation (autoradiography, FITC-staining) were routinely performed and have been previously described [1, 2].

Special experiments are explained later in this chapter. Cell counting after ³H-thymidine (³H-TdR)-labeling was carried out in relation to epidermal surface length on randomly selected specimens of wounded skin. In open wounds 0.5 mm. of both wound borders were analyzed. All values were calculated per mm. surface length. To assess cell migration in deep wounds, ³H-TdR was injected in one, two and three-day-old wounds which were excised 2–4 days after labeling.

NORMAL GUINEA PIG EAR EPIDERMIS

In previous studies some relevant physiological data have been worked out which shall be summarized briefly for better understanding. The epidermis on the average was 40 μ thick, the stratum corneum excluded. Hair growth is sparse and nonsynchronized. There are 10–12 layers of horny cells (Fig. 3-1), which show quite a variable architectural pattern [3]. Mainly depending on the thickness and on the rate of new cell production a highly ordered stratum corneum can be found in a thinner epidermis (below 40 μ average thickness), which changes stepwise to complete disorder in a thicker epidermis [3].

The normal rate of new cell production can be judged by compiling the following data: approximately 6% of the basal epidermal cells are involved in DNA synthesis. The living portion of the epidermis is renewed in about two weeks [4], whereas no direct measurements of the stratum corneum are available. However, the calculated value for the rate at which one new cell is being produced revealed that approximately one cell layer in the stratum corneum is formed in one day. Recent experiments using ³H-histidine incorporated into keratohyalin and electronmicroscopical autoradiography for detection have confirmed this value [5].

Fig. 3–1.—Normal guinea pig ear epidermis. The stratum corneum is about 10 cell layers thick and shows a fairly constant degree of cell overlap. Cell columns are not quite regular. FITC-stain.

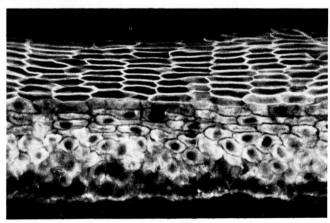

THE PROLIFERATIVE RESPONSE

In the guinea pig ear, a few firmly applied strips of adhesive tape will suffice to remove the major bulk of the stratum corneum (Fig. 3-2B). Further stripping produces a moist surface ("glistening") at which point the entire horny layer, eventually also the stratum granulosum is taken off (Fig. 3-2A). The histological features of the remaining epidermis as well as of the consecutive repair phases have been described several times [1, 6–9]. The proliferative response of the epidermis as revealed by the number of ^{3}H-TdR-labeled cells is shown in Figure 3-3. Similar response curves have been found by other investigators, differences mainly consisting in the absolute number of labeled cells [1, 6–10].

The results depicted in Figure 3-4 were obtained after vigorous stripping which resulted in two waves of labeled cells about 30 hrs. apart. Since it can be presumed from the position of labeled cells that daughter cells after a first division have again entered the S-phase, the difference in time between the two

Fig. 3–2.—Guinea pig ear epidermis after adhesive tape stripping. A, 15 times and B, 5 times. The specimens were taken immediately after removal of the last strip. C, 48 hrs. after stripping, 15 times. Necrotic tissue mass and serum are located above several layers of newly formed stratum corneum. FITC-stain.

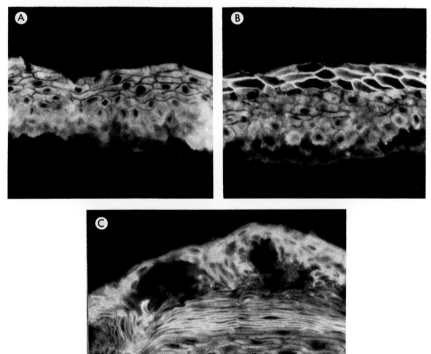

peaks of ³H-TdR-uptake represents the length of one cycle (which lasts nearly 30 hrs.). A very similar pattern of the proliferative activity has been found in wounds made by cutting [11–18]. It begins several cell diameters away from the wound margins and during repair it moves closer toward the defected zone [11, 12, 15]. It seems to be worth mentioning that 24–30 hrs. after stripping the highest number of labeled cells was observed whenever keratohyalin granules became visible in the uppermost epidermal cells. The full resumption of the tissue specific functions seems to occur very much at the same time.

A particular aspect in this kind of tissue reaction is the so-called lag phase.

Fig. 3–3.—Guinea pig ear epidermis 24 hrs. after adhesive tape stripping, 40 min. after intracutaneous injection of 10 µCi ³H-TdR/0.1 ml. saline. **A**, stripped 5 times, **B**, 8 times and **C**, 15 times. Note the number of labeled cells in B. When the entire stratum corneum is removed, the superficial cell portion becomes parakeratotic and invaded by leukocytes as shown in C. Comparatively little uptake of ³H-TdR is seen in the remaining epidermis.

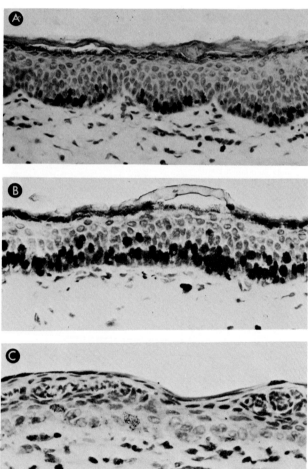

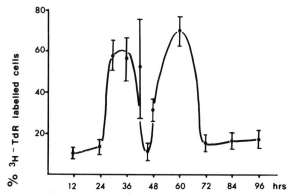

Fig. 3–4.—Labeling index in the guinea pig ear epidermis after removal of the horny layer with adhesive tape. Adhesive tape stripping was performed at 0 time until no more horny cells could be taken off by the tape. The values represent the averages plus SD of two experimental series, comprising 11 animals each. Both ears were injected with ³H-TdR and the specimens were excised 40 min. later.

This is the time between injury (stripping) and the onset of the proliferative activity. It lasts about 24 to 30 hrs. [1, 7–10] and ends with the sudden rise of a remarkably high synchrony of DNA-synthesis in the lower epidermal portion (Figs. 3-3, 3-4). It is believed by several authors that this phase is the interval necessary for the programming and the synthesis of enzymes involved in the subsequent production of DNA. In terms of cell kinetics, this is when the cells are entering the R-phase [19]. It cannot be overlooked however, that the exposure of epidermis devoid of its horny layer may cause serious harm to the remaining cells, so that recovery from injury at the cellular level must be included in this phase.

This question was investigated by stripping the epidermis to various degrees and determining the number of ³H-TdR-labeled cells at a fixed time, namely after 24 hrs. S-phase cells labeled with ³H-TdR 40 min. before excision were counted per standard surface length (5 mm.). The values in Figure 3-5 show that after 24 hrs. DNA synthesis was most active in the epidermis slightly damaged. Removal of more cells caused a delay in the uptake of ³H-TdR. Autoradiographs taken at later times showed a heavily labeled basal cell row in these specimens (Fig. 3-6), whereas sections prepared at earlier intervals (6 and 12 hrs.) did not reveal a considerable uptake of the label.

In the latter experiments (*Sm* and *Sh* in Fig. 3-5) there was a loss of viable epidermal cells which was due to parakeratotic necrosis (taking place in the first few hours after stripping [4]). This occurred whenever the granular layer became exposed (Fig. 3-5) or had been removed entirely (Fig. 3-5). Therefore, there is a greater response more quickly when the tissue is only slightly damaged whereas it takes longer to recover from more extensive cell loss. These observations indicate that the extent of damage has considerable effect on the subsequent proliferative response. Epithelium more damaged and more exposed to external and possibly also internal influence seems to be less readily able to participate in wound repair. This is supported by the observation that epithelization is con-

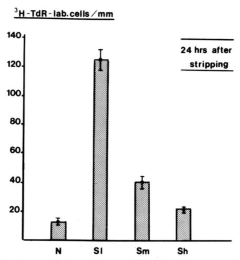

³H -TdR - lab.cells ⁄ mm

Fig. 3–5.—Quantitative analysis of the proliferative response of the guinea pig ear epidermis after stripping. ³H-TdR-labeled cells were counted per mm. surface length in specimens 24 hrs. after stripping, 40 min. after local injection of 10 μCi ³H-TdR/0.1 ml. saline. *N* = normal controls, *Sl* = slightly stripped (3 times), *Sm* = moderately stripped (8 times) and *Sh* = heavily stripped (more than 12 times).

siderably faster when wounds are protected and permitted to remain moist [20–24].

In deep wounds of the guinea pig ear epidermis, the initial repopulation is primarily accomplished by postdivisional daughter cells coming from the wound margins. Consecutively, a number of cells in this regenerating epithelium will undergo mitosis and thus further cells are added. In the autoradiographs pre-

Fig. 3–6.—Guinea pig ear epidermis 60 hrs. after stripping. Beneath a thin stratum corneum the granular layer is re-formed. Note highly synchronized uptake of ³H-TdR in the basal layer 40 min. after local injection of the precursor. *Inset,* cross section through entire ear with stripped, highly labeled side on top.

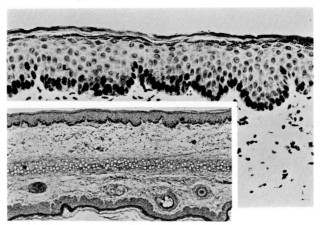

pared from wounds up to 7 days old and excised 40 min. after ³H-TdR injection, striking differences were found in the extent of cell proliferation between the wound margins and the wound epithelium itself (Fig. 3-7). The values shown in this figure are computed per standard epidermal surface length (1 mm.) for comparison. DNA-synthesis is quite low in the regenerating epithelium (day 3 in this wound model) and becomes higher on the following days. At this time several layers of cells are present in the wound and keratohyalin soon reappears (day 4). As seen in stripped epidermis, reappearance of keratohyalin and highest number of DNA-synthesizing cells occur very much at the same time.

The time between refilling of the wound floor by regenerating cells and full onset of cell proliferation within this cell portion (day 2–3) is of interest. It may be variable in wounds of different sizes, but seems to be a constantly occurring phenomenon. Several authors observed, that in larger wounds mitosis or DNA synthesis is low in the advancing epithelial tongue and becomes important only at a certain distance away from the protruding tip [12, 13, 15, 25, 26]. This would be comparable to the situation found in smaller wounds as described here. FITC-stained specimens demonstrated a considerable widening of the intercellular spaces (spongiosis) in this tissue portion (Fig. 3-9). It indicates that more fluid is present than normal. Also, cornification as seen in the appearance of membrane stained horny cells is not of considerable importance in this time period: the number of newly formed horny cells rarely exceeded 2 to 3. Taking these observations together there seems to be evidence, that during this phase in the life of the regenerating epidermal cell metabolic activities are comparatively low. It resembles the situation found one day after stripping.

Fig. 3–7.—The proliferative response of the two cell portions of a deep wound (marginal epidermis and regenerating wound floor epidermis). DNA synthesis of the marginal epidermis is rapidly increased within two days. In contrast, the regenerating wound floor epidermis shows delayed cell proliferation rising slowly from day 2 to 5. Closure of the wound is achieved by day 3 whereas the granular layer does not appear before day 4. Both events coincide with increasing DNA synthesis.

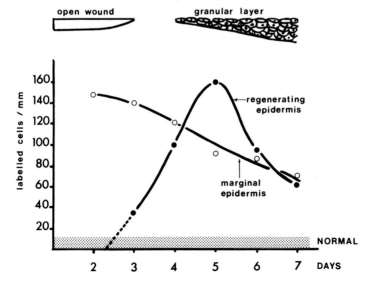

THE LENGTH OF THE DNA REDUPLICATIVE PHASE (S)

Reports dealing with labeling indices are necessarily conflicted because the indices can be influenced by the length of time which is spent in the DNA reduplicative phase (S-phase). The difficulty of measuring the length of S in wounded tissue is based on factors which expectedly will affect the movement of cells through the different phases of the cycle in a regenerating epithelium (cellular locomotion, dehydration, inflammation, exoserosis, etc.). Because of this the portions of the cell cycle were determined again after stripping, where fairly constant conditions together with a maximum tissue response are prevalent. Sixty hours after horny layer removal ³H-TdR was injected locally and the animals were sacrificed at hourly intervals up to 24 hrs. after injection of the tracer. The percentage of labeled mitosis allows a fairly good estimate of the length of S when drawn as a curve against the time of tissue excision [27]. Endpoints between the ascending and the descending side of the curve at the 50% level (Fig. 3-8) will give the respective values for S. The results show that the DNA replicative phase can be speeded up considerably. Under normal conditions in the guinea pig ear epidermis the S-phase has a length of 11.3 hrs. It becomes reduced to 9 hrs. after stripping.

Although restrictions could be made when using local injections of ³H-TdR instead of the systemic application, we have found this to be of no influence on the analysis because the availability of ³H-TdR is not longer after local injection than after parenteral application. It is natural for a wounded tissue to speed up the phases of the reduplicative cell cycle to a certain extent. The part of the cycle which is shortened most profoundly is the G 1-phase, which in our system is shortened to about 15 hrs. from approximately 5 days under normal conditions. Cell kinetics (meaning cell cycle timing) in epidermal wound healing seem to reflect the general principle of wound repair, namely rapid restoration

Fig. 3–8.—Labeled mitosis curve (%) obtained in guinea pig epidermis. ○ = normal epidermis, ● = after stimulation (60 and more hrs. after removal of the stratum corneum). The length of the S-phase as determined by the 50%-line is 11.3 hrs. in the normal epidermis and 9.1 hrs. in stripped epidermis.

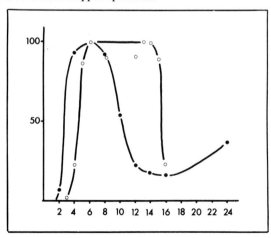

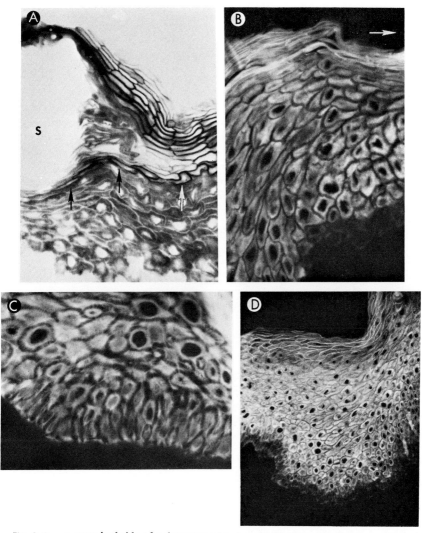

Fig. 3–9.—**A**, marginal side of a deep wound 1 day old. Epidermal cells have migrated into the defect. Beneath the old (stacked) stratum corneum and a necrotic zone one layer of horny cells has newly formed. *s* = scab. FITC-stain. **B**, marginal wound epithelium 2 days after wounding. The cells are elongated and appear to stream into the defect (*right*). Staining of the basal cell row is almost absent. FITC-stain. **C**, spongiosis with elongation of the intercellular bridges in the epithelium of the wound floor. No membrane stained horny cells can be detected at this time. FITC-stain. **D**, deep wound, day 4. The defect is filled with epithelial cells which are predominantly round. A few layers of membrane stained horny cells are present. FITC-stain.

of the depleted cell population by an increased rate of new cell production. The phase of the cycle most affected characteristically is G 1.

LOCOMOTION OF POSTMITOTIC CELLS

As shown by Winter [21] and more recently by Krawczyk [28] the advancing epithelial lips proceed into the defect by sliding of the cells over each other. It is still a matter of interest, however, how this is performed in the more distant portion of the regenerating epidermis where new cell production is highly increased and the signs of resumed cell differentiation (cornification and keratohyalin synthesis) become apparent. In Figure 3-9B it can be seen, that after 48 hrs. the cells in the wound margin have assumed an elongated shape with one extended process pointing toward the wound. Also, the stratum corneum formed by these cells shows a similar pattern (Fig. 3-9D).

Fig. 3–10.—A, section of an in vitro explant showing direction of epidermal growth on a semi-liquid medium. B, section of in vivo implant. *i*, implant; *e*, surface epidermis; *arrows* indicate epithelium of the cyst.

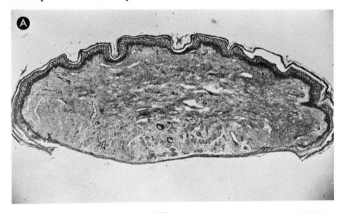

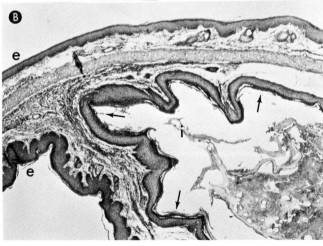

In the corresponding autoradiographs cell migration (2–4 days after labeling with ³H-TdR in 1–3-day-old wounds) was faster in the upper portions of the regenerating epidermis. It could be seen that cells originating at the wound margins had migrated into the re-epithelialized zone. They were located either in the granular layer, which was newly formed at the wound margins or in the mid-portion in the center of the wound. There is an increasing deflection from the vertical direction toward a more horizontal plane of epidermal cell movement from the wound margin toward the center of the wound with cells originating at the border zone becoming keratinized in the wound zone. The typical shape of the regenerating epidermal cells, together with the position of labelled daughter cells in the wound after two or three days labeling, indicate that the upper epithelial cell layers slide over the cells which are positioned closer to the dermis. Mitotically inactive cells therefore migrate faster and further. Full re-population of a wound then seems to be achieved basically by the same principle as shown by Winter [21] and Krawczyk [28] in the advancing epithelial tongue. Differences obviously exist in the number of cells involved in this process.

Besides this characteristic epidermal sideward growth, epithelial downgrowth along suture tracts has also been demonstrated [29]. It appears that distinct pre-conditions have to be fulfilled for the direction of movement chosen by the migrating cells. To determine what factors are involved in this process, the direction of epithelial outgrowth was compared in intradermally implanted skin pieces and skin explants maintained under tissue culture conditions. Pieces of guinea pig ear skin (5 × 5 mm.) including epidermis and dermis were excised from one ear after thorough local disinfection. In the other ear a spatula was pushed intradermally from the proximal to the distal border and the excised piece of ear skin was introduced into the pocket. In one group of 8 animals the skin pieces were inserted with the epidermis up, whereas in the other group of 5 animals the epidermis was facing the cartilage (Fig. 3-10). Histological specimens were observed after from 5 to 21 days. In this time period epidermal cells had migrated into the host dermis and after joining of the outgrowing lips a cyst

Fig. 3–11.—Diagrammatic representation of epidermal growth in in vivo implants, in vitro explants, and open wounds in situ. **A,** in vivo implants of skin into artificial ear pockets. Horny material always sheds into the lumen of the ensuing cyst. *e,* surface epidermis; *i,* implant; *arrows* indicate the direction of the epidermal cell movement. **B,** typical epibolies formed when explants of skin are maintained in vitro for 5 days. *Arrows* indicate the direction of epidermal migration. **C,** movement of open wound epidermis in situ.

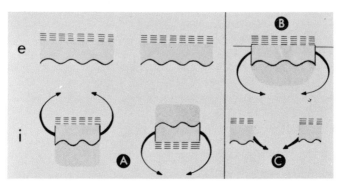

became formed. It was a constant observation that horny material was shed into the lumen of the cyst and in no instance could different patterns be found. Close contact between the dermis of the implant and the host connective tissue was always soon established. Heavy inflammatory reaction predominantly consisting of polymorphonuclear leukocytes was seen near or above the stratum corneum.

In the other series of experiments skin fragments were cultured on an agar medium containing 20% fetal calf serum, Hank's balanced salt solution and 100 μg./ml. streptomycin. The specimens had a size of approximately 1×1 mm. and were kept at 37°C and slightly gased with oxygen during the culture period. After 5 days of culture in most of nearly 50 explants the typical downward growth of epithelial cells along the dermal surface was seen. The migrating epithelial lips met at the under surface of the specimens. In all experiments the skin pieces were exposed to new conditions favorable for migration and growth. The direction of cell movement however differed fundamentally (Fig. 3-11). While sideward outgrowth in the "implants" led to the formation of cysts (meaning upward movement of epithelial cells away from the proper dermis), the tissue culture explants became typical epiboly structures. Possibly because of early connection between the dermal tissues of the host and the implant, the outgrowing epidermal cells moved along the roof of the host pocket, which in addition was heavily infiltrated by inflammatory cells. On the other hand, epiboly formation, which has been observed by various authors before, more readily seems to depend on environmental, e.g., substrate factors than space.

These experiments seem to show that the outgrowing epidermis becomes oriented by factors such as available space and suitable microenvironment including nutritional requirements. In general terms, suitability, but not the dependence upon its own connective tissue stroma, seems to be the predominating factor for the direction of epidermal locomotion. This also includes the availability of space (meaning points of least resistance). It is interesting to note, that such a simple factor as availability of space was found to be the most proper explanation for the phenomenon of epidermal cell column formation [2].

CELL TRANSITION IN STRIPPED EPIDERMIS

Onset of cell migration is known to be one of the earliest signs of epithelial repair in open epidermal wounds of mammals and even more so in amphibians or mammalian lens epithelium [25]. The cells are actively migrating into the defect before mitotic activity becomes important. In stripped skin however, this aspect is largely unknown. Does a similar release from contact inhibition possibly exist in stripped epidermis? When ³H-TdR is injected shortly after removal of the stratum corneum in autoradiographs, labeled daughter cells are observed slowly moving toward the keratogenous zone on the first 3 days and about the third day they are located in the reformed granular layer. In specimens which were heavily stripped, ³H-labeled nuclei were sometimes seen in the parakeratotic scale. It was a consistent observation however, that the transition time was not reduced beyond about 3 days.

On the other hand, when the newly formed stratum corneum was stripped for a second time (60 hrs. after the initial stripping), entirely different results were obtained in the autoradiographed specimens of the following days. Whenever

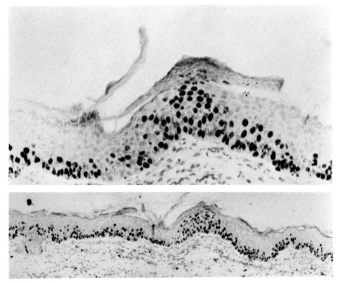

Fig. 3–12.—Guinea pig ear epidermis. Cell proliferation was stimulated by stripping 84 hrs. before the specimen was excised. At 60 hrs. the newly formed stratum corneum was stripped again with removal of the granular layer. In the central position ^{3}H-TdR was injected into the ears at this time. There is rapid migration of labeled daughter cells 24 hrs. after labeling into the area where the granular layer was removed. Adjacent portions of the epidermis show postdivisional daughter cells still located in the lower cell layers.

the stratum granulosum was removed, there was a rapid upward movement of labeled cells in 24 hours after the second horny layer stripping. This happened only after removal of the entire horny layer, whereas slight stripping did not reveal an increased speed in epidermal cell transition. In sections, where the horny layer was completely removed only in small areas, labeled cells were seen funneling into the defect (Fig. 3-12). Since, in the autoradiographs, this rapid movement of daughter cells occurred only when the granular layer was completely absent or severely damaged, this phenomenon is likely to be comparable to cellular migration in a cut wound. Only presence of both factors, namely, high cell proliferation and loss of viable cells in the superficial layers, resulted in highly accelerated cell migration. Therefore in stripped skin it does not seem to be a matter of population pressure alone to force a cell into a different position.

CORNIFICATION

Essential for epidermal wound repair is the process of cornification. The time sequence at which this specific tissue function is carried out in relation to wounding has not been analyzed before. It is facilitated by the technique of demonstrating cornified cells by means of the fluorescent staining technique [2]. The typical staining pattern obtained by this method in cornified cells served as a

Table 3-1
Criteria of Healing* Based on the Degree of Differentiation

	Normal Epidermis	Wound Margin (2–3 Days Old)	Center	Stripped Epidermis (1 Day)
Presence of keratohyalin	+	+	−	−
Cornification	+	+	−	−
Disintegration of nuclei	+	+	−	−
Spongiosis	−	−	+	+
Cell columns	+	−	−	−

*Synthetic activity of regenerating epidermis—wound covered by epithelial cells.

criterion for the identification of normal or abnormal horny layer formation. The two parameters readily assessible were parakeratosis and the presence of a granular layer. Using these parameters the tissue specimens obtained after cutting as well as after stripping were examined.

The results are given in Table 3-1 which shows the differentiative activity of the regenerating epidermal cells at the two sides of the wound at a time when the defect is covered by the cells and during the lag phase after stripping. Obviously in both types of tissue injury the process of differentiation has not become a proper cell function yet. It seems then that re-population is not at all sufficient to call a wound healed. The various signs of cornification as presented in Table 3-1 are resumed at later times. Interestingly enough one notices that nearly identical situations exist in both types of wounds, namely after cutting as well as after stripping. Membrane stained horny cells as well as keratohyalin granules reappeared first at the wound margins (Fig. 3-9A). They were seen in the wound center later. Compared to the highly increased number of replicating cells in this portion, their numbers were small. Cell loss (due to keratinization) therefore is lagging behind considerably at this phase.

CONCLUSIONS

Both types of tissue injury as demonstrated in this study have in common that they stimulated the remaining cells to respond. Stripping as well as deeper wounding produced cell loss, be it in the living or in the dead portion of the epidermis. Obviously tissue homeostasis is not limited to the living epidermis alone but involves the stratum corneum as well.

The highly increased number of DNA-synthesizing cells seen on the day following injury shows, that a certain proportion of cells normally at rest has entered the cell cycle. Together with this event the time necessary for the production of daughter cells is considerably reduced. Increase of the proliferative pool size and concomitant reduction of the cell cycle time therefore seem to be prerequisites for rapid new cell production. The first point has been studied by a number of investigators [1, 6–9, 12–16, 18]. The differences in the absolute numbers of replicating cells as well as the exact timing in different animals, sometimes in the same epidermis, are described. They do not influence the general mode of response, however, and are more likely to be due to technical variations.

The tissue specific functions of the epidermis, namely, new cell production and the formation of an effective barrier, can be speeded up considerably when stimulated. This is shown to occur after local application of various hyperplasia inducing agents [4]. An epidermis exercising its normal functions seems to be necessary. In wound healing, however, cornification and reconstruction of the barrier are delayed and take place after a minimal number of newly formed daughter cells has re-filled the lost portion.

The dissociation of the two main organ functions obviously is typical in wound repair. It has been shown before in the guinea pig ear epidermis, that on a quantitative basis the number of normally proliferating cells is correlated to the size of entire epidermal cell population, e.g., thickness [3]. It remains an interesting question then how much the normal proliferative pool size does affect the speed of epithelial repair.

Besides the loss of cells, injury of the living cells also appears to initiate subsequent repair activities. This has been clearly pointed out by Tsanev [30]. It seems interesting, furthermore, to consider the amount of damage inflicted to the epidermal cells. Our observations indicate that there is a gradient of cell injury with a maximum at the wound margins, which decreases toward the normal epidermis. It is reflected by the different metabolic activities the epidermal cells are able to perform after the insult:

1. While a considerable proportion of the upper Malpighian cells becomes necrotic in the wound margin, the basal cells belonging to this area start to exert migratory activities. They do not synthesize DNA however, nor do they go into mitosis.

2. Basal cells located more distant from the wound start to newly synthesize DNA after a relatively short pre-S-phase and give rise to daughter cells.

3. With recovery and repopulation first new cell production is resumed, while the synthesis of keratin precursors (differentiation) is retarded.

4. The reappearance of the granular layer and of horny cells (indicating resumption of normal keratinization) starts at the sides of the wound and is noticed latest in the center.

Cellular damage as a consequence of organ damage explains a number of phenomena, especially the sequence of repair activities. The findings apply for cut wounds as well as for stripped epidermis.

The heavily damaged cells at the wound margin (like the cells in vigorously stripped skin) are unable to perform reduplication and leave this to cells located more distally from the zone of tissue loss. The distribution of cells performing replication then does reflect a dose response of the amount of damage given to the cells and their ability to respond. Certainly, one of the main factors leading to epidermal cell damage is simple exposure to a strange environment. This is exemplified by the formation of a parakeratotic scale after stripping [4]. Also, in electronmicroscopic studies [28, 31] of wound healing dead epidermal cells were seen in the protruding epithelial lip, possibly as an effect of this foreign milieu. Exposure of the regenerating cells to an unfavorable environment also seems to influence their proliferative activity. In this study DNA-synthesis was only seen in cells located at least 4–5 cell positions away from the advancing lip.

Table 3-2
Epidermal Cell Activity During Wound Healing

Degree of Reconstruction	Open Wound	Stripped Epidermis
1–2 cell layers	migration	—
2 cell layers	DNA-synthesis +	DNA-synthesis +
3–4 cell layers	DNA-synthesis + + cornification +	DNA-synthesis + + cornification +
4–5 cell layers	DNA-synthesis + + + cornification + + keratohyalin +	DNA-synthesis + + + cornification + + keratohyalin +

These labeled cells were surrounded by neighboring basal cells and covered by not less than 1–2 layers of migrating cells. Also, as seen in the stripping experiments, removal of too large a portion of the epidermis causes delay in the onset of the proliferative response. These observations indicate that the ability of the cells to synthesize specific molecules is strongly influenced by the local environment. Detectable signs of resumption of normally occurring metabolic accomplishments were visible when more than a few cells were grouped together possibly by re-establishment of minimal suitable conditions (Table 3-2). In other words, the sequence of metabolic performances seems to depend upon how much the single cell is exposed. Recovery from nonepithelial and obviously harmful influences allows return to more specialized tissue functions.

The matter of epithelial wound repair has been confused by the sole restriction to the timing of kinetic events. It is important for the understanding of the physiologic response of epithelial cells to also evaluate factors which are important in influencing repair processes—extent of cell loss and cell injury, local microenvironments, proliferative pool size, and dermal interaction.

Wound healing is a subject which has attracted many students of biology. However, there are still quite a number of topics to be considered for future work. This has been tentatively demonstrated in the present paper.

ACKNOWLEDGMENTS

I wish to thank Miss Brigitte Klahre for skillful technical assistance and Mr. Bilek for help in photography.

REFERENCES

1. Christophers, E., and Braun-Falco, O.: Epidermale Regeneration am Meerschweinchenohr nach Hornschichtabriss, Arch. klin. exper. Dermat. 231:85, 1968.
2. Christophers, E.: Die epidermale Columnärstruktur, Ztschr. Zellforsch. u. mikr. Anat. 114:441, 1971.
3. Christophers, E.: Correlation between new cell production and the formation of cell columns in the normal guinea pig ear epidermis. First Annual Meeting, European Society for Dermatological Research, Nordwijk-aan-Zee April 20–21, 1971.
4. Christophers, E., and Braun-Falco, O.: Mechanisms of parakeratosis, Brit. J. Dermat. 82:268, 1970.

5. Christophers, E., Wolf, H. H., and Braun-Falco, O.: In preparation.
6. Brophy, D., and Lobitz, W. C.: Injury and re-injury to the human epidermis. II. Epidermal basal cell response, J. Invest. Dermat. 32:495, 1959.
7. Pinkus, H.: Examination of the epidermis by the strip method of removing horny layers. Observations on thickness of the horny layer and on mitotic activity after stripping, J. Invest. Dermat. 16:383, 1951.
8. Pinkus, H.: Examination of the epidermis by the strip method. II. Biometric data on regeneration of the human epidermis, J. Invest. Dermat. 19:431, 1952.
9. Schellander, F.: Reaktion von Epidermis und subepidermalem Bindegewebe auf Hornschichtabrisse, Arch. klin. exper. Dermat. 234:158, 1969.
10. Hennings, H., and Elgjo, K.: Epidermal regeneration after cellophane tape stripping of hairless mouse skin, Cell Tissue Kinet. 3:243, 1970.
11. Arey, L. B.: Wound healing, Physiol. Rev. 16:327, 1936.
12. Bullough, W. S.: Epithelial Repair, in Dunphy, J. E., and van Winkle, W. (eds.): *Repair and Regeneration* (New York: McGraw-Hill Book Co., Inc., 1969).
13. Hell, E., and Cruickshank, C. N. D.: The effect of injury upon the uptake of ^{3}H-thymidine by guinea pig epidermis, Exper. Cell Res. 31:128, 1963.
14. Hell, E.: The effect of injury upon epidermal mitotic indices in guinea pigs, Exper. Cell Res. 32:354, 1963.
15. Oehlert, W.: Die Zellneubildung im Epithel und im Granulationsgewebe bei der Wundheilung, Symposium d. Vereinigung d. Deutschen Katgut Industrie e. V. S. 22 (1966).
16. Oehlert, W.: Die Steuerung der Regeneration am mehrschichtigen Plattenepithel, Verhandl. deutsch. Gesellsch. Path. 50:90, 1966.
17. Sullivan, B. S., and Epstein, W. L.: Mitotic activity of wounded human epidermis, J. Invest. Dermat. 41:39, 1963.
18. Viziam, C. B.: Epithelialization of small wounds, J. Invest. Dermat. 43:499, 1964.
19. Frankfurt, O. S.: Effect of hydrocortisone, adrenalin and actinomycin D on transition of cells to the DNA synthesis phase, Exper. Cell Res. 52:222, 1968.
20. Hinman, C. D., Maibach, H., and Winter, G. D.: Effect of air exposure and occlusion on experimental human skin wounds, Nature 200:377, 1963.
21. Winter, G. D.: Movement of epidermal cells over the wound surface, in Montagna, W., and Billingham, R. E. (eds.): *Advances in Biology of the Skin,* Vol. 5, *Wound Healing* (New York: The Macmillan Company, 1963).
22. Winter, G. D.: Regeneration of epidermis, in Rook, A., and Champion, R. H. (eds.): *Progress in the Biological Sciences in Relation to Dermatology* (London: The Syndics of the Cambridge University Press, 1964).
23. Winter, G. D.: Formation of the scab and the rate of epithelization of superficial wounds in the skin of the young domestic pig, Nature 193:293, 1962.
24. Winter, G. D., and Scales, J. T.: Effect of air drying and dressings on the surface of a wound, Nature 197:91, 1963.
25. Friedenwald, J. S., and Buschke, E.: The influence of some experimental variables on the epithelial movements in the healing of corneal wounds, J. Cell. Comp. Physiol. 23:95, 1944.
26. Giacometti, L.: The healing of skin wounds in primates. I. The kinetics of cell proliferation, J. Invest. Dermat. 48:133, 1967.
27. Sherman, F. G., Quastler, H., and Wimber, D. R.: Cell population kinetics in the ear epidermis of mice, Exper. Cell Res. 25:114, 1961.
28. Krawczyk, W. S.: A pattern of epidermal cell migration during wound healing, J. Cell Biol. 49:247, 1971.
29. Gillman, T., and Penn, J.: Studies on the repair of cutaneous wounds, Med. Proc. 2, Suppl. 1956.
30. Tsanev, R.: Role of nucleic acids in the wound healing process, Symp. Biol. Hung. 3:55, 1963.
31. Odland, G., and Ross, R.: Human wound repair. I. Epidermal regeneration, J. Cell Biol. 39:135, 1968.

This work was supported by the Deutsche Forschungsgemeinschaft.

4

Epidermal Regeneration Studied in the Domestic Pig

George D. Winter, Ph.D. *

There were good reasons for choosing to use the domestic pig to study wound healing. To begin with it was necessary to obtain a clear picture of the normal structure of the skin in the backs of young Large White pigs where the wounds were to be made. Figure 4-1 illustrates the general character of skin from this region.

In basic architecture it resembles human skin in the relative thicknesses of the epidermis and dermis, the presence of epidermal ridges and a distinct dermal papillary layer, relative sparsity of hairs and deep layer of subdermal fat. These morphological similarities can be traced to the fact that both man and the pig rely for insulation on fat not fur. As Hartwell [1] said, porcine skin resembles human skin more closely than does the skin of any of the common small laboratory animals. Nevertheless, there are many differences as Montagna and Yun [2] point out. These mostly reflect the fact that porcine skin is less important as an organ for regulating body temperature than is human skin.

In skin on the back of a pig the only epidermal appendages are the hair follicles, sebaceous glands and apocrine glands (Fig. 4-2). The underside of the surface epidermis is formed into a well developed system of intersecting ridges enclosing small irregularly shaped dermal papillae. Figure 4-3 illustrates the general form of the epidermis which, between the ridges consists in depth of about six living cells and a moderately thick cornified layer. The basal cells have branched cytoplasmic processes embedded in the collagenous tissue of the dermal papillary layer which are reinforced by spiral filaments (Fig. 4-4).

The dermis is about 2 mm. thick in the 15-week-old Large White strain pigs. Its lower surface is perforated at intervals by sloping cone-shaped spaces filled with hypodermal fatty tissue reaching up into the lower third of the dermis (Fig. 4-5). These spaces accommodate part of the apocrine glands and are permanent capsules of fatty tissue within which the lower two thirds of the hair follicles move up and down in the catagen and early anagen stages of the hair growth

*Department of Biomedical Engineering, Institute of Orthopaedics (University of London), Royal National Orthopaedic Hospital, Brockley Hill, Stanmore, Middlesex, England.

71

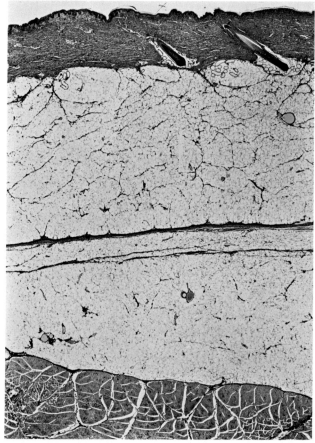

Fig. 4–1.—Cross-section showing the general character of porcine skin from the back of a young, Large White strain pig.

cycle. The spatial relationships of hair follicles in skin from the back of a 14-week-old Large White pig are illustrated in Figure 4-6. There are about 25 hair follicles/cm.^{2} grouped in threes, as pairs or singly. There are never more than three follicles to a group. Groups of three form a triangle with the apical hair ventrad. The follicles occupy spaces up to 0.5 mm. wide in the dermis and the greatest distance between adjacent follicles near the surface is about 2.0 mm. These facts are significant when it comes to analyzing the regeneration of the epidermis following injury. Hair follicles in the skin of these pigs appear to go through their phases of growth and quiescence independently of one another, that is there is a mosaic pattern of hair replacement as in man.

There are numerous tubular apocrine glands closely associated with the hair follicles. They have ducts opening to the surface immediately ventral to the follicles, but no eccrine glands and the pig does not regulate body heat by sweating on the general body surface. The sebaceous glands are small compared with those in human skin from the same region.

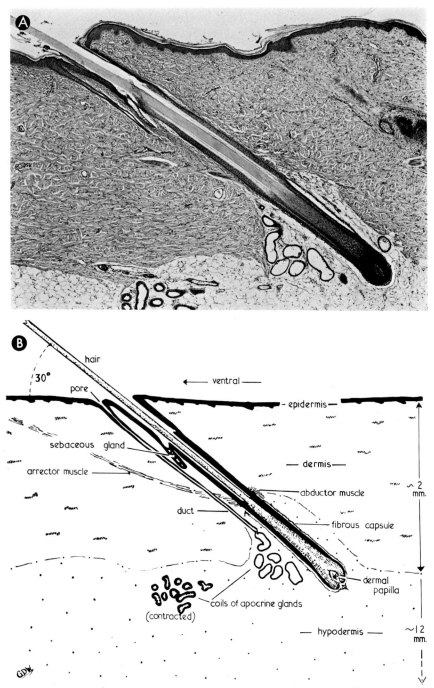

Fig. 4–2.—A, cross-section showing a hair follicle and apocrine glands. B, diagrammatic representation of skin structure around a hair follicle in the pig.

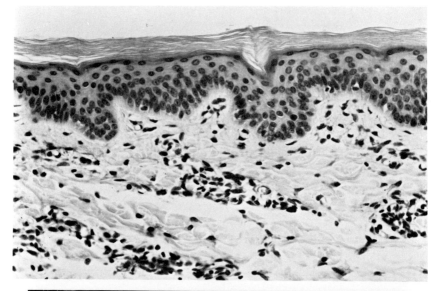

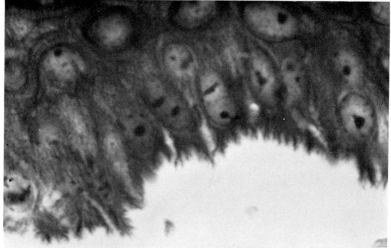

Fig. 4–3 (top).—Cross-section of interfollicular epidermis showing thick stratum corneum.

Fig. 4–4 (bottom).—Cross-section illustrating cytoplasmic processes of basal cells embedded in the collagenous tissue of the papillary dermis.

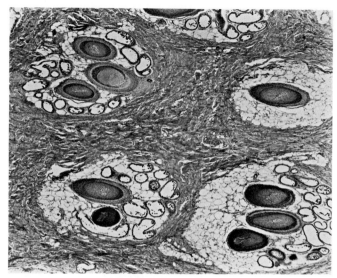

Fig. 4–5.—Oblique section showing fatty spaces and distribution of hair follicles in the lower dermis.

Fig. 4–6.—Diagram of the distribution of hair follicles on the skin surface. Hairs occur singly or in groups of 2 or 3.

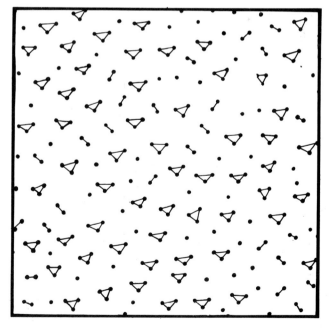

METHODS FOR THE STUDY OF SHALLOW WOUNDS

most cells of hair follicles and ducts of apocrine glands dehydrate and die. About White strain pigs, 15–20 weeks old, all from the same pedigreed herd. Special precautions were taken by the use of a guard strapped to the pigs which protected the wounds against damage that otherwise would have confused the histological picture [3]. Three days before the wounds were to be made, the hairs on the back of a pig were clipped short with electric clippers and the protective guard was put on the animal. For the sake of uniformity all experiments were begun between 10.00 and 12.00 hours. Operations were performed in a well equipped animal operating theater; sterile gowns, gloves and face masks were worn and all towels and instruments were sterilized. The skin was not prepared with antiseptics as this might have modified the course of wound healing.

To make standard shallow wounds, which measured 2.5 × 2.5 cm., a scalpel was drawn over the skin against a 'Perspex' template to mark the wound outline with shallow incisions, then with the scalpel blade held in the plane of the skin, the dermal tissue was cut through just below the epidermis. The freshly made wounds were not swabbed or interfered with in any way. When all the wounds were made the pig was allowed to recover from the anesthetic, returned to its pen wearing its guard and isolated from other animals.

Fig. 4–7.—Surface and side views of the polythene dressing. Dimensions are indicated on the diagram.

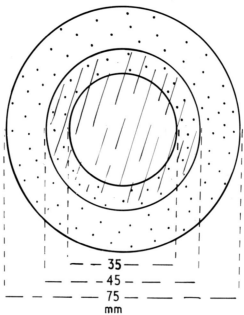

Biopsy specimens of healing wounds were obtained immediately after wounding, after 8, 12 and 18 hours, daily up to 35 days and at less frequent intervals until 731 days. Altogether several hundred wounds were studied. The pigs were anesthetized to take biopsy specimens. Only one specimen was taken from each wound which was then sutured, covered with a dressing and dismissed from the experiment. Specimens for histological examination were taken across the entire width of the wounds and included some of the undamaged skin at the sides of the wounds. The specimens were cut in the dorsovertical direction so that the hair follicles could be cut longitudinally, aiding histological interpretation. They were dehydrated in alcohol, cleared in benzene or chloroform and embedded in paraffin wax. Serial sections were cut on a rotary microtome at 10 μm. to provide vertical sections of the skin and healing wounds. Some duplicate specimens were serially sectioned in the horizontal plane of the skin.

To study the effects of covering wounds, polythene film was used, held in place by a ring of elastic adhesive plaster. The dimensions of the dressing are shown in Figure 4-7. The film was 0.0015 inch thick, natural grade, low density polyethylene (British Cellophane Ltd.). It was cleaned by soaking in a 1% solution of a nonionic detergent, washed thoroughly in running water, rinsed in distilled water, blotted dry with clean filter paper, sealed in polythene bags and sterilized by ultraviolet radiation.

To investigate the effects of drying wound surfaces more extensively than occurs when a wound is merely exposed to the air, wounds were made as described above and the pigs floated on the levitation apparatus described by Scales [4] and Scales and Winter [5]. Air at 45°C (arbitrarily found to be the temperature of moving air necessary to maintain body temperature of a pig constant at 38°C on this version of the levitation apparatus) was blown over the wounds for 30 minutes after wound making and a further 30 minutes, 5 hours later. The air flowed at 1,350 ft.^{3}/minute. Biopsy specimens were obtained after blowing on the wounds and 3 and 7 days later.

OBSERVATIONS ON THE HEALING OF SHALLOW WOUNDS IN THE SKIN OF THE PIG

Gross Appearances

There is only slight bleeding when the wounds are made and the blood soon coagulates. Within a few minutes, droplets of straw colored fluid appear on the surface and coalesce, covering the wound with a moist layer which gradually dries. After 24 hours there is a thin rigid yellowish scab. There are no gross signs of inflammation; the skin around the wound does not become reddened or noticeably swollen. There has been no sepsis. Once covered by a dry scab the wounds do not alter in appearance until, about three weeks after the injury is inflicted, the scab loosens and is shed.

The Extent of the Wound

The epidermis and the papillary layer of the dermis are cut away and the upper part of the reticular layer of the dermis is exposed (Fig. 4-8). Included in each 6.25 cm.^{2} wound area are approximately 160 hair follicles and the ducts of the apocrine glands associated with them. Each hair follicle is damaged to the extent that the outer 1/50th of its total length is excised, its connection with the

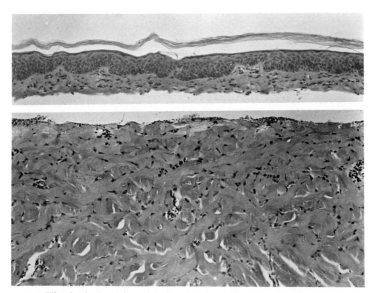

Fig. 4–8.—Histological section showing depth of the partial-thickness excision in the study. *Upper,* epidermis and superficial dermis removed by wounding; *lower,* wound bed after wounding.

surface epidermis is severed and the outer root sheath in the pilary canal region of the follicle is exposed. Similarly the terminal portions of the ducts of apocrine glands are destroyed. The wound is about 0.2 mm. deep. Such a shallow wound scarcely disturbs the mechanical integrity of the skin, but the protection normally afforded to the dermis by the epidermis is wholly lacking.

General Pattern of Healing

The missing epidermis is replaced by regeneration from the epidermis at the wound margins, the outer root sheaths of hair follicles and the walls of the ducts of apocrine glands. Epidermal regeneration begins within 24 hours and the wound is resurfaced by new epidermis by the sixth or seventh day after injury. New connective tissue is formed under the new epidermis, the most vigorous growth occurring between about the fifth and twelfth days, at which time the epidermis is hyperplastic. From about the twelfth day there is gradual reorganization and maturation of the newly formed tissues, culminating in near perfect regeneration of the epidermis and the dermal papillary layer.

Inflammatory Reaction

The injury invokes a vigorous local inflammatory reaction, the histological manifestations being: swelling, extravasation of leukocytes, and the presence of a serous exudate. Early in the course of the inflammatory reaction the injured tissue swells (see Fig. 4-8) and fills the shallow defect in the skin. As a result, the dermal surface of the wound is brought level with the surface of the surrounding epidermis. The swelling is due to fluid between the collagen fibers and perhaps to swelling of the collagen itself. Histologically the bundles of fibers are more closely packed than normal. Swelling affects the dermis for about 1.5 mm. around the wound.

In the same area the small blood vessels are dilated and filled with leukocytes. Many leukocytes are free in the tissues and evidently move among the swollen fibrous tissue. They collect in a band of tissue about 0.2 mm. deep immediately below the wound surface. Covering the wound is a thin blood clot which later dissolves in the serous fluid that oozes out of the dermis. The fluid is an exudate filtered through the walls of abnormally permeable blood vessels just beneath the wound surface. Erythrocytes in the blood clot are lysed and are represented in sections by clumps of eosinophilic material. Some leukocytes move into the exudate from the dermis.

Formation of the Scab

The changes thus far described occur within eight hours. Ten hours later, that is 18 hours after injury, there is evidence that the acute inflammatory reaction is over. Many of the blood vessels are now filled with erythrocytes and the swelling of the fibrous tissue is subsiding. Lymphatic vessels are dilated and filled with fluid. The most significant change visible in histological sections at this time is the evidence that the exudate and some of the fibrous tissue beneath it is becoming dried (Fig. 4-9). The numerous leukocytes concentrated in the drying layer of dermis are shriveled and pale staining. Collagen bundles and fibers can still be recognized in the dehydrated tissue. The fibers remain birefringent and still stain readily with eosin or acid fuchsin. Parts of blood vessels and fragments of arrector pili muscles in the affected tissue are dried and shrunken. The upper-

Fig. 4–9.—Cross-section of a 24-hour, air exposed wound showing surface drying.

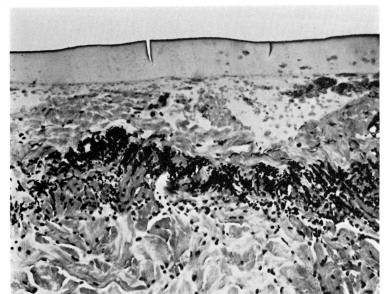

most cells of hair follicles and ducts of apocrine glands dehydrate and die. About 0.1 mm. depth of the superficial dermal tissue is dried by 24 hours. No more tissue is affected after this time and it is probable that at this level there is an equilibrium between the rate of water loss by evaporation and the rate at which the tissue is re-wetted from below. If a cooled glass plate is held over the dry surface of a wound at this stage, moisture rapidly condenses on the glass showing that water vapor passes freely through the scab. Drying is accompanied by considerable compaction of the tissues and the 0.1 mm. deep layer measured in histological sections may represent 0.3 mm. or so of the dermis in its normal hydrated state.

Regeneration of Epidermis

The regenerating epidermis moves through the moist dermal fibrous tissue under the dry layer (Fig. 4-10). Ahead of the epidermis are collagen bundles running uninterruptedly into the scab. The epidermis cleaves a way through them and separates the dry scab from the remainder of the dermis.

Grossly, epidermal migration may be said to begin about 24 hours after the injury is inflicted, but it is possible to detect the movement of one or two epidermal cells in some areas of the wound by eight hours and there may be up to 0.1 mm. of new epidermis extended from the wound edge in 18 hours. On the other hand, there is usually no movement of cells from some of the hair follicles until after more than 24 hours have elapsed. The determining factor seems to be the progressive dehydration of the exposed tissues which immobilizes epidermal cells that might otherwise have started to move across the wound.

As remarked above there are some 160 hair follicles in the wound; new epidermis spreads radially from each of these sources of epidermal cells, from the

Fig. 4–10.—Section of an advancing tip of migrating epidermis moving through the dermis.

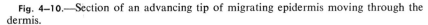

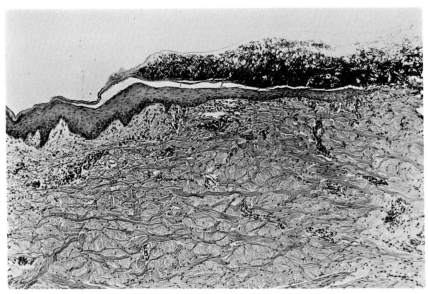

apocrine gland ducts associated with them and from the epidermis at the wound edges. In a wound of this size over 90% of the new epidermis derives from the epidermal appendages within the wound. Nowhere has the epidermis further than 1.0 mm. to move before meeting with another sheet of cells moving in the opposite direction. It is six days from the time epidermal regeneration begins that the wound is fully covered by new epidermis and the overall average speed of epidermal cell movement works out on this basis at 7 μm./hour or roughly one cell diameter in an hour.

Two changes in the epidermis around the wound are worthy of note. Within 18 hours it is slightly swollen due to enlargement of the cells. Also, it stains quite heavily for glycogen over an area about 3 mm. back from the wound. The migrating epidermal cells contain glycogen which can be detected in them in lesser quantities throughout the 30- to 35-day period of healing. Similar changes are seen in the outer root sheaths of hair follicles and in the walls of the ducts of apocrine glands in the wound.

Leap-Frog Hypothesis of Epidermal Regeneration

Considerable interest attaches to how the epidermis spreads across the wound. The basal cells of the epidermis adjacent to the wound do not become detached from the papillary layer and it is certain that the epidermis as a whole does not move bodily across the wound. It is unlikely too that the cells above the basal layer crawl en masse out of the epidermis bordering the wound and continue on across the wound until halted by contact with other epidermal cells. On the contrary it is probable that no single epidermal cell moves more than two or three cell lengths from its original position. The new epidermis is built up by successive implantation of cells on the wound surface [6, 7]. The first cell to move out of the parent epidermis promptly rounds up and becomes the first of the basal cells of the new epidermis. The cell above and behind it stretches over the new basal cell and comes to lie on the wound surface ahead of it where it too rounds up and becomes stationary. Thus is the new epidermis built up, each forward movement taking about one hour. Simultaneously other cells extend over the basal cells and others above them so that the new epidermis is four to six cells deep at the outset. Moreover, only a few cell diameters back from the leading edge the new epidermis is seven to eight cells deep in less than 48 hours and is stratified in the normal way. There is a distinct basal layer, the more superficial cells are progressively more flattened, there is a layer of cells that contain keratohyalin granules and the most superficial cells are scale like and have lost their nuclei. These uppermost cells adhere to the scab. It appears that the cells just behind the advancing border of epidermis, those that lie between the leading edge and the original wound edge, are not moving laterally over the wound but are moving upwards towards the surface as in the normal epidermis. If cells are not flowing through from the old epidermis it follows that the slow advance of the epidermis must be sustained by the production of cells in the new epidermis itself. It is found that the new basal cells begin to divide within about 24 hours of their having settled down on the wound surface.

Regeneration of the Papillary Layer

It will be recalled that the epidermis moves through the dermis. In so doing it creates a new surface comprising the highly collagenous tissue of the upper reticular layer of the dermis interrupted here and there by spaces filled with loose connective tissue, blood vessels and perivascular cells. These are the vascular compartments of the subpapillary plexus. It is from them that new connective tissue originates.

After the acute inflammatory reactions are over, the number of polymorphonuclear leukocytes declines and they no longer accumulate near the wound surface. Mononuclear cells now become predominant. These new arrivals have a small intensely basophilic nucleus, often slightly indented, and a narrow ring of faintly basophilic cytoplasm. These characteristics suggest that they are lymphocytes or other mononuclear cells presumably migrated from nearby blood vessels. Similar cells are seen in unusually large numbers inside the blood vessels near the wound at this time. Owing to the presence of these mononuclear cells and some granulocytes there is a moderate increase in the population of perivascular cells. About 48 hours after wounding, some mitotic figures are seen in cells around the vessels and in endothelial cells of the blood vessels. Apart from this there is little morphological evidence of regenerative activity on the part of the

Fig. 4–11.—Seven-day wound showing regeneration of the papillary layer; note the ridges forming at the dermal surface of the epidermis.

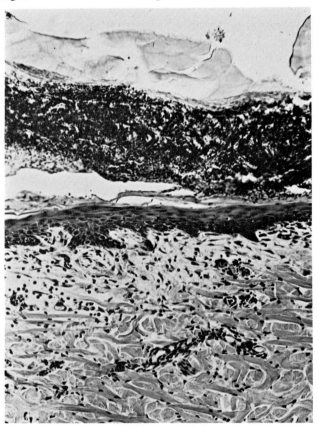

connective tissue until the fifth day when a fluid exudate collects under the older parts of the new epidermis adjacent to the margins of the wound and near the hair follicles which lifts the epidermis away from the dermal tissue (Fig. 4-11). Blood vessels, regenerating from the subpapillary plexus, grow into the exudate accompanied by the perivascular cells whose origins have just been discussed. Within 48 hours after the start of connective tissue regeneration, that is about seven days after injury, fibroblasts are becoming plentiful and the mononuclear cells begin to disappear. This suggests that the mononuclear cells, tentatively identified as cells from the blood, become fibroblasts.

Changes in the Epidermis

As new tissue accumulates under the epidermis, the undersurface of the epidermis, which until now was flat, begins to develop irregularities (see Fig. 4-11). In ordinary vertical sections the epidermal outgrowths are like greatly attenuated epidermal ridges (Fig. 4-12). Reconstruction in wax from serial sections showing the three-dimensional form of the epidermis at this stage reveals that the projections are the walls of pockets of epidermal tissue dividing the developing connective tissue into numerous separate compartments [6]. They slope at an angle of approximately 30° to the horizontal as though the epidermis has flopped towards the ground under its own weight. Each pocket surrounds one or two growing blood vessels and the associated papilla of developing connective tissue (Fig. 4-13).

Fibrogenesis

The first new collagen fibers are visible as straight thin fuchsinophilic threads on the eighth or ninth day. At first they are sparsely scattered but by the tenth day they are more numerous and mostly orientated perpendicular to the dermis. The free ends of the coarse bundles of fibers in the dermis adjoining the new tissues have a frayed appearance and the new fibers merge into them, the new fibrous tissue seemingly becoming physically continuous with the old.

As the new tissue becomes more fibrous the cell population wanes. The subepidermal layer is deepest about 10–15 days after injury and then begins to shrink in volume. Contraction of the connective tissue brings the epidermis close to the original dermal tissue. At the same time the walls of the pockets of epidermal tissue on the underside of the epidermis are reduced to shallow ridges. There is no sign of a foreign body type reaction on the part of the connective tissue which might account for the elimination of the epidermal spurs.

After contraction the collagen fibers mostly lie horizontally in the plane of the skin and are densely packed. The tissue has the fine texture characteristic of the normal papillary layer. By this time, 30–40 days after the injury was inflicted, the wounded area of skin cannot easily be distinguished from normal skin in histological sections and the wound may be said to be fully healed.

The Effects of Covering Shallow Wounds

The wounds covered with polythene film are protected from dehydration and this alters the pattern of healing in its early stages and affects the speed of epithelization and of connective tissue formation. The tissue fluid oozing from the injured dermis remains in a fluid state on the wound surface. Leukocytes do not

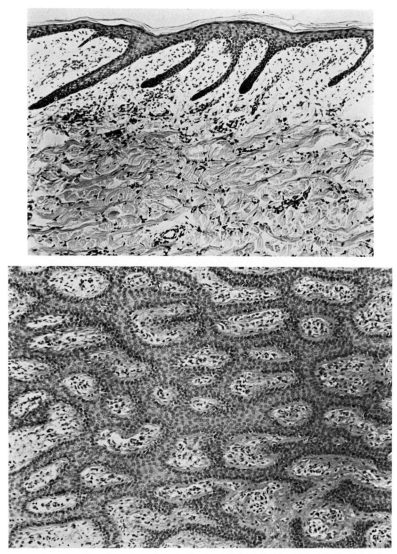

Fig. 4–12 (top).—Ten-day wound; note the protrusion of the epidermis into the dermis.
Fig. 4–13 (bottom).—Tangential section of a 15-day wound illustrating the epidermal ridges and blood vessels within the dermal papillae.

accumulate in the fibrous tissue but migrate out of the dermis into the moist serous layer beneath the polythene film (Fig. 4-14).

The regenerating epidermis moves through the moist exudate traveling either directly upon the dermal fibrous tissue, or just above it. In the latter instance it looks as if it is moving upon relatively coarse fibers, perhaps of fibrin, but certain confirmation of the nature of these fibers has not been made. The migrating epi-

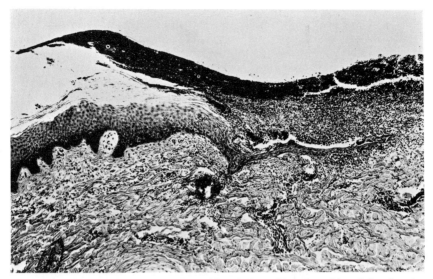

Fig. 4–14.—Two-day wound covered with polythene film; the epidermis is migrating through the moist exudate on wound surface.

dermal cells are markedly flattened and elongated and the moving sheet of cells is sometimes only two or three cells thick over a considerable area. The wounds are fully covered by new epidermis in 72 hours, three days earlier than normal. The new epidermis by the end of the third day is 6–8 cells deep and the cells are already organized in characteristic layers. Projections are beginning to be formed on its undersurface. New blood vessels begin to grow into fluid under the epidermis 48 hours after the injury was inflicted. Thus connective tissue regeneration begins about 3 days earlier than normal. Large numbers of mononuclear cells are seen in the subepidermal layer on the third day. There are a few fibroblasts by this time, many on the fifth day and by the seventh day there is a mass of new collagen fibers. Maturation of the new tissue takes the same course as in normal wounds and by about day 20 there is no difference in the histological appearance of covered wounds and wounds exposed to the air.

Epidermal and Connective Tissue Interaction

The speedier growth of new connective tissue when wounds are covered and kept moist might suggest that the presence of epidermis has some inductive effect on the growth of connective tissue, but this is unlikely, since connective tissue grows in the base of a deep wound before the epidermis has moved across the surface. The logical explanation is that as new connective tissue can only grow into a space filled with a suitable exudate and since in normal wounds the dehydrated dermal tissue is continuous with the remainder of the dermis until the epidermis has passed across and separated it, there is no space to accommodate an exudate and new connective tissue. The subepidermal layer can only develop when a sufficient length of scab is detached from the dermis and can then be floated away by fluid welling up from the subjacent dermal tissue.

The origin of the subepidermal exudate is important, since its formation is apparently a decisive first step in the genesis of new connective tissue. It is partly an inflammatory exudate due primarily to increased permeability of the walls of the vessels in the subpapillary plexus. It seems likely that the vessel walls remain abnormally permeable even after seven days since cells evidently leave the vessels at this time. In any case the regenerating blood vessels will be very leaky [8]. It may also in part be due to seepage of tissue fluid from the adjacent tissues. Thirdly, if the epidermis secretes a collagenolytic enzyme in moving through the fibrous tissue, some of the subepidermal fluid may arise from solubilization of the existing collagen. Histological sections parallel to the surface show that in the tissue recently traversed by migrating epidermis the collagen fibers are scattered and partly disintegrated.

The growth of blood vessels undoubtedly has a bearing on the morphology of repair and where a skin wound is quite shallow, as were these wounds, and where the subpapillary plexus is intact, there still exists the anatomical basis for the normal pattern of papillary blood vessels and this may be one of the reasons for the perfect repair of these wounds. As a small group of blood vessels grows up into the subepidermal exudate, the epidermis over the top of the vessels recedes away from them, simply because the pressure of exudation from the vessels floats the epidermis away, or through some more subtle interaction between growing blood vessels and epidermis. The intriguing question is: what stops the blood vessels and connective tissue from growing indefinitely? Probably beyond a certain point the weight of the epidermis and the scab, and the elastic tension of the epidermal layer which is pinned down by the hair follicles, prevent the accumulation of more fluid substrate and automatically halts further growth.

Around the sides of the growing papilla of blood vessels and connective tissue cells the epidermal cells do not float upwards but proliferate and remain relatively static so that walls of epidermal tissue are built up around the papillae and form pockets on the underside of the epidermis.

Conversion of the dilute subepidermal tissue with its scattered fibers of collagen into a compact papillary layer with a fine texture of fibers is mainly due to contraction of the newly formed tissue. Contraction of newly formed connective tissue, therefore, has in shallow wounds, as in deep wounds, a definite morphogenic function.

As the subepidermal tissue slowly contracts the deep epidermal ridges are reduced to normal proportions. In man, according to Gillman and Penn [9] the pseudopegs, as they called them, break up into small internally keratinizing cysts and are attacked and eliminated by foreign body type reaction (macrophage and giant cell activity) on the part of the connective tissue. There is no evidence for this in the present material. The ridges simply melt away. The probable explanation is that the cells continue to move towards the skin surface where they desquamate, but cell proliferation slows down or ceases entirely in the ridges so that they are gradually depleted of cells. There is a similar problem in the disappearance of the lower third of a hair follicle in the catagen stage of the hair growth cycle which may be explained in the same way.

By the fortieth day, or thereabout, the regenerated epidermis has regained a normal structure and the papillary layer is likewise normal. Regeneration following the infliction of a clean shallow wound in the skin of young Large White strain pigs is perfect. In man, rodents and the rabbit, it has been said that regeneration is always less than perfect and so far as present knowledge goes, the pig is unique in this respect. It is possible, but unlikely, that perfection of repair in the animals investigated is due to their relative immaturity. Perhaps the wounds were shallower than those studied by others. It is also possible that this is a genuine difference from other animals so far investigated, and that for some reason good skin healing has some special evolutionary advantage in the species.

Observations on Very Dry Wounds

Blowing air over wounds shortly after the injury is inflicted creates a dry scab that is deeper than normal. From the wound edges the epidermis migrates vertically downwards before moving horizontally through the dermis under the dehydrated tissue. The upper parts of the hair follicles are dried, and the cells killed, and it is the uppermost surviving cells that move out from the follicles and form a new epidermis, separating the thick scab from the remainder of the dermal tissue.

Epidermal regeneration is delayed when the wound surface is extensively dehydrated, there being only about half as much new epidermis on these wounds after 3 days as on wounds with normal thin dry scabs [10].

Effects of Pricking Through the Epidermis

The skin surface was disturbed by multiple pin pricks to stimulate an inflammatory reaction in the papillary layer and accumulation of fluid under the epidermis. As Figure 4-15 shows, the epidermis after three days is lifted by a fluid exudate and the epidermal ridges have elongated. There is a similarity between the bloated dermal papillae and attenuated ridges produced in this way and the

Fig. 4–15.—Section showing changes in papillary dermis and hypertrophy of epidermis 3 days after injuring tissues by pricking through the epidermis.

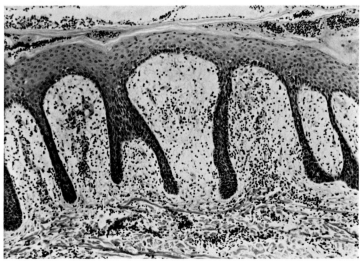

developing connective tissue papillae, partly enclosed by pockets of epidermal tissue, at a stage in the healing of a shallow wound, illustrated in Figure 4-12.

Additional Observations on Epidermal Cell Migration

The following four observations show that where there is a suitable moist exudate for the epidermis to grow into, epidermal cells from all levels below the horny layer may move out onto adjacent surfaces of keratinous or collagenous tissue.

First, when shallow incisions are made in the surface of the epidermis alongside wounds—the cuts just perforating the horny and granular layers, the cells from the prickle cell layer promptly move out of the epidermis into the serous exudate on the skin surface (Fig. 4-16).

Second, it occasionally happened that in making the wounds a short length of epidermis at the edge was turned back on itself so that the epidermal ridges were

Fig. 4–16.—A, 18-hour wound showing epidermal cells migrating out of the skin surface. B, diagrammatic representation of wound site and migrating cells.

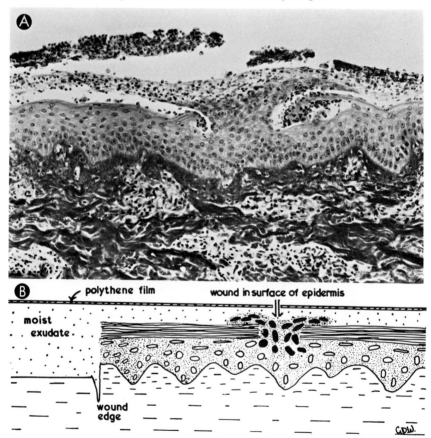

uppermost and epidermal cells moved out from the ridge into the exudate bathing the surface as shown in Figure 4-17.

Third, it is often found that in those wounds kept moist on the surface by covering them with polythene film, epidermal cell migration from the wound edges begins with cells moving back over the surface of the epidermis as well as forward across the wound surface.

Finally, also on covered wounds it is found that the cut ends of hair follicles are sealed over by migrating epidermis as shown in Figure 4-18. This behavior is consistent with the leap frog hypothesis of epidermal cell migration.

Fig. 4–17.—A, everted epidermis at wound edge showing epithelial migration from an excised epidermal ridge. B, edge of a wound covered by polythene film, 18 hours after injury. Epidermis is migrating back over skin surface as well as across the wound.

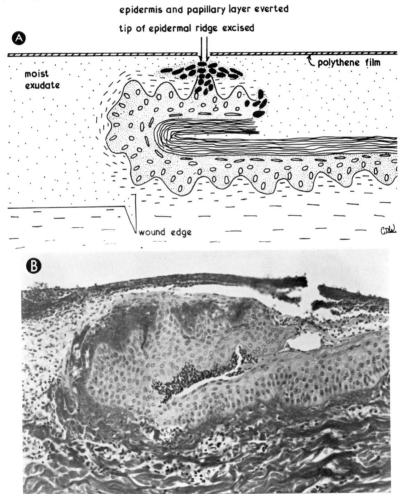

epidermis and papillary layer everted

tip of epidermal ridge excised

A

moist
exudate

polythene film

wound edge

B

epidermal cells moving out of

outer root sheath

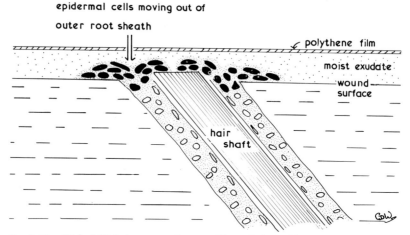

Fig. 4–18.—Hair follicle in a wound covered by polythene film, 18 hours after injury. The cells from the outer root sheath migrate over the cut hair as well as out across the wound surface.

Absence of Effect of Wounds on Hair Growth

In view of the mosaic pattern of hair replacement in the pig it would be difficult to detect any subtle effects the presence of a wound might have on the duration and rate of hair growth. It is found that throughout healing there are some follicles under the wound in the anagen stage of the hair growth cycle and some in the telogen stage. It is certain therefore that excision of the outer 1/50th of a hair follicle and trauma and inflammation near the skin surface do not cause all the hairs to stop growing and the follicles to enter catagen, nor apparently does the injury stimulate all quiescent follicles into activity.

Measurement of the Speed of Regeneration of Epidermis

Observations of the speed of healing of wounds depending on simple inspection of the wound surface, upon photography and planimetry or on qualitative assessment from histological sections were judged to be too imprecise for the present purpose which is to define as accurately as possible the normal growth curve of epidermal regeneration after injury. Such data, based on normal wounds, are necessary basic information when subsequently the effects of experimental treatments on epidermal growth is investigated.

On shallow wounds the new epidermis grows from many sources, so it is necessary to cut serial sections and examine a sufficient area of the wound surface and include a representative sample of the hair follicles.

Method. Shallow wounds were made and serial sections prepared as already described. Every fifth section in a series was examined under the microscope at ×80 magnification and the separate lengths of epidermis grown from the wound edges and the epidermal appendages in the wound were measured to within 0.01 mm. The total length of the wound surface in each section was also measured. About 400 sections across the full width of each wound were sampled; the sum

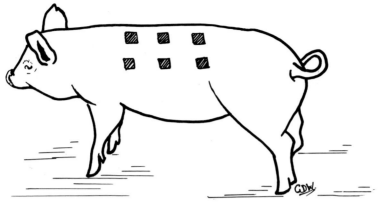

Fig. 4-19.—Diagram showing the position of the wounds.

of the separate lengths of epidermis was found and the amount of new epidermis expressed as a percentage of the total wound surface.

To make measurements a dial gauge was used against the moving stage of the microscope and the microscope was equipped with a cross-hair graticule in the eyepiece.

Usually 12 wounds were made on one animal, six on either side of the back, spaced well apart (Fig. 4-19). In a preliminary experiment six wounds were exposed to the air and six were covered with polythene film. Biopsy specimens of each type of wound were taken after 1, 3, 5, 7, 9 and 11 days, to establish the

Table 4-1
Summary of Data on the Speed of Epidermal Regeneration

Normal Wounds

Time after Injury	Proportion of Wound Surface Covered by Regenerated Epidermis	Variation
18 hours	0.7%	0– 6%
24 hours	3.0%	2– 11%
2 days	18.0%	10– 28%
3 days	38.0%	21– 58%
4 days	about 55.0%	
5 days	78.0%	61– 95%
6 days	99.0%	95–100%

Covered Wounds

Time after Injury	Proportion of Wound Surface Covered by Regenerated Epidermis	Variation
18 hours	0.5%	0– 1.6%
24 hours	9.0%	6– 16.0%
2 days	50.0%	33– 73.0%
3 days	92.0%	62–100.0%

general pattern of growth of the epidermis when the wound surface is dry and moist respectively. In a separate experiment six wounds exposed to the air were compared with six wounds covered with polythene film, biopsy specimens being taken from all the wounds after 3 days. Further experiments were conducted to establish the amount of epidermis after 18 hours, 1 day, 3, 4, 5 and 6 days.

There will be a small error if the widths of cut surfaces of hair follicles and the ducts of apocrine glands are counted as new epidermis. In the results for 18 hours, only the migrated epidermis either side of the epidermal appendages has been measured; at later times the proportionate error introduced by including the width of the epidermal appendages is small and has been ignored.

Results. Preliminary experiments showed that epidermal regeneration was faster under polythene film than when the wounds were exposed to the air [11]. The results of the measurement to establish the normal speed of healing are given in Table 4-1.

Effects of Covering Wounds with Other Plastic Films. Employing similar techniques, the speed of epithelization of wounds covered by polyester and polypropylene films was measured, with the following results:

Polypropylene film
0.0005 inch thick, type T.R.B./5 (Shorks Metal Box Ltd).
Number of wounds: 7
Total length of wound surface examined: approx. 646 cm.
Total length of new epidermis: "   454 cm.
Proportion of wound surface covered by new epidermis after 72 hours:
Mean and standard error: 70% ± 5.1%

Polyester film
0.00025 inch thick, Grade 0, Melinex (I.C.I. Ltd).
Number of wounds: 19
Total length of wound surface examined: approx. 1,790 cm.
Total length of new epidermis: "   937 cm.
Proportion of wound surface covered by new epidermis after 72 hours:
Mean and standard error: 52% ± 4.4%

Polythene film (Control, same animals)
0.0015 inch thick, natural grade, low density
(British Cellophane Ltd).
Number of wounds: 12
Total length of wound surface examined: approx. 1,200 cm.
Total length of new epidermis: "   1,080 cm.
Proportion of wound surface covered by new epidermis after 72 hours:
Mean and standard error: 90 % ± 3.7%.

After three days there is 20% less new epidermis on polypropylene covered wounds and 40% less on polyester covered wounds than on similar wounds covered with polythene film, differences which are statistically highly significant (Students t test, $p < 0.005$ in either case).

Oxygen Tension and Epidermal Regeneration

Intermittent treatment with 100% oxygen at a pressure of 2 atmospheres absolute accelerated epidermal regeneration on both exposed and covered wounds by about 30% [12]. Probably the oxygen tension in the tissue fluid bathing the migrating epidermal cells was raised and the cells made use of this increased fuel supply to move faster. That epidermal regeneration can be accelerated in this way demonstrates that during normal wound healing the quantity of oxygen available is a critical rate limiting factor.

Of the three plastic films the polythene film has the highest oxygen permeability. Polypropylene allows the passage of about 60% less oxygen and the polyester film has only 1% of the oxygen permeability of low density polythene. These facts, together with the results of the hyperbaric oxygen experiments, suggest that the more rapid epidermal regeneration observed under polythene film (90%), than under polypropylene (70%) and polyester (52%), is directly related to the oxygen permeabilities of these films. During occlusive therapy of wounds oxygen from the air, passing through the film, dissolves in the serous exudate and can be utilized by the migrating epidermal cells. Hence for most rapid healing a film of high oxygen permeability should be used.

Mitotic Activity in the Epidermis

To study the pattern of cell division, an adaptation of the colchicine method was used. The technique, using pigs weighing about 50 lbs., was to inject 1 ml. of colchicine solution containing 2 mg. Colcemid per 1 ml. of 0.9% saline, intravenously, 4 hours and again 2 hours prior to taking biopsy specimens of the skin for histological evaluation. The injections were given in the ear vein, the animals being quieted by brief light anesthesia induced by a mixture of nitrous oxide, oxygen and fluothane given through a face mask. The dose of colchicine was divided in order to maintain a sufficient concentration in the serum to arrest mitosis in the epidermis for 4 hours while avoiding possible toxic amounts. Skin specimens were immediately fixed in Zenker formaldehyde solution and subsequently embedded in wax and cut 10 μm. thick into a continuous series of sections. Every fifth section of a series of 100 sections was mounted in series, stained with hematoxylin and eosin and examined through a ×40 (N.A.O. 75) microscope objective at a magnification of ×400. The number of mitotic figures in each unit length of 0.33 mm. of epidermis was counted and an average obtained for 10 sections in series. Counts were made in this way on 1 cm. of skin from the back of each of 12 animals.

On examination there were numerous typical "colchicine metaphase" nuclei and no telophase figures. It is estimated that the average mitotic count in epidermis on the backs of these pigs at 1400 hours is 0.76 ± 0.13 dividing cells/unit length (0.33 mm.) epidermis, under the given experimental conditions.

Mitotic Activity in Epidermis at the Edge of a Shallow Wound

It was planned to determine the mitotic activity in epidermis at the edge of shallow wounds after 12 hours, 1–7 days, 9, 11, 15, 20, 25, 30 and 40 days. Two pigs were studied at each time interval. The animals were all young female large white pigs from the same pedigreed herd weighing approximately 50 lbs. Twenty

1 cm. × 1 cm. shallow wounds were made on the backs of each animal as described earlier. Ten of these wounds on one side were covered with polythene film and the other ten were exposed to the air. The colchicine technique was used and biopsy specimens of all twenty wounds were obtained at the appropriate time. Serial sections were prepared and the number of mitotic figures counted in every 0.33 mm. unit length of epidermis from the wound edge to a point 5 mm. away from the wound. This was done in ten sections at 50 μm. intervals on both dorsal and ventral edges of all twenty wounds in each animal. The mean number of dividing cells was calculated from the sum of the 200 counts for each of the 15 unit lengths of epidermis adjacent to the ten wounds. Figure 4-20 illustrates the pattern of cell proliferation at the edge of a wound 48 hours old, when no dressing is used and will serve to demonstrate to the reader how the mitotic counts are related to the wound edge. The results of the experiment are given in a series of histograms (Fig. 4-21).

It is found that under normal conditions, when no dressing is used and a dry scab forms there is, at first, some inhibition of mitosis (Fig. 4-22). Peak activity

Fig. 4–20.—Part of a normal shallow wound exposed to the air, 48 hours after injury. **A**, bar graph in which the figures given are averages from counts of ten sections at two edges of each of ten wounds on one animal. **B**, composite histological section demonstrating the pattern of epidermal cell proliferation at the wound edge.

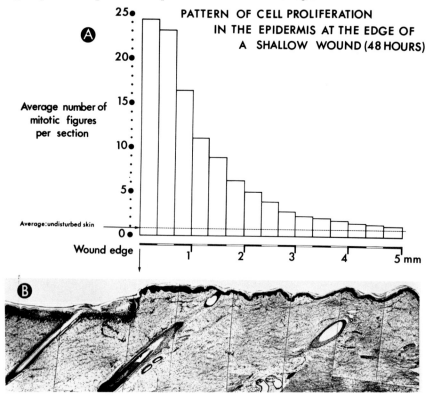

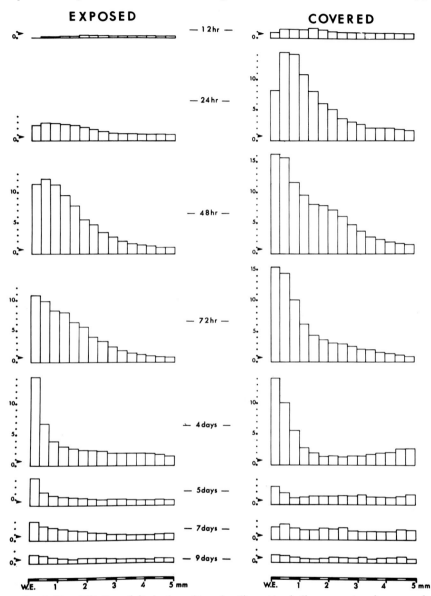

Fig. 4–21.—Mitotic activity in the epidermis adjacent to shallow wounds, when wounds are exposed to the air **(left)** and are covered with polythene film **(right)**. *W.E.*, wound edge. *Arrow,* normal level of mitotic activity in undisturbed skin under same experimental conditions. Ordinates: arithmetical mean number of mitotic figures per section in each unit length of epidermis (0.33 mm.) from counts of 10 sections at two edges of each of 10 wounds in 2 animals.

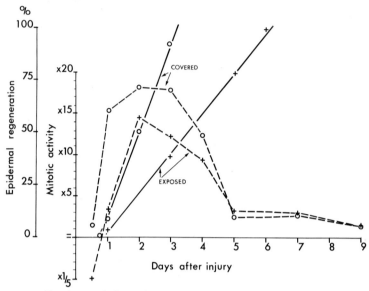

Fig. 4–22.—Graph correlating epidermal regeneration and mitotic activity in the epidermis at the margins of the wounds. Epidermal regeneration (*solid lines*), data from Table 4-1, showing proportion of wound surface covered by new epidermis. Mitotic activity (*broken lines*), data from Figure 4-21. Wounds covered by polythene film (∘). Wounds exposed to the air (+).

is recorded after 48 hours when in the millimeter of epidermis adjacent to the wound edge there is about seventeen times more activity than in the undisturbed epidermis. Activity then declines sharply while the epidermis is still migrating across the wound surface and by the time epithelization is complete, mitotic activity in the epidermis at the wound edge has fallen to about 3 or 4 times its normal level. It remains slightly elevated for at least three more days.

There is a similar pattern of mitotic activity at the edges of shallow wounds covered with polythene film. The epidermis migrates across the wound more rapidly, the burst of mitotic activity begins earlier and there is more intensive mitotic activity in the millimeter wide band of epidermis adjacent to the wound.

Plainly the epidermis does not react in an all-or-none fashion when injured and its full mitotic potential is not realized under normal conditions of healing. These findings are consistent with the idea that mitosis in the epidermis is at least in part a reaction to epidermal cell migration. The point is not conclusively proved because it is possible that covering the wound creates better conditions for mitosis as it does for cell migration.

The chalone theory developed by Bullough and Lawrence [13–17] explains the burst of mitotic activity at the margins of the wound. As in the mouse, there is a marked gradient of mitotic activity adjacent to wounds in porcine skin, which is greatest near the wound edge and falls away gradually. Raised activity is confined to within one millimeter from the wound in the mouse, but extends at least 5 mm. in the pig. Within the first 24 hours the highest mitotic activity was a third of a millimeter away from the edge of the wound, probably because ‚those cells nearest the wound are programmed for movement, which excludes mitosis.

Epidermal Regeneration After the Skin Is Injured by Burning

Scalds, 3.8 cm. in diameter, were made by running water at 60°C through a 'Perspex' tube placed on the shaved skin surface for 60 seconds. The epidermis was killed and the blood vessels on the upper two thirds of the dermis coagulated. The dead epidermis protects the underlying tissue from dehydration and if the epidermal blister is scraped off the underlying dermal tissue forms a dry eschar. With or without the dead epidermal blister the eschar remains attached and continuous with the underlying viable dermis and is only separated from it by migration of the epidermis through the dermis below the nonviable fibrous tissue. This is similar to the healing of a shallow wound when scab formation is allowed to take place naturally. The eschar may separate with the formation of a fluid layer of inflammatory exudate if deep sepsis supervenes.

The most remarkable observation on burns is that tissue regeneration is so long delayed. No epidermal regeneration takes place for 8–10 days after the injury is inflicted. This is not because the epidermis at the edge of the burn is immobilized by the thermal injury, as can be demonstrated by making an incision immediately adjacent to the lesion when the epidermis promptly heals by migration and mitosis within 48 hours, showing that these cells can respond to a normal stimulus.

When regeneration starts after this long lag period, epidermal cells move out from the edges of the lesion and from the remains of the severely damaged hair follicles deep in the dermis. Scalds, as described, are completely epithelized by the fifteenth day.

Epidermal Reactions Around Transcutaneous Implants

It is well known that epidermal tissue grows down around a skin suture and by about the tenth day the implant is completely invested in a tube of epidermis. In a recent experiment small sheets of various plastics, including polythene film, P.T.F.E. film, 0.45 μm Millipore, polyhydroxyethyl methacrylate (Poly-HEMA) gel, Poly-HEMA sponge and porous P.T.F.E. film, measuring approximately 3 mm. × 1 mm. × 0.2 mm., were inserted through small incisions into the skin on the back of young Large White pigs leaving about 0.5 mm. protruding through the skin surface, then covered with an occlusive film to minimize dehydration around the point of entry. Specimens have been studied histologically to 15 days of implantation.

As expected the epidermis migrates alongside the nonporous implants, P.T.F.E. film, polythene film, Poly-HEMA gel and the microporous Millipore. By the tenth day the epidermis, moving down each side of the implant, has united in the dermis under the implant 2 mm. below the surface (Fig. 4-23).

The epidermis did not migrate around the porous implants, Poly-HEMA sponge and porous P.T.F.E. (Fig. 4-24). The sponge has interconnecting tunnels running through it and the holes are of the order of 40–60 μm in diameter. When implanted in the skin, blood vessels penetrate into the interior of the im-

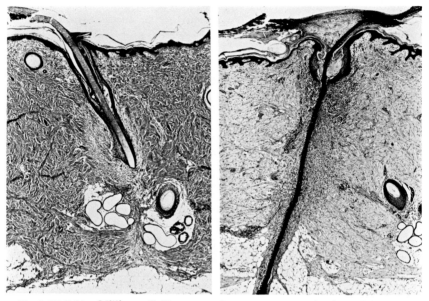

Fig. 4–23 (left).—Millipore, 0.45 μm pore size, transcutaneous implant. Epidermis has grown around the implant in 10 days.

Fig. 4–24 (right).—No migration around porous P.T.F.E. implant, 15 days.

plant and fibrous tissue fills the sponge. The pores in the P.T.F.E. film are of the same order of size and they too became filled with fibrous tissue.

Locke [18] said that when strips of Millipore filter were inserted in Rhodnius larvae through a slit in the integument, cell migration did not occur around the porous implant as it did around nonporous implants of glass or Teflon. Mizuno and Fujii [19] repeated this experiment with mice and report that the epidermis does not grow around implants of Millipore sheets having pores 0.01 μm–1.0 μm. They conclude that epidermal cells can communicate by chemical means and that physical contact is not essential for contact inhibition to occur.

Preliminary studies using the pig do not wholly confirm these findings. The epidermis grew around the implants of Millipore filter which had a pore size of 0.45 μm. It is true that no growth took place around implants with much larger pores which became filled with collagenous tissue continuous with the surrounding connective tissue, but it is likely that epidermal migration was brought to a halt because the epidermis was unable to migrate through the newly formed collagen bundles.

DISCUSSION

Formation of the Scab and the Level of Epidermal Migration

In this investigation wounds were exposed to the air as in nature and care was taken to protect the wounds from damage and to retain the scab during processing for histological examination. The findings on the way in which the scab is formed and the level at which the epidermis migrates differ from the usual description of the healing of shallow wounds and this forms the first topic for discussion.

One function of the epidermis is protection of the underlying tissues against dehydration and when an area of epidermis is lost water vapor begins at once to evaporate from the exposed dermal tissue. The exudate on the wound surface dries and becomes the outer layer of the scab, but this does not stop water from evaporating from the dermis underneath. The surface of the dermis itself is progressively dried over a period of about 18 hours and a water table is established approximately 0.3 mm. below the surface.

It is shown that if conditions at the skin surface are more severe than normal as when warm air is blown rapidly over the wounds, considerably more dermal tissue may be dehydrated.

Epidermal migration is affected because conditions at the wound surface are constantly changing and are unsuitable in the first 12 hours or so and because the epidermal cells, particularly those in the exposed ends of transected hair follicles, are themselves killed by dehydration. When conditions become stabilized the uppermost level at which the epidermis can migrate, where enough moisture remains to support the life of these cells, is beneath the dried dermal tissue, and so migration takes place through the fibrous tissue of the upper reticular layer of the dermis.

In the earlier literature on wound healing, it was held that connective tissue grows in the blood clot on a wound surface and the epidermis later migrates over the surface of the new tissue. Gillman and Penn [9] showed that in shallow wounds the epidermis is the first tissue to be regenerated. They describe the epidermis moving on the wound surface, that is the cut surface of the dermis, through a blood clot. The observations reported here that most nearly agree with theirs are those for covered wounds. In this instance, however, the epidermis does not move through a blood clot, but through a layer of serous exudate that collects on the wound surface in the first few hours and, being protected by the polythene film, remains fluid. The blood clot in both normal wounds exposed to the air and wounds covered by polythene film, plays an insignificant role beyond its function in the first few minutes after injury of plugging the leak of blood from the cut ends of the blood vessels.

The Epidermal Collagenase

Gillman and Penn deduce that the epidermis secretes a proteolytic enzyme which enables it to burrow through the blood clot [9] but this raises certain problems. If the epidermis passes over the wound surface through a moist exudate, there seems no need to postulate that it secretes a proteolytic enzyme because the exudate, being fluid, offers no resistance to the cells. If the exudate is dry, the epidermis must burrow beneath it. In this latter instance, it is necessary to explain how the epidermis cleaves a way through the collagenous fibers in the dermis. It suggests that the epidermis secretes a collagenolytic enzyme which is more likely to come from the epidermis than from leukocytes or other cells in the vicinity, because the collagen bundles remain histologically intact in the scab even though surrounded by large numbers of leukocytes and because the scab is attached to the dermis and bundles of collagen fibers pass uninterruptedly into the scab until the epidermis has passed across. No fluid layer develops ahead of the regenerating epidermis; it is its passage across the wound that separates the

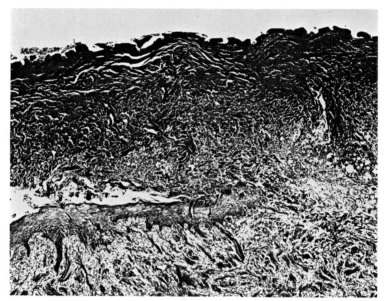

Fig. 4–25.—Burn in human skin, 38 days. Epidermis migrating under eschar. Note undigested collagen within epidermis.

scab from the dermal tissue. Of great interest in this connection is the demonstration by Gross and Lapiere [20] that the tip of the regenerating stump of the amputated fore limb of an amphibian will dissolve collagen in vitro. It is known that in amphibians regeneration depends in some way on the prior appearance of the epidermis. Eisen and Gross [21] found that the collagenolytic enzyme originated from the epithelial cells and that the mesenchymal cells produced a hyaluronidase and suggested that both tissues cooperate in the destruction of extracellular structures. Injured corneal epithelium produces collagenase on the second day after wounding [22] and collagenolytic activity present in mammalian skin increases markedly after wounding [23].

The probable function of the epidermal collagenase in the healing of surgical wounds and burns is to enable the epidermis to cleave a path through the dermal fibrous tissue beneath the scab or eschar. Figure 4-25 shows fragments of undigested collagen within the epidermis migrating beneath the eschar of a burn in human skin, 37 days after injury. A possible explanation for the long delay preceding epidermal regeneration when the skin is injured by burning is that the heated collagen cannot be attacked by the epidermal collagenase.

Owing to its method of formation, the scab has a high content of collagen and there are references to collagen in the scabs of skin wounds of rats [24–27], rabbits [28], pigs [11] and man [29]. It may reasonably be concluded that migration of the epidermis through the dermis and the incorporation of a superficial layer of dermis into the scab is the normal pattern of healing of shallow wounds in the skin of terrestrial mammals.

The Inflammatory Reaction and Formation of a Leukocytic Layer

Dehydration adequately explains the presence of a dense layer of leukocytes, many of them polymorphonuclear leukocytes, near the wound surface. When the wound surface is kept moist artificially, these cells migrate completely out of the dermis and collect in the fluid layer under the polythene film where they remain alive. Evidently, in normal wounds they also move towards the wound surface in the first few hours after injury, but only a few of them gain access to the serous layer before it dries and the majority is trapped in the upper part of the dermis where they are overtaken by the progressive dehydration of this tissue and die. In the dry conditions they shrink but do not autolyse and are readily stainable in histological sections for many days. Probably they form a powerful barrier layer against the ingress of microorganisms which would be of particular significance in the first few hours, when the surface is still moist and most suitable for the establishment of sepsis.

Initiation of Movement

With regard to the initiation of epidermal migration, according to Weiss [30] the creation of a defect is itself the stimulus for repair in that it releases the cells at the margins of the defect, unilaterally, from contact inhibition. The argument runs: a capacity for movement is a pristine property of cells, movement does not have to be stimulated, it is automatic and the integrity of tissues is normally assured by a built-in mechanism to inhibit movement. A similar argument is applied to another basic cell function, that of mitosis [15]. Apparently contact inhibition is also inoperative when other cells are still present, but dead, since in ordinary circumstances the free edge of epidermis becomes dehydrated and regeneration begins a short distance back from the original edge behind the dry layer, the migrating cells becoming disentangled from their dry and immobilized neighbors.

A number of reports in the literature describe a period varying from 24 hours to 5 days before epidermis begins to migrate. Some of these are rather crude observations depending on recognition of the epidermis with the naked eye. In the cornea it is reported that the cells begin to migrate almost at once [31]. From our investigation it looks as if this is true of the surface epidermis also. It was found that some cells had moved from hair follicles and the wound edges in eight hours. Epidermal cells move very slowly and it takes about 24 hours for them to spread 0.5 mm. under the best conditions.

The Speed of Epidermal Regeneration

The speed of epithelization depends basically on two factors, the speed of displacement of the epidermal cells and the distance apart of the separate sources of new epidermis. The data obtained apply strictly to animals about 15–20 weeks old. Probably the regenerative power of the epidermis does not vary with age (except perhaps in old age) since the epidermis is regenerating throughout life, but theoretically epithelization should be faster in younger animals because the full complement of hair follicles is present within a few weeks of birth and in the adult the follicles become further apart as the skin surface area increases

[32]. Thus the older the animal, the greater the distance to be covered by epidermal migration.

The size of the wound should make no difference to the speed of epithelization unless the wound is very small so that the continuous epidermis in the wound margins contributes a significant proportion of the new epidermis. A large shallow wound in the skin may be regarded as a series of micro-wounds stretching from one hair follicle to the next. The maximum distance over which a sheet of new epidermis must be constructed is half the distance between adjacent follicles and this takes six days.

Covering wounds doubles the speed of epithelization and this has also been found to be true in man [33]. The reason is that when wounds are covered and the surface remains moist, epidermal cells move directly over the wound surface without obstruction in conditions akin to those of a tissue culture experiment. Under normal circumstances the epidermis moves through fibrous tissue which is evidently a slower process since there are collagen bundles in the path of the migrating cells.

To appraise movement fully one needs to know the scale of movement relative to the size of the moving object. The free edge of regenerating epidermis advances a mere one cell diameter an hour. Comparing this with amoeboid movement, the fresh water protozoan *(Amoeba proteus)* covers the same distance in about one second, traveling about 50 times its own length in an hour [34]. Granular leukocytes may be even faster, size for size, for it is said that they can travel 20μm in one minute [35]. Even the regeneration of peripheral nerve which clinically is a very slow event is, at the cellular level, about eight times faster than the regeneration of epidermis. The axon protoplasm flows outward at about 4 mm. per day [36]. Significantly, perhaps, the speed of epidermal regeneration, between 0.25 mm. and 0.5 mm. a day, is of the same order of magnitude as another example of conjoint movement and mitosis in epidermal cells, the production of hair, which grows about 0.3–0.5 mm. a day [37–40].

An advance of one cell an hour is well within the proliferative capabilities of the epidermis; it means that for each cell in front line there should be one new cell produced each hour to maintain the rate of advance of a sheet of epidermis. Any cells produced in excess of this will add to the thickness of the new epidermis.

Mechanisms of Epidermal Regeneration

There is no dispute about the origin of the reparative cells; new epidermis arises only from existing epidermis. In this connection it may be noted that epidermal cells retain the potential to develop along several different lines. Cells which normally form the walls of hair follicles and sweat gland ducts are competent to form surface epidermis [39].

An important generalization is that epidermal regeneration is primarily a matter of cell movement [41]. The evidence for this was reviewed by Arey [42]. The pertinent observations were made on injuries to the epidermis of chick embryos and larval and adult amphibia; the epithelium of the gills of fish, and the cornea of the rat, and in all cases it was found that epidermal cells began to move across the wound surface before the cells at the margins of the wound began to proliferate. Arey and Covode [43] made trench like wounds measuring 3 mm. × 0.5 mm. in the cornea of rats and counted the number of mitotic figures in the corneal cells around the wound. They found that although cell division was depressed for three days, the wounds were fully covered by the movement of cells over the wound floor in 12 hours. Friedenwald and Bushke [31] made multiple needle injuries in rat corneas, estimating that each wound measured about 30μm. in diameter. Mitotic division in the cornea was inhibited for at least four hours after the injury but the cells bordering the wounds had completely covered the denuded surfaces in three hours. Weiss and Matoltsy [44] discovered that cell movement and mitosis are independent of one another in the cornea and the epidermis of chick embryos before the tenth day of incubation. Cells at the edges of wounds divided but did not move to cover the defect until the tenth day when migration started spontaneously. It is well established, too, that epidermal cells will grow out as a sheet of cells from an explant of skin in tissue culture before there is any sign of cell division taking place. These studies make it clear that defects in the epidermis are healed primarily by cell movement.

In amphibian larvae the epidermal cells move in ranks, each cell moving independently, but all of them keeping a constant station in line [45]. The question is whether in mammals the migrating epidermis is also a thin sheet of cells, all of them moving. It is often assumed that it is [30, 46–48]. But regeneration in the dry multistratified epidermis of mammals is not necessarily the same as in amphibians.

It has been pointed out that epidermal cells in amphibian skin move across a wound ten times faster than in mammals [6]. Similarly epidermal healing in fish is said to be an extremely rapid event [49, 50]. In these water animals the consequences of injuring the epidermis are likely to be especially serious because of the risk of dilution of the body fluids. It may be that extra rapid healing has evolved in response to the need for quickly restoring the normal barrier layer on the body surface.

Abercrombie says that one of the special problems of epithelial movement is ". . . how the whole sheet stops and starts. . . .", and he also says "they (epithelial cells) do not move over each other's surfaces."

On the contrary, in wounds in pig's skin the new epidermis does appear to be built up by cells moving over one another and becoming implanted one after another on the wound surface. In rabbit skin, too, epithelization involves mitosis and differentiation as well as cell migration [51].

Where epithelial cells do move over a wound surface in line there are certain problems of interpretation [47]. It must be postulated either that the cells in the free edge of the sheet drag the remainder of the cells behind it, like a locomotive and a chain of coaches, or that some or all of the cells behind the free edge move individually, "much as a herd of animals" [30]. Abercrombie and Weiss deduce that the latter explanation is probably the correct one. There is then the problem how, when the free edge of the sheet meets another migrating sheet and stops immediately, information about the meeting is conveyed to all of the moving cells to bring them simultaneously to a halt.

There has been speculation about which of the layers of epidermal cells in the wound edge is mobilized and moves out across the wound. Hartwell [1] thought that the majority of cells came from the middle and uppermost living layers of the epithelium adjacent to the wound. Gillman and Penn [9] said that the new epidermis was derived from the upper layers of the stratum Malpighi. Bishop [52] thought that the migrating cells may have been those cells in the old epidermis that were about to transform into the granular layer. Uhlenhuth [53] said that only the basal cells participated in the healing, in vitro, of skin epithelium from the adult frog, and Matoltsy [54] reached the same conclusion about the in vitro repair of adult human skin. Viziam, Matoltsy and Mescon [51] state firmly that migration begins with the displacement of basal cells from the wound edge. However, their diagram seems to indicate that they include all the cell layers beneath the stratum granulosum as basal cells.

Arising from this discussion two propositions can be put forward about epidermal regeneration:

1) cells which meet in the center of the wound are the very same cells that lay originally at the periphery of the defect.

2) cells at the wound edge are displaced only a few cell diameters from their original position and it is their progeny, several generations removed, that finish up in the middle of the wound.

The first proposition may be correct for larval Ambyostoma, as shown by Lash [45], who marked cells by pushing carbon particles into them and then watched their displacement under the microscope.

The second proposition is probably true of epithelization in mammalian skin, but the evidence is indirect. That the cells behind the free edge of regenerating epidermis round up, divide and differentiate, strongly suggests that the sheet of new epidermis is stationary except at its extreme tip. Probably any of the living cells in the epidermis of the skin surface, the outer root sheath of a hair follicle or the wall of an epidermal duct can move laterally and participate in the formation of a new epidermal layer. If there is a suitable moist exudate for them to grow into, basal cells will move out from the tip of an epidermal ridge, cells from the upper layers of the epidermis will move out of the surface of the epidermis and cells will move from the cut edge of epidermis at the border of a wound back over the epidermis as well as forward across the wound surface. Similarly cells from the outer root sheath will move over the cut surface of a hair follicle. They move over each other's surfaces and the position adopted by the first few cells, determined by the shape of the cut edge of epidermis and the physical conditions of the adjacent tissue determines the orientation of the migrating epidermis.

Epidermal Morphogenesis

Surely the behavior of normal surface epidermis, so-called physiological regeneration, bears a close relation to the regeneration of epidermis following injury. But here is a dilemma, for on the one hand it is thought that in the normal epidermis the morphogenic force is the pressure of mitosis, but it is firmly established that following injury the epidermis is regenerated primarily by cell movement.

If, as Medawar [41] has said, "the tactics of regeneration as of embryonic development, is primarily and fundamentally a matter of the movement of cell substance, cells and cell groups, it is not primarily a matter of cell division, nor of synthesis in general, though in due course these are called upon to play their part." It is very likely that the everyday physiological regeneration of epidermis is primarily a matter of cell movement.

A difficulty in accepting the idea of movement of cells in the intact epidermal layer is too literal application of the theory of contact inhibition which cannot strictly apply to normal stratified epidermis without some qualifications. It must be postulated that melanocytes have similar surface configuration to epidermal cells since they live symbiotically. Basal cells seem to be in an anomalous position because they are contacted by epidermal cells on three sides only. If cells are rigorously excluded from moving relative to one another, they should rise from the basal layer to the surface simultaneously, in successive sheets spread out in the plane of the skin, which is certainly not how the epidermis behaves.

If epidermis grew by cells budding off from the basal layer and being pushed to the surface by mitotic pressure, one might reasonably expect the division of a basal cell to take place in such a way that one of the daughter cells is thrust upwards, the other remaining in the basal layer to maintain the stock of germinal cells. But a simple mechanism of this kind does not provide for increase of surface area, and it is well known that in the later telophase stage of mitosis the daughter cells are mostly found side by side in the basal layer, not one above the other.

Pinkus [55, 56] wounded the epidermis by stripping the horny layers with adhesive tape and then studied the reactions of the remaining live cells. He made the very interesting comment that there were indications of another mechanism of direct conversion of basal cells into prickle cells, even before mitosis set in. He noticed that after 24 hours many of the basal cells, identified by their supranuclear cap of pigment, had moved upwards towards the surface. He suggested that the basal cells were squeezed into the prickle cell layer, but did not say how this could have been brought about.

Leblond, Greulich and Pereira [57] and Greulich [58] reported a careful study of the relationship between cell formation and cell migration in mouse esophageal epithelium. They labeled the epidermal cells with tritiated thymidine and identified paired daughter nuclei on the autoradiographs. They found that the daughter cells remained in the basal layer for at least 24 hours and that by 48 hours they were both still in the basal layer, were both in the spinous layer, or lay one in each layer. They concluded that mitosis and migration of cells in the epithelium are largely independent of one another. In order to maintain a steady state it follows that, on average, for each cell that divides, one moves from the basal layer to the spinous layer. They suggest that cells may be displaced from the basal layer by the indirect pressure of mitosis. A cell may be squeezed between a dividing cell and a nearby resting cell and pushed in a superficial direction. Bullough and Laurence [16] came to a similar conclusion about the surface epidermis.

Three hypotheses can therefore be stated regarding the mechanism of cell movement in the normal epidermis.

Direct mitotic pressure. Cells are budded off from a germinal layer and pushed upwards by a vertical force generated by mitosis. This hypothesis is probably no longer tenable for reasons already discussed.

Indirect mitotic pressure. Cells are pushed upwards by a lateral force in the basal layer, generated by mitosis, which squeezes cells from the basal layer.

As Van Scott [59] points out a proliferating cell population must generate expansion forces equal in all directions; forces opposed by equal and opposite forces in the surrounding tissues. In the epidermis it must be presumed that the weakest opposing force, the path of least resistance, is in the outward direction against the substance of the overlying epidermal layers.

This does not adequately explain the displacement of cells from the basal layer. The very fact that a cell moves out of this layer implies that it, or the cell above it, differs from the others or the postulated lateral expansion force should simply compress all the cells equally. Random weaknesses can conceivably occur but this seems too haphazard a mechanism for the maintenance of homeostasis in the epidermis. Another objection to this hypothesis is that it would act indiscriminately, cells preparing for mitosis or undergoing mitosis would be dislodged as readily as cells programmed to begin differentiation.

Furthermore, there are mechanical considerations against it. Basal cells are quite firmly attached to the dermis by delicate cytoplasmic processes and specialized attachment plaques and are also fixed to their neighbors. An unmodified basal cell squeezed away from the basal layer would be torn apart. Clearly, it must be postulated that changes take place at the cell surface prior to its displacement.

Active cell movement. Cells actively move out of the basal layer toward the surface and the potential space is filled by division of one of the basal cells.

Having deduced that some changes must take place to a cell before it leaves the basal layer, it is implied that the cell takes an active rather than a passive role in its displacement. This hypothesis fits the observations made by Pinkus and by Leblond, Greulich and Pereira. It equates regeneration following injury with physiological regeneration in the epidermis. It can explain those instances when epidermis 'melts away', as in the disappearance of the lower third of a hair follicle in the catagen stage of the growth cycle and in the reduction of the walls of pockets of epidermal tissue to short ridges in the later stages of healing of shallow wounds.

Unfortunately, it is not known how epidermal cells move. It has been found that their movements are extremely slow, equivalent to about one, or at the most two cell diameters an hour. In the regenerating epidermis and probably in the normal surface epidermis the cells move over each other's surfaces.

Since for a cell to leave the basal layer, it must be unzipped from the 'basement membrane' and from its neighbors, it is suggested that active epidermal cell movement is primarily a matter of cell elongation assisted by temporary anchorages provided by the desmosomes. The following sequence of events may be visualized.

First, the cell attachments at the prospective forward end are dissolved. The cell then elongates and makes new forward attachments. The attachments at the tail end are then broken down and the tail of the cell is drawn up. The cell will then have moved effectively about one cell diameter. New attachments are formed between the displaced cell and its new neighbors and between the cells it formerly separated. Thus, the cell may employ the desmosomes to move among its neighbors in much the same way as a mountaineer uses scaling irons to draw himself upward.

Epidermal cells may migrate over a wound surface in the same manner. Similarly this may be how they move in the hair follicle.

Clinical Application—Wound Dressings and Epidermal Regeneration

Wounds vary so much in depth and area, in degree of contamination by dirt or microorganisms, in the presence of devitalized tissue and in other ways, that it is not possible to design a dressing to perform optimally under all the varied conditions. Dressings are therapeutic agents differing in properties and should be selected for the task in hand. To make an intelligent choice demands knowledge of the functions of a dressing and its effects on healing.

Dressings divide into two groups, those that prevent or delay evaporation of water from the wound surface enough to permit epidermal migration through a moist exudate over the original damaged surface of dermis, and those that allow of drying so that the regenerating epidermis is orientated below a scab through the dermal fibrous tissue [10]. Under the better dressings in the first category epithelization is more rapid and no extra tissue is sacrificed (Fig. 4-26). At face value the occlusive dressing seems to be the best treatment but in practice there are complications. A fully occlusive dressing is difficult to keep in place on wounds that produce excessive exudate. There is a risk of sepsis since the dilute serous exudate, which provides an ideal medium for the growth of the epidermis, is also a suitable milieu for rapid multiplication of microorganisms.

One unsatisfactory feature of all commonly used dressings is that they cause fresh damage to the wound when removed because they adhere to the wound surface. The problem was investigated both in the laboratory and on wounds in the skin of pigs using the shallow wound model. Tests of a range of materials, of dressings in everyday use and of experimental ones, using a tensiometer to measure the adhesion of a standard strip of material to reconstituted human serum dried on hardboard under controlled conditions of humidity and temperature, indicated that there is little hope of finding a material, suitable in other ways as a dressing, that will not adhere to drying serum [60]. One of the important properties of an ideal dressing is that it shall have high absorbency, a property incompatible with nonadhesion since the serous exudate, as it dries and is concentrated is a coherent and powerful glue which forms a mechanical key with the dressings.

In animal experiments concerned with this problem various materials were compared with a control dressing of cotton lint on standard shallow wounds, the dressings being removed daily and recordings made of the amount of fresh damage caused by changing the dressings. All materials tested adhered to the wounds, including some advertised as being nonadherent, confirming the laboratory findings. Histological sections prepared from wounds with the dressing in place show the serous exudate in the fabric of the dressing, dried in the interstices (Fig. 4-27). The migrating epidermis adheres to the underside of the scab and is only lightly adherent to the wound, and sections cut from wounds from which dressings have been removed show that the scab and much of the new epidermis are removed with the dressing.

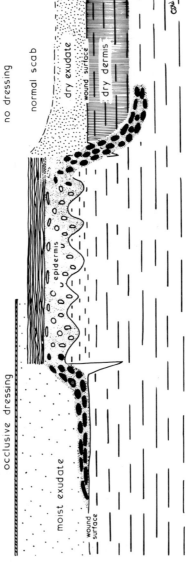

Fig. 4–26.—Comparison of the mode of epidermal regeneration in shallow skin wounds under exposed and occlusive conditions.

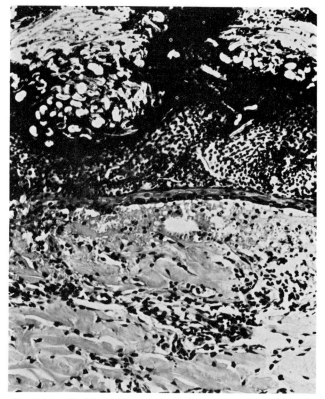

Fig. 4–27.—Position of dressing relative to migrating epidermis.

One approach to this problem is the tulle-gras type dressing and more recent developments using polyethylene glycol instead of soft paraffin as the impregnant. Studies of these dressings show that the impregnant tends to melt away and the coarse fabric lies directly on the wound surface. The migrating epidermis is irregular and bizarre, tending to wander into the fabric, and on removing these dressings, fresh damage is caused to the wound.

Another approach is the film type dressing with holes to permit drainage into an absorbent backing fabric. These also become strongly adherent due to columns of exudate drying in the holes in the film and there is considerable fresh bleeding when the dressing is removed. Histological sections of wounds covered by such dressings show regularly spaced areas of dehydrated dermis corresponding to the holes in the film [61]. These dressings are usually made from polyester film which because of its low oxygen permeability is less suitable than many other films available.

The ideal dressing for most purposes should keep the wound surfaces just damp [3]. There should be no free standing fluid between the dressing and the wound. It will also be advantageous if an exchange of gases can take place between the atmosphere and the wound surface. The dressing should consist of an absorbent portion to disperse the exudate and provide some mechanical protection and have a microporous surface, imitating some of the important functions of the epidermis, namely, waterproofing and prevention of ingress of foreign bodies and bacteria, but allowing the passage of water vapour and oxygen molecules.

Finally, it may be commented that appraisal of the facts of wound healing does not encourage hope that it may be speeded up to any significant extent to produce "super normal" healing, despite the efforts expended to this end. It is important to analyze healing closely to define the optima of temperature, pH and like factors, but radically altering the physical conditions for epidermal migration by occlusion is likely to be the most significant factor in determining the speed of healing.

ACKNOWLEDGMENTS

I thank Dr. John T. Scales for his constant help and encouragement. Much of the material for this paper has been taken from the writer's Ph.D. thesis: "A Study of Wound Healing in the Domestic Pig", and acknowledgment is made to the University of London. I am grateful to the Zoological Society of London for the Thomas Henry Huxley award, 1966, in connection with this thesis and to the Governors of Birkbeck College, University of London, for the Armitage Smith Memorial Prize. I thank Professor Bullough and Dr. Edna Laurence for much useful advice and discussion, and D. W. Clarke, S. E. Barnett, M. E. Wait and S. J. Varley for skilful technical assistance. I am grateful to Courtaulds Limited and the Medical Research Council for financial assistance towards the costs of this investigation.

REFERENCES

1. Hartwell, S. W.: *The Mechanism of Healing in Human Wounds* (Springfield, Ill.: Charles C Thomas, Publisher, 1955).
2. Montagna, W., and Yun, J.: The skin of the domestic pig, J. Invest. Dermat. 43: 11, 1964.
3. Winter, G. D.: Healing of Skin Wounds and Effect of Dressings in the Repair Process, in *Surgical Dressings and Wound Healing* (In press).
4. Scales, J. T.: Levitation, Lancet 2:1181, 1961.
5. Scales, J. T., and Winter, G. D.: "Levitation". A Possible Means of Treating Burns, in *"La Cicatrization."* (Paris: Centre Nationale de la Recherche Scientifique, 1964).
6. Winter, G. D.: Movement of Epidermal Cells over the Wound Surface, in Montagna, W., and Billingham, R. E. (eds.): *Advances in Biology of Skin*, Vol. 5, *Wound Healing* (Oxford: Pergamon Press, 1964).
7. Winter, G. D.: Regeneration of Epidermis, in Rook, A., and Champion, R. H. (eds.): *Progress in Biological Sciences in Relation to Dermatology* (Cambridge: Cambridge University Press, 1964).
8. Schoefl, G. I.: Studies of inflammation. III. Growing capillaries: their structure and permeability. Virchows Arch. Path. Anat. 337:97, 1963.
9. Gillman, T., and Penn, J.: Studies on the repair of cutaneous wounds. I. Healing of incised wounds—epidermal reactions to sutures. II. Healing of wounds—loss of superficial portions of the skin, Med. Proc. 2:121, 1956.
10. Winter, G. D., and Scales, J. T.: Effect of air drying and dressings on the surface of a wound, Nature 197:91, 1963.

11. Winter, G. D.: Formation of the scab and the rate of epithelization of superficial wounds in the skin of the young domestic pig, Nature 193:293, 1962.
12. Winter, G. D., and Perrins, D. J.: Effects of Hyperbaric Oxygen Treatment on Epidermal Regeneration, in Wada, J., and Iwa, T. (eds.): *Proceedings of the Fourth International Congress on Hyperbaric Medicine* (Tokyo: Igaku Shoin Ltd., 1970).
13. Bullough, W. S., and Laurence, E. B.: A technique for the study of small epidermal wounds, Brit. J. Exper. Path. 38:273, 1957.
14. Bullough, W. S., and Laurence, E. B.: The energy relations of epidermal mitotic activity adjacent to small wounds, Brit. J. Exper. Path. 38:278, 1957.
15. Bullough, W. S.: The control of mitotic activity in adult mammalian tissues, Biol. Rev. 37:307, 1962.
16. Bullough, W. S., and Laurence, E. B.: The production of epidermal cells, Symp. Zool. Soc. London 12:1, 1964.
17. Bullough, W. S.: Epithelial Repair, in Dunphy, T. E., and Van Winkle, H. W. (eds.): *Repair and Regeneration* (New York: McGraw-Hill Book Company, Inc., 1969).
18. Locke, M.: The development of patterns in the integument of insects, Advances Morphogenesis 6:33, 1967.
19. Mizuno, T., and Fujii, T.: Analysis of the two processes, Wound repair and early changes in carcinogenesis, by use of Millipore filter implanting: The possible role of heparin-like compound in cell interactions, J. Fac. Sci. Univ. Tokyo Sec. IV. 11: 475, 1969.
20. Gross, J., and Lapiere, C.: A collagenolytic activity in amphibian tissues. A tissue culture assay, Proc. Nat. Acad. Sc. 48:1014, 1962.
21. Eisen, A. Z., and Gross, J.: The role of epithelium and mesenchyme in the production of a collagenolytic enzyme and a hyaluronidase in the anuran tadpole, Developmental Biol. 12:408, 1965.
22. Brown, S. I., and Weller, C. A.: Cell origin of collagenase in normal and wounded corneas, Arch. Ophth. 83:74, 1970.
23. Grillo, H. C., and Gross, J.: Collogenolytic activity during mammalian wound repair, Developmental Biol. 15:300, 1967.
24. Devenyi, I., and Holczinger, L.: The morphology of wound healing under crusts, Acta morphol. 4:447, 1954.
25. James, D. W.: A connective tissue constituent in the scab formed over cutaneous wounds, J. Path. & Bact. 69:33, 1955.
26. Zahir, M.: Hydroxyproline in scabs, J. Path. & Bact. 84:79, 1962.
27. Hadfield, G.: The tissue of origin of the fibroblasts of granulation tissue, Brit. J. Surg. 50:807, 1963.
28. Braun, A. A., and Magazanik, G. L.: The effect of paraffin wax application of long and short duration on the epithelisation of skin wounds in experiments. Vop. Kurort. 4:349, 1959.
29. Forage, A. V.: The effects of removing epidermis from burnt skin, Lancet 2:690, 1962.
30. Weiss, P.: The biological foundations of wound repair, The Harvey Lectures Series 55:13, 1959–60.
31. Friedenwald, J. S., and Bushke, W.: The influence of some experimental variables on the epithelial movements in the healing of corneal wounds, J. Cell. & Comp. Physiol. 23:95, 1944.
32. Szabo, G. L.: The Regional Frequency and Distribution of Hair Follicles in Human Skin, in Montagna, W., and Ellis, R. A. (eds.): *Biology of Hair Growth* (New York: Academic Press, Inc., 1958).
33. Hinman, C. D., and Maibach, H.: Effect of air exposure and occlusion on experimental human skin wounds, Nature 200:377, 1963.
34. Spector, W. S.: *Handbook of Biological Data* (Philadelphia: W. B. Saunders Co., 1956).
35. Florey, H. W.: Inflammation, in Florey, H. W. (ed.): *General Pathology,* 3d ed. (London: Lloyd-Luke [Medical Books] Ltd., 1962).
36. Young, J. Z.: The History of the Shape of a Nerve Fibre, in Le Gros Clark, W. E.,

and Medawar, P. B. (eds.): *Essays on Growth and Form* (Oxford: Oxford University Press, 1945).

37. Myers, R. J., and Hamilton, J. B.: Regeneration and rate of growth of hairs in man, Ann. New York Acad. Sci. 53:562, 1951.

38. Flesch, P.: Hair Growth, in Rothman, S. (ed.): *Physiology and Biochemistry of Skin* (Chicago: University of Chicago Press, 1954).

39. Montagna, W.: *The Structure and Function of Skin,* 2d ed. (New York: Academic Press, Inc., 1962).

40. Side, M. J., and Rudall, K. M.: Rates of Hair Growth, in Rook, A., and Champion, R. H. (eds.): *Progress in the Biological Sciences in Relation to Dermatology,* Vol. 2 (Cambridge: Cambridge University Press, 1964).

41. Medawar, P. B.: Biological aspects of the repair process, Brit. M. Bull. 3:70, 1945.

42. Arey, L. B.: Wound healing, Physiol. Rev. 16:327, 1936.

43. Arey, L. B., and Covode, W. M.: The method of repair in epithelial wounds of the cornea, Anat. Rec. 85:75, 1943.

44. Weiss, P., and Matoltsy, A. G.: Absence of wound healing in young chick embryos, Nature 180:854, 1957.

45. Lash, J. W.: Studies on wound closure in urodeles, J. Exper. Zool. 128:13, 1955.

46. Weiss, P.: Biological aspects of wound healing, in Patterson, B. W. (ed.): *Wound Healing and Tissue Repair* (Chicago: University of Chicago Press, 1959).

47. Abercrombie, M.: The bases of the locomotory behaviour of fibroblasts, Exper. Cell Res. Suppl. 8:188, 1961.

48. Abercrombie, M.: Behaviour of Cells towards One Another, in Montagna, W., and Billingham, R. E. (eds.): *Advances in Biology of Skin,* Vol. 5, *Wound Healing* (Oxford: Pergamon Press, 1964).

49. Harabath, R.: Über die Heilung von Schnittwunden der Haut bei Fischen, Virchows Arch. path. Anat. 268:794, 1928.

50. Szanto, G., Szekely, O., and Szonyi, S.: Regional differences (axial gradients) in wound healing, Symp. Biol. (Hung.) 3:101, 1963.

51. Viziam, C. B., Matoltsy, A. G., and Mescon, H.: Epithelization of small wounds, J. Invest. Dermat. 43:499, 1964.

52. Bishop, G. H.: Regeneration after experimental removal of skin in man, Am. J. Anat. 76:153, 1945.

53. Uhlenhuth, E.: Cultivation of the skin epithelium of the adult frog. Rana pipiens, J. Exper. Med. 20:614, 1914.

54. Matoltsy, A. G.: In vitro wound repair of adult human skin, Anat. Rec. 122:581, 1955.

55. Pinkus, H.: Examination of the epidermis by the strip method of removing horny layers. I. Observations on thickness of the horny layer and mitotic activity after stripping. J. Invest. Dermat. 16:383, 1951.

56. Pinkus, H.: Examination of the epidermis by the strip method. II. Biometric data on regeneration of the human epidermis, J. Invest. Dermat. 19:431, 1952.

57. Leblond, C. P., Greulich, R. C., and Pereira, J. P. M.: Relationship of Cell Formation and Cell Migration in the Renewal of Stratified Squamous Epithelia, in Montagna, W., and Billingham, R. E. (eds.): *Advances in Biology of Skin,* Vol. 5, *Wound Healing* (Oxford: Pergamon Press, 1964).

58. Greulich, R. C.: Aspects of Cell Individuality in the Renewal of Stratified Squamous Epithelia, in Montagna, W., and Lobitz, W. C. (eds.): *The Epidermis* (New York: Academic Press, Inc., 1964).

59. Van Scott, E. J.: Definition of epidermal cancer, in Montagna, W., and Lobitz, W. C. (eds.): *The Epidermis* (New York: Academic Press, Inc., 1964).

60. Scales, J. T., and Winter, G. D.: The Adhesion of Wound Dressings. An Experimental Study, in Slome, D. (ed.): *Wound Healing* (Oxford: Pergamon Press, 1961).

61. Winter, G. D.: A note on wound healing under dressings with special reference to perforated film dressings. J. Invest. Dermat. 45:299, 1965.

5

The Effect of Occlusive and Semipermeable Dressings on the Cell Kinetics of Normal and Wounded Human Epidermis

Louis B. Fisher, Ph.D.* and Howard I. Maibach, M.D.†

Scales [1] suggested that with our present knowledge, an ideal wound dressing would require a compromise between occlusion and nonocclusion. It should absorb exudate, thus removing bacteria; permit evaporation of fluid; and either should be not incorporated into the eschar or should be sufficiently fragile to allow its removal without compromising the healing wound. This conclusion was based on the accumulated evidence that although occlusive dressings produce quicker and stronger healing of relatively superficial wounds [2, 3, 4], they also promote infection [5], while dressings of cotton gauze or lint adhere to the eschar. Considerable experimentation has shown that for superficial wounds tape closure of incised and excised wounds produces better results than sutures. The reaction to the suture is absent, contracture and granulation tissue are reduced with plastic dressings [3, 6] and hyperplasia of the renewing epithelium is reduced [2, 6]. It was further noted that provided the tape remained in place for at least ten days the tensile strength of the wound was equal to or greater than suture closed wounds [2]. Forrester *et al.* [7, 8] concluded, however, that these wounds were more brittle so that in spite of increase in tensile strength they showed no greater ability to resist rupture. Brunius and Ahren [9] concluded that a taped wound resulted in a more rapid maturation of scar tissue.

The increased rate of closure under occlusion is seemingly due to an increase in cell migration both from the wound edge and from any appendages in excised wounds. This has now been demonstrated on many occasions [10–12]. These authors showed that under occlusion no eschar was formed, and as a result, epithelialization could occur directly across the wound surface. Winter and Scales [13] demonstrated that this effect of occlusion was due to the maintenance of a moist environment. The use of a perforated plastic dressing (Telfa) has been shown to result in "occlusive" healing beneath the plastic and "non-occlusive"

---

*Research Fellow, Division of Dermatology, Scripps Clinic and Research Foundation, La Jolla, California.

†Associate Professor, Department of Dermatology, University of California (San Francisco) School of Medicine, San Francisco, California.

healing beneath the pores, i.e., crust formation and epithelialization beneath the eschar [14] and yet Knudsen and Snitker [15] were unable to show any advantage over open wounds using this same material. However, Ordman and Gillman [16] obtained good closure of surgical wounds using a porous, rayon fiber tape (Micropore). These results suggest that maybe a microporous dressing in which the pores exist as minute spaces within the weave of the material may have many of the properties of the compromise suggested by Scales.

The disadvantage of complete occlusion with polyethylene film was well demonstrated by Smith *et al.* [17] where infection prevented healing of ulcers. On the other hand, Harris and Keefe [18] obtained faster healing of wounds, with no infection, in pig skin, under similar conditions. However, these animals are apparently more resistant than humans to infection [1]. The evidence, as cited above, that occlusion promotes healing of superficial wounds is strong. In this light the isolated reports of occlusion inhibiting cell division seem curious.

Fry *et al.* [19] using plastic film and Baxter and Stoughton [20] using Blenderm tape showed that occlusion of psoriatic lesions would significantly reduce the mitotic activity of this hyperplastic epidermis. Petzoldt *et al.* [21] showed that occlusion with plastic film would also reduce much of the increased enzymatic activity found in these lesions. These results may, of course, be due to a peculiarity of the psoriatic epidermis, but Williams and Hunter [22] showed inhibition of mitotic activity in skin stripped with cellophane tape followed by occlusion with the same tape; and Born [23] demonstrated inhibition of DNA synthesis in normal skin after occlusion with plastic film. The present investigation was undertaken to clarify the action of occlusive dressings on cell division in the normal and wounded epidermis. Such quantitative kinetic information should lead to a better understanding of wound healing and possibly some insight into the role of wound dressings in the maintenance of skin function.

MATERIALS AND METHODS

The basic technique used was that previously described by Fisher and Maibach [24]. The subjects used were normal adult males. Since several biopsies were required from each individual, investigation was confined to the back. Four different dressings were used: an adhesive, occlusive tape (Blenderm); the adhesive alone from this tape, presumably nonocclusive; an adhesive, less occlusive porous tape (Micropore); and a nonadhesive, occlusive plastic film (Saran wrap—a chlorinated hydrocarbon polymer). These dressings were applied for 2–6 days, being carefully removed and a fresh dressing applied daily. On the morning of the last day the dressings were removed, 0.5% Colcemid cream (N-desacetyl methyl colchicine) applied under an occlusive patch test plaster, for 6 hours, and 3 mm. punch biopsies taken. Colcemid was employed to arrest cells at metaphase so that the greater number of mitoses present would simplify the counting and decrease the number of biopsies required. This basic experimental design allowed the use of each subject as his own control, which made the use of small groups of volunteers practical. The specimens were fixed in Davidson's fixative, embedded, cut at 7μ and stained with the Feulgen reaction for DNA. Counts of dividing cells were made from twelve separate sections for each specimen and the mean mitotic rate expressed as mitoses per thousand viable epidermal cells. Statistical significance was determined by the F test for analysis of variance [25].

In the studies on wounded epidermis, cellophane tape was repeatedly applied to the area until glistening was noted uniformly through the treated site.

In the punch biopsy studies, the sites were anesthetized with 1% lidocaine solution (without epinephrine) and full thickness skin removed with a 1 mm. punch. Hemostasis was obtained with pressure. When the area was dry (usually one hour later), the dressings were applied.

EXPERIMENTS AND RESULTS

Occlusive Tape

The occlusive adhesive tape was arbitrarily chosen as the standard dressing and its effect on the mitotic activity of both normal and stripped skin investigated with respect to time. As noted in Table 5-1 occlusive tape applied to normal skin showed a decrease in mitotic rate at 3 days which was not statistically significant ($P > 0.05$). However, at 4 days there was a significant doubling of the mitotic rate at the occluded site compared to the normal skin ($P < 0.005$). This was re-checked in additional experiments not employing Colcemid. An increase in mitotic count was again observed although on this occasion it was not significant, possibly due to the smaller numbers involved since fewer mitoses are seen without Colcemid. At 6 days of application the mitotic rates of occluded and unoccluded skin were identical.

Quite a different effect occurred in skin whose mitotic rate was greatly increased by removal of the stratum corneum with cellophane tape stripping to glistening (Table 5-1). When examined at 2, 3 and 4 days after stripping, the stripped untreated sites had a 17-fold or greater mitotic rate than normal skin. Occlusive tape application markedly decreased the mitotic rate to much closer to normal levels ($P < 0.005$ for all time periods). Six days after stripping the mitotic rate of the untreated sites was still approximately five times higher than normal skin but that of the occluded sites was now reduced to normal levels ($P < 0.005$). In other words the very high rate of cell division induced by stripping is, in the main, inhibited.

On examining these sections we noted that the epidermal thickness seemed to be different under the occlusive tape. Consequently, epidermal thickness was measured using an eye piece micrometer. An arbitrary unit length of epidermis was taken as that length found between the borders of an eye piece grid. All viable cells were then counted under oil immersion, throughout the depth of the epidermis, but within the lateral boundaries of the grid. This type of measurement is greatly dependent upon the ability to obtain perfectly transverse sections. Care was taken in this regard and since the material was prepared without knowledge of the identity of each specimen bias was unlikely to enter into the procedure. Furthermore, since quantitative measurements were not required but only a comparison between different treatments, use of a good statistical method [25] would identify any significant change in epidermal thickness. As can be seen from Table 5-2 there is a minimal but definite increase in the thickness of normal skin ($P < 0.025$ to <0.005) that has been occluded with tape. A greater

Table 5-1

The Effect of an Occlusive Adhesive Tape on the Mitotic Activity of Normal and Stripped Skin

	Normal					Stripped				
	Treated		Control			Treated		Control		
Time	N*	Mitotic Index ± SD	N*	Mitotic Index ± SD	P	N*	Mitotic Index ± SD	N*	Mitotic Index ± SD	P
2 days	—	—	78	1.06 ± 1.30	—	43	3.36 ± 1.39	48	18.65 ± 14.18	<0.005
3 days	78	0.75 ± 1.28	191	0.62 ± 0.78	>0.05	48	3.91 ± 4.05	48	19.60 ± 6.26	<0.005
4 days	192	1.24 ± 1.63	48	0.07 ± 0.14	<0.005	48	9.62 ± 8.31	48	17.30 ± 6.49	<0.005
No colcemid	48	0.15 ± 0.25	—	—	>0.05	—	—	—	—	—
6 days	78	0.65 ± 0.71	78	0.65 ± 0.59	>0.05	48	1.04 ± 1.11	47	5.15 ± 5.20	<0.005

*N = total number of individual slides counted—usually 6 per biopsy.

Table 5-2

The Effect of Occlusive Adhesive Tape on the Epidermal Depth* of Normal and Stripped Skin

	Normal					Stripped				
	Treated		Control			Treated		Control		
Time	N†	Cells/Unit Length ± SD	N†	Cells/Unit Length ± SD	P	N†	Cells/Unit Length ± SD	N†	Cells/Unit Length ± SD	P
2 days	—	—	—	—	—	86	89.0 ± 24.0	96	87.1 ± 19.7	<0.05
3 days	156	78.1 ± 23.8	156	72.0 ± 18.8	<0.025	96	102.6 ± 27.4	96	79.9 ± 17.1	<0.005
4 days	480	81.9 ± 21.8	478	76.1 ± 24.0	<0.005	96	127.1 ± 49.6	96	91.5 ± 22.5	<0.005
6 days	156	76.4 ± 22.9	155	58.8 ± 45.2	<0.005	96	89.0 ± 27.4	94	83.1 ± 27.4	<0.005

*The epidermal depth was measured in terms of viable cells per unit length of epidermis. The unit of length was arbitrarily taken as the width of an eyepiece grid. Cells were counted throughout the complete epidermal depth staying within these lateral borders.

†N = total number of counts made—usually 12 per biopsy.

increase in thickness occurred in stripped skin that had been so treated (P < 0.05 to 0.005).

Other Dressings

These effects on cell kinetics were then compared with similar applications of the other dressings at 3 and 6 days. These data are presented in Table 5-3. At 3 days on normal skin the adhesive mass from the occlusive tape showed no appreciable effect (P > 0.05). However, the less occlusive "porous" tape and the occlusive plastic film showed definite reductions in mitotic rate (P < 0.025 and 0.005). Similar effects were found after 6 days. At both 3 and 6 days the greatest reduction in mitotic rate occurred with the less occlusive "porous" tape (P < 0.005).

On stripped skin all materials (including the adhesive mass) produced a significant reduction in mitotic rate at 3 days. Generally a greater inhibition was observed under the less occlusive dressings (adhesive mass and "porous" tape) than under the occlusive dressings (adhesive occlusive tape and occlusive film)— P < 0.005. The reduction under the porous tape was significantly greater than under the adhesive mass (P = 0.025), while no difference was observed between the occlusive dressings. However, at 6 days, when the mitotic rate of the control sites was returning toward normal those sites covered with the "porous" tape

Table 5-3
The Effect of Various Dressings on the Mitotic Activity of Normal and Stripped Skin

Time	Dressing	N*	Normal Mitotic Index ± SD	P	N*	Stripped Mitotic Index ± SD	P
3 days	Occlusive adhesive tape	78	0.75 ± 1.28	>0.05	48	3.91 ± 4.05	<0.005
	Plastic film (No adhesive)	71	0.65 ± 0.65	>0.025	48	4.93 ± 4.32	<0.005
	"Porous" tape	78	0.22 ± 0.27	<0.005	44	0.91 ± 1.14	<0.005
	Adhesive mass (Without occlusion)	78	0.92 ± 1.60	>0.05	48	2.11 ± 3.25	<0.005
	Control (Untreated skin	78	1.06 ± 1.30	—	48	19.60 ± 6.26	—
6 days	Occlusive adhesive tape	78	0.65 ± 0.71	>0.05	48	1.04 ± 1.11	<0.005
	Plastic film (No adhesive)	78	0.44 ± 0.42	<0.025	47	1.87 ± 1.06	<0.005
	"Porous" tape	72	0.29 ± 0.38	<0.005	46	10.56 ± 10.21	<0.005
	Adhesive mass (Without occlusion)	74	0.67 ± 0.76	>0.05	46	2.51 ± 4.24	<0.01
	Control (Untreated skin	78	0.65 ± 0.59	—	47	5.15 ± 5.20	—

*N = total number of counts made.

Table 5-4
The Effect of Various Dressings on the Epidermal Depth* of Normal and Stripped Skin

Time	Dressing	N†	Normal Cells/Unit Length ± SD	P	N†	Stripped Cells/Unit Length ± SD	P
3 days	Occlusive adhesive tape	156	78.1 ± 23.8	<0.025	96	102.6 ± 27.4	<0.005
	Plastic film (No adhesive)	142	87.4 ± 39.0	<0.005	96	105.8 ± 25.9	<0.005
	"Porous" tape	156	76.1 ± 23.5	>0.05	88	99.4 ± 30.7	<0.005
	Adhesive mass (Without occlusion)	156	84.9 ± 29.3	<0.005	96	98.6 ± 25.5	<0.005
	Control (Untreated skin	156	72.0 ± 18.8	—	96	79.9 ± 17.1	—
6 days	Occlusive adhesive tape	156	76.4 ± 22.9	=0.05	96	89.0 ± 27.4	<0.005
	Plastic film (No adhesive	156	81.2 ± 23.8	<0.005	94	100.4 ± 28.3	<0.005
	"Porous" tape	144	76.3 ± 20.4	<0.05	94	119.0 ± 37.1	<0.005
	Adhesive mass (Without occlusion)	148	85.5 ± 29.0	<0.005	94	105.5 ± 31.5	<0.005
	Control (Untreated skin	155	71.7 ± 18.7	—	94	83.1 ± 27.4	—

*The epidermal depth was measured in terms of viable cells per unit length of epidermis.
†N = total number of counts made.

once more showed high counts (P < 0.005). The other treated sites still remained lower than the controls (P < 0.01 and 0.005).

As can be seen from Table 5-4 there was minimal but significant increase in thickness of normal skin from these dressings and a much bigger increase after application to stripped skin.

Punch Biopsy Wounds

Since the results on normal and stripped skin were to some extent inconsistent, this raised the possibility of there being some chemical inhibitor in the adhesive which was not penetrating the intact normal skin. To test this possibility circular wounds were made with a 1 mm. punch biopsy. These were then covered with one of three dressings: occlusive film, occlusive tape and "porous" tape. Biopsies were taken with a 4 mm. punch at 3 days. As can be seen from Table 5-5 a minimal increase in mitotic activity was found with the occlusive tape, when compared with the effect on normal skin, but otherwise there was no effect.

In the same experiment, the rate of epithelialization was noted by measuring the distance between the two opposing epithelial edges. As can be seen from Table 5-5 the rate of closure under each of the three dressings was approximately

Table 5-5
The Effect of Various Dressings on 1 mm. Punch Biopsy Wounds

Time	Dressing	N*	Mitotic Index ± SD	P	N*	Wound Size† ± SD	P
3 days	Occlusive adhesive tape	45	9.04 ± 6.27	>0.05	84	1.06 ± 0.50	<0.005
	Plastic film (No adhesive	43	7.34 ± 4.11	>0.05	73	1.21 ± 0.43	<0.005
	"Porous" tape	35	7.65 ± 8.84	>0.05	82	1.23 ± 0.44	<0.005
	Control (Untreated skin)	43	7.18 ± 4.26	—	81	1.85 ± 0.65	—

*N = total number of counts made.

†This was measured in terms of micrometer eyepiece units as the distance between the opposing epithelial edges.

NOTE: The occlusive tape shows a significantly smaller wound size than either the plastic film or "porous" tape P < 0.005.

double that of the control (P < 0.005). However, the occlusive tape also showed a significantly smaller wound size than either the plastic film or the "porous" tape (P < 0.005).

DISCUSSION

Since these dressings had basically no effect on the mitotic activity at the edge of a circular punch biopsy wound after three days it is not likely that there is any chemical inhibitor present in these tapes. It is interesting to note that occlusion does indeed decrease the time required for wound closure as already shown by Winter in the pig [11] and Hinman and Maibach in man [12], but a similar effect is also found using a relatively nonocclusive tape. This is the porous, rayon fiber tape shown by Ordman and Gillman [16] to be particularly effective in closing surgical wounds. The pores in this tape are only those found within the weave of the material. Since these are particularly small one might suggest a "partial occlusion"—something between a polyethylene film and the perforated plastic dressing investigated by Winter [14]. However, when a dressing of this type is covering wounded skin, absorption of the exudate would probably make it more occlusive.

On investigating the effects of essential fatty acid (EFA) deficiency, Menton [26] suggested that the resultant epidermal hyperplasia may have been due to an abnormal stratum corneum and hence an abnormal water barrier, with increased epidermal permeability. On putting EFA deficient mice, with their abnormal stratum corneum, into a humid environment he did indeed show that the degree of hyperplasia was reduced. Since water loss is also excessive in stripped skin, any type of covering will reduce this. Consequently if there is a connection between the integrity of the epidermal water barrier and epidermal proliferation one might expect the results demonstrated in these presentations.

A second possibility is that there is a negative feedback existing between the keratinized layers and the basal layer so as to maintain a steady state in epidermal depth. This has been suggested many times in theory, and in practice Born and Bickhardt [27] demonstrated inhibition of DNA synthesis in the epidermis by extracts of the stratum corneum. This could suggest that exposure of stripped skin to the environment might increase the rate of keratinization, due to cellular dehydration, which would in turn decrease the mitotic rate. A mechanism such as this might explain the significantly greater fall in mitosis seen under the less occlusive dressings. Although the keratin found on these specimens did not seem any thicker than under the occlusive dressings, neither the histological techniques used nor the micrometer were sufficiently sensitive to detect small changes in the depth of the stratum corneum. Thus in excised wounds one would expect increased epithelialization under occlusion but since the water loss across the new epithelium is reduced the subsequent mitotic activity and the resultant epidermal thickening would also be reduced. This is in accord with the results shown by Gillman [2]. The return of stripped skin to high levels of mitotic activity after 6 days covering only with the "porous" tape is difficult to explain. However, since the dressings were changed daily it is possible that there was a renewed stripping effect if insufficient care was taken, and absorption of exudate by the porous tape might result in greater adherence to the wound surface. Pinkus [28] showed that very little stripping is needed to increase mitotic activity. In fact the extraordinarily wide range of results in this particular instance (0.23–24.21) might support such an explanation.

Since the reduction in mitotic activity is particularly marked in stripped skin which has been covered, how does one explain the equally marked increase in epidermal thickness under identical circumstances? A possible explanation is that since keratinization requires exposure to the ambient environment and as this is excluded by the dressing, the increased thickness is simply representative of viable cells which under other conditions would have formed part of the stratum corneum. On this basis one might expect increased thickness in the stripped covered skin, since even the reduced mitotic rate is still above normal. In fact one can see a smaller increase in epidermal thickness of stripped skin under the "porous" tape or the adhesive backing, both of which produce a slightly greater fall in mitotic activity than the occlusive dressings. It is also interesting to note that in normal skin under the "porous" tape where mitotic activity is reduced below normal levels there is no increase in thickness.

These results suggest that all the types of dressing used in this study produce a change in the microenvironment such as to decrease the transepidermal water loss, increase cellular migration and possibly decrease keratinization. These factors in turn are probably affecting cell division by some indirect mechanism as yet unknown.

In conclusion, one can see that all the types of dressings investigated in this report produce a decrease in the epidermal mitotic response after wounding and an increased rate of epithelial migration. Since this is so, one might suggest that the porous, rayon fiber tape would be the wound dressing of choice. The microenvironmental conditions developing beneath it might be less than ideal for bacterial growth resulting in a decreased risk of infection seen with the occlusive dressings. Furthermore, these systems may be of value in decreasing the abnormally high mitotic rates seen in diseases like psoriasis and some of the ichthyotic states.

SUMMARY

Tape closure of superficial wounds has been shown to have certain advantages over sutures. Among these are absence of a reaction to the suture and more rapid healing. However, occlusion has been shown to inhibit cell division both of psoriatic lesions and stripped skin. This work was undertaken to further investigate this apparent anomaly. Four dressings: an occlusive, adhesive tape, the adhesive backing from this tape, a less occlusive adhesive tape and an occlusive nonadhesive film, were used to cover regions of normal and stripped skin for periods from 2 to 6 days. The results show a slight increase in mitotic rate and epidermal thickness of normal skin but a decreased mitotic rate and increased thickness of stripped skin, under all dressings. These results are discussed and it is suggested that the less occlusive tape might be of benefit in accelerating the healing of wounds without adding the risk of infection seen under complete occlusion.

ACKNOWLEDGMENTS

Drs. Lester Pope and Eugene Prout, California Department of Corrections, cooperated in this study. Sally Ronquillo and Ann Stafford expertly prepared the histological sections.

REFERENCES

1. Scales, J. T.: Wound healing and the dressing, Brit. J. Indust. Med. 20:82, 1963.
2. Gillman, T.: Healing of cutaneous abrasion and of incisions closed with sutures or plastic adhesive tape, South African Med. Proc. 4:751, 1958.
3. Gillman, T.: Some aspects of the healing and treatment of wounds, Triangle 4:68, 1959.
4. Gillman, T., et al.: Closure of wounds and incisions with adhesive tape, Lancet 2:945, 1955.
5. Scales, J. T., et al.: Development and evaluation of a porous surgical dressing, Brit. M. J. 2:962, 1956.
6. Gillman, T., et al.: Is skin homografting necessary? A reexamination of the rationale for auto- or homografting of cutaneous injuries and a preliminary report on the action of plastic dressings, Plast. & Reconstruct. Surg. 18:260, 1956.
7. Forrester, J. C., et al.: Tape closed and sutured wounds. A comparison by tensiometry and scanning electron microscopy, Brit. J. Surg. 57:729, 1970.
8. Forrester, J. C., et al.: The tape closed wound—a bioengineering analysis, J. S. Res. 9:537, 1969.
9. Brunius, U., and Ahren, C.: Healing during the cicatrization phase of skin incisions closed by non-suture technique, Acta chir. scandinav. 135:289, 1969.
10. Winter, G. D.: Formation of the scab and the rate of epithelization of superficial wounds in the skin of the young domestic pig, Nature 193:293, 1962.
11. Winter, G. D.: Movement of epidermal cells over the wound surface, in Montagna, W., and Billingham, R. E. (ed.): *Advances in Biology of the Skin,* Vol. 5, *Wound Healing* (New York: The MacMillan Company, 1964).
12. Hinman, C. D., and Maibach, H.: Effect of air exposure and occlusion on experimental human skin wounds, Nature 200:377, 1963.
13. Winter, G. D., and Scales, J. T.: Effect of air drying and dressings on the surface of a wound, Nature 197:91, 1963.
14. Winter, G. D.: A note on wound healing under dressings with special reference to perforated film dressings, J. Invest. Dermat. 45:299, 1965.
15. Knudsen, E. A., and Snitker, G.: Wound healing under plastic coated pads, Acta Dermato.-venereol. 49:438, 1969.

16. Ordman, L. J., and Gillman, T.: Studies in the healing of cutaneous wounds. III. A critical comparison in the pig of the healing of surgical incisions closed with sutures or adhesive tape based on tensile strength and clinical and histological criteria, Arch. Surg. 93:911, 1966.
17. Smith, K. W., *et al.*: A comparison of gold leaf and other occlusive therapy, Arch. Dermat. 96:703, 1967.
18. Harris, D. R., and Keefe, R. L.: A histologic study of gold leaf treated experimental wounds, J. Invest. Dermat. 52:487, 1969.
19. Fry, L., *et al.*: Effect of plastic occlusive dressings on psoriatic epidermis, Brit. J. Dermat. 82:458, 1970.
20. Baxter, D. L., and Stoughton, R. B.: Mitotic index of psoriatic lesions treated with anthralin, glucocorticosteroids and occlusion only, J. Invest. Dermat. 54:410, 1970.
21. Petzoldt, D. G., *et al.*: Effects of plastic foil occlusion on psoriatic lesions, Arch. klin. u. exper. Dermat. 238:160, 1970.
22. Williams, M. G., and Hunter, R.: Studies on epidermal regeneration by means of the strip method, J. Invest. Dermat. 29:407, 1957.
23. Born, W.: Epidermale DNS Synthese unter occlusiv Verbänden in tritium thymidin Autoradiogram. Ztschr. Haut. Geschlechtskr. 44:305, 1969.
24. Fisher, L. B., and Maibach, H. I.: The effect of corticosteroids on human epidermal mitotic activity, Arch. Dermat. 102:39, 1971.
25. Goldstein, A.: *Biostatics: An Introductory Text* (New York: The Macmillan Company, 1964).
26. Menton, D. N.: The effects of essential fatty acid deficiency on the skin of the mouse, Am. J. Anat. 122:337, 1968.
27. Born, W., and Bickhardt, R.: Zur Regelung des Zellnachschubs in der Epidermis, Klin. Wchnschr. 46:1312, 1968.
28. Pinkus, H.: Examination of the epidermis by the strip method. II. Biometric data on the regeneration of the human epidermis, J. Invest. Dermat. 19:431, 1952.

The study was supported by a special appropriation from the State of California and by Research Grant No. AM 11649 and Training Grant No. AM 05566 from the National Institutes of Health.

6

Some Ultrastructural Aspects of Epidermal Repair in Two Model Wound Healing Systems

*Walter S. Krawczyk, D.D.S.**

In the progression of events leading to epidermal repair after wounding, two major components can be distinguished: an early stage which results in the restoration of epidermal continuity and a later stage during which restoration of normal epidermal architecture occurs. Important in effecting the completion of each of these stages are the cellular and subcellular mechanisms responsible for such basic phenomena as cell migration, mitosis and differentiation [1–9]. To study and better understand the role these mechanisms play in the reparative process two complementary wound healing models have been developed in our laboratory [7]. These two model systems consist of (1) *Intact* suction induced subepidermal blisters and (2) *Opened* subepidermal blisters (the blister roof was removed immediately after induction leaving an open wound). Certain of the aforementioned phenomena are being studied at both the light and electron microscopic levels.

During the early stages of the repair process questions concerning the relative involvement of epidermal cell division and/or epidermal cell migration have arisen. Is restoration of epidermal continuity dependent upon: division of epidermal cells, whereby daughter cells are "squeezed-out" over the denuded dermal surface; epidermal cell migration independent of cell division; or a combination of both, that is, epidermal cell division with subsequent migration by the daughter cells?

In the later stages of epidermal wound healing we have directed our research interests toward a small lamellated organelle called a keratinosome [10] to determine its role in epidermal morphogenesis and renewal. Unique to epidermal cells, keratinosomes† are approximately 300–350 mμ in length and 150–200 mμ in width. These organelles are most abundant in the upper layers of the stratum

---

*Department of Oral Histopathology and Periodontology, School of Dental Medicine, Harvard University, and Department of Dermatologic Genetics, New England Medical Center Hospitals, Boston, Massachusetts.

†Other terms used to describe these bodies are Membrane Coating Granules [11], and Odland Bodies [9, 12].

spinosum and the stratum granulosum. In the stratum granulosum, keratinosomes are mainly found between the distal plasma membrane and the central
portion of the cell. At the interface of the stratum corneum and the stratum
granulosum, numbers of keratinosomes can be observed fused to the plasma
membranes of granular cells with subsequent extrusion or "secretion" of the
keratinosome and its lamellar contents into the intercellular space. The function
of these epidermal organelles at this time still remains obscure.

To date these studies have provided information on the preeminent role of
epidermal cell migration during the early stages of epidermal repair and, from
sequential observations during restoration of epidermal continuity in the two
model wound healing systems, a pattern of epidermal cell movement has been
proposed [7]. During the later stages of epidermal wound healing it is possible to
study the initial appearance and fate of organelles such as keratinosomes, to determine their role in the conversion of granular epidermal cells to horny cells.
In this chapter we will discuss some of the observations we have made. Except
for a brief description of our method of wounding, no attempt will be made to
detail the techniques used since these can be found elsewhere.

WOUNDING

To obtain the two model wound healing systems used for these studies, subepidermal blisters were induced in the skin of young mice with a suction device
[7]. Subsequent to wounding the blisters on selected animals were allowed to remain intact, while on other animals the blister roof was immediately removed
leaving an opened wound. Intact and opened subepidermal blisters were biopsied
at sequential periods of time following induction, and prepared for light and
electron microscopic observation.

EPIDERMAL REPAIR

Intact Subepidermal Blisters

Histological examination of biopsies removed immediately after blister induction reveals that these wounds are subepidermal blisters (Fig. 6-1). Twelve hours
after wounding, epidermal cell movement can be observed as a wedge-like pro-

Fig. 6–1.—Intact blister removed immediately after induction. The epidermis has been
completely lifted away from the dermis (*d*) and forms the blister roof (*br*) of a subepidermal blister. Borate buffered toluidine blue stain. Formaldehyde-glutaraldehyde/
osmium fixation. ×72.

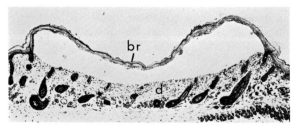

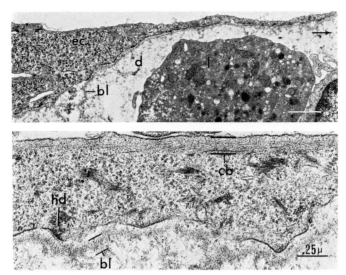

Fig. 6–2 (top).—Twelve hour biopsy of an intact subepidermal blister. The narrow elongated extension of a leading epidermal cell (*ec*) out over the denuded dermal surface is depicted. The basal lamina (*bl*) forms the uppermost boundary of the dermis (*d*). The direction of epidermal cell movement is indicated by the *arrow*. Leukocyte (*l*). Formaldehyde-glutaraldehyde/osmium fixation. ×13,800. Scale line = 1 micron.

Fig. 6–3 (bottom).—An area on a foremost epidermal cell further back from the free epidermal margin shows hemidesmosomal (*hd*) attachment of the epidermal cell to the "old" basal lamina (*bl*). In the cytoplasm, adjacent to the upper plasma membrane of the cell, a cortical band (*cb*) of fine fibers extends from the body of the cell out into the cellular extension. Formaldehyde-glutaraldehyde/osmium fixation. ×50,400. Scale line = 0.25 micron.

Fig. 6-4.—Twenty-four hour biopsy of an opened blister. An epidermal cell (*ec*) at the leading edge of the stratified sheet of epidermal cells contacts both fibrin (*f*) and surrounding mesenchymal cells (*double arrows*). No basal lamina is present and areas of the epidermal cell membrane are exposed to the dermal milieu (*single arrows*). Fine fibers cortically positioned (*cb*) can also be observed. Formaldehyde-glutaraldehyde/osmium fixation. ×16,200. Scale line = 1 micron.

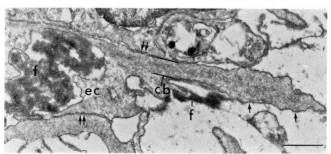

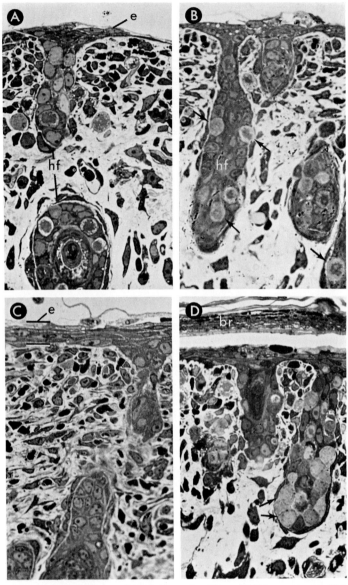

Fig. 6–5.—**A,** control biopsy of an intact subepidermal blister removed 12 hours following blister induction. Immediately following blister induction the animal received an intraperitoneal injection of saline. Epidermal cells (*e*) can be observed migrating out over the denuded dermal surface from the hair follicle root sheath (*hf*). **B,** twelve hour biopsy of an intact subepidermal blister from an animal receiving 0.1 mg./kg. body wt. of vinblastine sulfate, intraperitoneally, immediately after blister induction. Some epithelial cells of the hair follicle root sheath (*hf*) have been arrested in metaphase (*arrows*). Migration of epidermal cells can still be observed. **C,** control biopsy of an intact subepidermal blister removed 24 hours following blister induction. Twelve hours

jection from the epithelial root sheath of hair follicles out over the denuded dermal surface. This projection of epidermal cells is usually two to three cells deep nearest the follicle and tapers to one elongated cell at the free epidermal margin. At this time the blister roof is still intact but epidermal cells of the blister roof display signs of degeneration.

Ultrastructurally, the most advanced epidermal cell extends a pseudopodial extension out over the denuded dermal surface (Fig. 6-2). This cellular extension is in close proximity to the "old" basal lamina, which has remained as the uppermost boundary of the dermis following blister induction. At selected points along the basal plasma membrane of this foremost epidermal cell the sequential development of hemidesmosomes can be observed (Fig. 6-3). Cells in this position possess a cortically oriented band of fine fibers that extend from the main part of the cell out into the narrow cellular process. Occasionally, at the free epidermal edge, the foremost extension of one epidermal cell can be observed overlapping the extended process of another epidermal cell.

Eighteen hours after wounding epidermal repair has proceeded further, but the epidermal hiatus has not yet been closed. Basally positioned epidermal cells distal to the free edge have changed shape from low and elongated to an oval or round form. These basal epidermal cells also display a greater inter-digitation with the basal lamina compared with cells at the free epidermal margin. Epidermal cells superiorly positioned to these basal cells have a flattened and elongated appearance. The cortical band of fine fibers can still be seen in superiorly oriented cells but this cortical band is not observed in the oval or round basal cells.

Twenty-four hours after wounding, the original blister roof is still intact but the dermis is now completely covered by a noncornified epidermis 3–4 cells thick.

Opened Subepidermal Blisters

Removing the blister roof immediately after subepidermal induction exposes the denuded dermal surface. A biopsy at this time reveals that no epidermal cells have remained, and that the superior border of the dermis is formed by the basal lamina. At increasing periods of time after blister roof removal the exposed dermis displays signs of degeneration as a result of desiccation. The basal lamina is not evident one hour after the removal of the blister roof and the superior border of the dermis has an amorphous appearance.

Twenty-four hours after wounding a coagulum composed of degenerated leukocytes and mesenchymal cells covers the wound area. Extending from the peripheral epidermis beneath this coagulum is a stratified sheet of epidermal cells, 3–4 cells deep at the peripheral epidermis and tapering to one or two elongated cells at the free epidermal margin. The foremost cell of this stratified sheet is touching strands of fibrin and other cells of the dermis (Fig. 6-4). Since a basal

---

following blister induction the animal received an intraperitoneal injection of saline. A noncornified epidermis (*e*) 2–3 cells thick now covers the dermis. **D**, twenty-four hour biopsy of an intact subepidermal blister from an animal receiving 0.1 mg./kg. body wt. of vinblastine sulfate, intraperitoneally, 12 hours after blister induction. Groups of epithelial cells of the hair follicle root sheath are arrested in metaphase (*arrows*). The blister roof (*br*) is still intact and the dermis is covered by a noncornified epidermis 2–3 cells thick. All micrographs—borate buffered toluidine blue stain, formaldehyde-glutaraldehyde/osmium fixation. ×960.

lamina is not present, areas of the basal plasma membrane are exposed to the dermal milieu. A cortically positioned band of fine fibers can also be seen in this epidermal cell at the free margin of the stratified sheet. Vacuoles located within the cytoplasm of these epidermal cells contain an amorphous electron dense material similar in appearance to extracellular fibrin. Such deposits probably represent fibrin that has been phagocytized by the epidermal cells [5, 13].

Basally positioned epidermal cells further back from the advancing edge have a more oval or cuboidal appearance. Cells superior to these still have a low and extended profile.

Speed of Epidermal Repair

Epidermal repair takes place sooner in the intact subepidermal blisters than in the opened subepidermal blisters. At 24 hours after wounding, for example, the dermis of the intact subepidermal blisters is completely covered by a noncornified epidermis 3–4 cells thick. Whereas, 24 hours after wounding in the opened blisters initiation of epidermal repair is observed only at the lateral border of the wound. This appears as the extension of a stratified sheet of epidermal cells from the peripheral epidermis beneath the coagulum.

CELLULAR MIGRATION AND MITOSIS

To determine in intact subepidermal blisters the involvement of epidermal cell migration and/or mitosis during the early stages of epidermal wound healing, several different mitotic inhibitors were administered intraperitoneally immediately after wounding or at 12 hours after wounding. Interrupting mitotic activity by the administrations of colchicine or vinblastine sulfate produced no difference in epidermal cell migration at 12, 18 or 24 hours after wounding. Arrests in metaphase, however, were observed at 12 hours in hair follicle root sheaths (Fig. 6-5A and B) and at 24 hours in the root sheaths and the "new" basal epidermal layer (Fig. 6-5C and D). Application of the mitotic inhibitors had no effect on the morphologic integrity of the cortically positioned fine fibers.

KERATINOSOME APPEARANCE IN EPIDERMAL CELLS*

In intact subepidermal blisters, 18 hours after wounding, no keratinosomes can be observed in epidermal cells participating in the repair process. At 24 hours after subepidermal blister induction, however, keratinosomes are present in superiorly positioned epidermal cells of the noncornified epidermis that completely covers the dermis. These organelles can be easily seen after routine fixation for electron microscopic observation, or after prolonged incubation in a mixture of osmium tetroxide and zinc iodide (OZI) (prepared according to Niebauer et al. [14]). This latter technique results in a selective deposition of osmium black with keratinosomes thus permitting an easier visualization of these organelles (Fig. 6-6).

---

*The study on keratinosome appearance in epidermal wound healing was conducted in collaboration with Dr. George F. Wilgram and Mr. Joseph E. Connolly and their permission to use some previously unpublished micrographs is gratefully acknowledged.

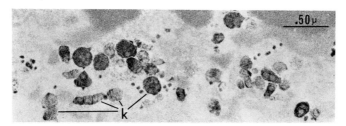

Fig. 6–6.—Twenty-four hour biopsy of an intact subepidermal blister prefixed in a mixture of formaldehyde-glutaraldehyde and then incubated at room temperature for 24 hours in an OZI mixture. Keratinosomes (k) in a most superior epidermal cell of the four cell thick noncornified epidermis display a selective deposition of osmium black. Section unstained. ×37,800. Scale line = 0.50 micron.

Thirty to thirty-six hours after wounding de novo formation of a stratum corneum has taken place resulting in the final stage of epidermal wound healing in the intact subepidermal blisters. At these times keratinosomes can be observed intracellularly, fused to the plasmalemma, and extracellularly at the granular-horny layer interface (Fig. 6-7).

DISCUSSION

While restoration of normal epidermal architecture during wound healing results from both mitosis and migration of epidermal cells, cellular migration is the primary biologic phenomenon responsible for closing the epidermal hiatus. This can be seen from the studies employing stathmokinetic agents during the early stages of epidermal repair of the intact subepidermal blisters. Furthermore, it would appear that cellular migration is independent of mitotic activity.

Results of these studies with mitotic inhibitors and those of other investigators [8] emphasize the preeminent role of epidermal cell migration in restoring epidermal continuity during wound healing. Though the environment of epidermal

Fig. 6–7.—Thirty hour biopsy of an intact subepidermal blister prefixed in a mixture of formaldehyde-glutaraldehyde and then incubated at room temperature for 24 hours in an OZI mixture. The extracellular lamellar remnants of two keratinosomes (*brackets*) show a selective deposition of osmium black. Area depicted is at the junction of the stratum granulosum (*sg*) and the stratum corneum (*sc*). Section unstained. ×60,000. Scale line = 0.25 micron.

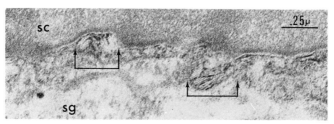

cells in intact subepidermal blisters differs from that of the opened subepidermal blisters, the pattern of epidermal cell movement appears the same. Epidermal cells appear to move by rolling or sliding over one another. Instrumental in mediating this movement are the intercellular junctions (desmosomes) and a firm attachment to a substrate through the hemidesmosomes. In the intact subepidermal blisters epidermal cells closely follow and attach to a continuous and homogeneous substrate, the retained basal lamina. In the opened subepidermal blisters attachment of epidermal cells is made to sporadic areas of fibrin and underlying mesenchymal cells.

These observations on a pattern of epidermal cell movement are in agreement with earlier light microscopic studies conducted on cutaneous porcine wounds [15].

The intracytoplasmic biomolecular mechanisms which effect the movement of epidermal cells during the early stages of wound healing have not been defined. From our observations we have been able to follow the de novo formation of hemidesmosomes along the basal plasma membrane of foremost epidermal cells in both systems. Since hemidesmosomes are considered to have a major role in mediating the attachment of the epidermis to the connective tissue [16, 17], the formation of these organelles during the early stage of epidermal repair would assign a new role to them in facilitating the movement of epidermal cells. The cortical band of fine fibers that we have consistently observed in both the intact and opened subepidermal blisters may have a significant role in the mechanisms of epidermal cell movement. Suggestions have been advanced that fibers similar in position and appearance may have a role during the morphogenesis of various tissues [18].

In the restoration of normal epidermal architecture during wound healing the appearance of keratinosomes 6 hours prior to the de novo formation of the stratum corneum could suggest an important role for keratinosomes in the conversion of granular epidermal cells to horny cells. From previous studies these organelles and their intercellular lamellar remnants have been shown to contain acid phosphatase [19, 20]. The presence of this hydrolytic enzyme has prompted some investigators to suggest a role for these bodies in the morphogenesis of the stratum corneum [9, 10, 19, 20]. In studies conducted on rats raised on an essential fatty acid (linoleic acid) deficient diet [21], increased numbers of keratinosomes were observed within the cytoplasm and extracellular spaces of the acanthotic and hyperkeratotic epidermis. From these findings it was suggested that keratinosomes were involved in the increased turnover of epidermal cells in essential fatty acid deficient rats. In other studies, the preferential deposition of osmium black following prolonged incubation of normal epidermis in the OZI mixture has been shown to be the result of substantial amounts of lipids within keratinosomes. Extraction with a variety of lipid solvents prior to incubation in the OZI mixture abolishes the selective deposition of osmium black within the keratinosome [22].

Present and future investigations into epidermal wound healing employing intact and opened suction induced subepidermal blisters will hopefully provide an insight into the complex integrated mechanisms effecting restoration of epidermal continuity and normal epidermal architecture.

REFERENCES

1. Arey, L. B.: Wound healing, Physiol. Rev. 16:327, 1936.
2. Bullough, W. S.: Epithelial Repair, in Dunphy, J. E., and Van Winkle, W. (eds.): *Repair and Regeneration* (New York: McGraw-Hill Book Company, Inc., 1969).
3. Croft, C. B., and Tarina, D.: Ultrastructural studies of wound healing in mouse skin. I. Epithelial behavior, J. Anat. 106:63, 1970.
4. Giacometti, L., and Montagna, W.: Healing of Skin Wounds in Primates, in Dunphy, J. E., and Van Winkle, W. (eds.): *Repair and Regeneration* (New York: McGraw-Hill Book Company, Inc., 1969).
5. Gibbins, J. R.: Migration of stratified squamous epithelium *in vivo*. The development of phagocytic ability, Am. J. Pathol. 53:929, 1968.
6. Kischer, C. W.: Epithelization, in *Immunopathology of Inflammation*, Proceedings of a symposium of the International Inflammation Club (Excerpta Medica International Congress Series No. 229).
7. Krawczyk, W. S.: A pattern of epidermal cell migration during wound healing, J. Cell Biol. 49:247, 1971.
8. Rafferty, N. S.: Mechanism of repair of lenticular wounds in *Rana pipiens*. I. Role of cell migration, J. Morph. 133:409, 1971.
9. Wilgram, G. F., *et al.*: A possible role of the desmosome in the process of keratinization, in Montagna, W., and Lobitz, W. C. (eds.): *The Epidermis* (New York: Academic Press, Inc., 1964).
10. Wilgram, G. F.: Das Keratinosome: Ein Faktor im Verhornungprozess der Haut, Hautarzt 16:377, 1965.
11. Matoltsy, A. G., and Parakkal, P. F.: Membrane coating granules of keratinizing epithelia, J. Cell Biol. 24:297, 1965.
12. Odland, G. F.: A submicroscopic granular component in human epidermis, J. Invest. Dermat. 34:11, 1960.
13. Odland, G., and Ross, R.: Human wound repair. I. Epidermal regeneration, J. Cell Biol. 39:135, 1968.
14. Niebauer, G., *et al.*: Osmium zinc iodide reactive sites in the epidermal Langerhans cell, J. Cell Biol. 43:80, 1969.
15. Winter, G. F.: Movement of Epidermal Cells over the Wound Surface, in Montagna, W., and Billingham, R. E. (eds.): *Advances in Biology of the Skin*, Vol. 5, *Wound Healing* (Oxford: Pergamon Press, 1964).
16. Brody, I.: An electronmicroscopic study of the junctional and regular desmosomes in normal human epidermis, Acta dermat.-venereol. 48:290, 1968.
17. Odland, G.: The fine structure of the interrelationship of cells in the human epidermis, J. Biophys. & Biochem. Cytol. 4:529, 1958.
18. Wessels, N. K., *et al.*: Microfilaments in cellular and developmental processes. Science 171:135, 1971.
19. Weinstock, M., and Wilgram, G. F.: Fine structural observations on the formation and enzymatic activity of keratinosomes in mouse tongue filiform papillae, J. Ultrastruct. Res. 30:262, 1970.
20. Wolff, K., and Holubar, K.: Okland-Körper (Membrane Coating Granules, Keratinosomen) als epidermale Lysosomen, Arch. Klin. exper. dermat. 231:1, 1967.
21. Menton, D. N.: The effects of essential fatty acid deficiency on the fine structure of mouse skin, J. Morph. 132:181, 1970.
22. Connolly, J. E., *et al.*: In preparation.

Part III

Quantification of Repair

Introduction

*Howard I. Maibach, M.D.**

Therapeutic efforts aimed at increasing the speed of wound healing in man have interested numerous surgeons, dermatologists and basic scientists. A considerable literature exists to document these activities. Yet many practical questions on the care of epidermal wounds require delineation, for much of this literature is more testimonial than documentary.

The basic reason for the lack of a consensus as to the proper methods to treat wounds is that the published literature often fails to present convincing data. Experimental design or execution may be at fault; more often the problem has been that a good quantitative method for determining wound healing kinetics has not been available.

The authors in this section seriously examine wound healing in relationship to its mensuration. This approach allowed them to draw firm conclusions of the parameters examined.

David Spruit utilized measurement of transepidermal water loss (WVL) as an index of skin function in normal and wounded skin. WVL refers to skin water loss not related to sweating. Several technological advances of the last decade allowed production of sensitive equipment for quantitating water that has finally made this approach practical. WVL amounts to less than one mg. per square cm. per hour in normal skin, necessitating great sensitivity of method. Spruit has admirably accomplished this and presents much valuable basic information for those utilizing or interpreting WVL data as an index of skin integrity.

David Rovee and his associates utilize migratory patterns and epidermal mitotic activity as their index of skin function. With the aid of colcemid to produce metaphase arrest, they demonstrate statistical differences in mitotic activity in several environmental situations. This method appears practical and efficient for quantitating this important aspect of wound repair.

Hopefully, these excellent papers will stimulate further work in the development of quantitative methods for measuring wound healing; these methods should stimulate development of better means of promoting wound healing.

---

*Associate Professor and Vice-Chairman, Department of Dermatology, University of California School of Medicine, San Francisco, California.

7

The Water Barrier and Its Repair

David Spruit, Ph.D. *

LOCATION OF THE WATER BARRIER

The human body maintains about 65% water in its tissues. Somewhere there has to be a barrier which allows water to escape from the body to the environment only with difficulty. The skin, the body's outer organ, logically provides the barrier which separates the moist inner milieu from the relatively dry outer environment and this barrier has been shown to be located only in the outer part of the skin—the 0.02 mm. thick horny layer. This part can be gradually removed by repeatedly fixing adhesive tape to the skin and removing the tape after a minute, when some horny layer cells have adhered to it. This stripping technique, originally employed by Wolf [1], has been applied frequently in the study of the water barrier of human skin. Applying the technique of gradual removal of the outer horny layer cells, Blank [2] originally argued that the water barrier was located principally in the deepest layers of the stratum corneum. More than 10 years later he gave the correct interpretation of his earlier experiments [3]; every cell layer of the stratum corneum probably contributes equally to the barrier properties of the skin. This is a remarkable result as the composition and structure of inner and outer horny cell layers differ [4]. The water content of the inner layers is higher, which can be expected to be associated with a higher water permeation. However, the mutual adherence of these cells is better which may well have the opposite effect. Until now the problem of the exact contribution of the various horny cell layers has not really been solved in detail.

The location of the water barrier in the stratum corneum implies that water evaporates freely from the body after this layer has been removed. This stratum corneum is formed from the underlying stratum granulosum. The growth of the stratum corneum is very slow; a horny cell is not removed by scaling until at least two weeks after its formation [5]. The stage of growth of a granulosum cell determines whether its contribution to the barrier properties is already present or not. The exact frontier of the water barrier is located in this transition; the barrier may include some granulosum cells. None of the deeper layers of the epi-

---

*Department of Dermatology, University of Nijmegen, The Netherlands.

dermis (stratum spinosum, stratum basale) have any water barrier properties [6]. This certainly does not exclude the possibility that they may function as barrier against the permeation of other substances.

QUALITY OF THE WATER BARRIER

The quality of the water barrier varies; it is not dependent on the thickness of the horny layer. The water vapor loss from scrotal skin is 2–20 times as high as the water vapor loss from the equally thick horny layer of abdominal skin [7]. The horny layer of the palm of the hand is about ten times as thick as the horny layer of forearm skin, yet the water loss from the skin of the palm is about 7 times as high as the water loss from forearm skin [8]. The thicker horny layer of the palm is a very poor water barrier in spite of its thickness.

When the water vapor loss is high, the water barrier is not functioning efficiently. A "good" or "high" barrier means a high resistance against water vapor loss, and thus low water permeability. The resistance of the water barrier is reciprocal to the water vapor loss; in practice the water vapor loss is measured. Usually water vapor loss measurements are not converted into units of resistance against water loss. Results expressed in units of water vapor loss are sufficiently clearly interpretable in practice as they usually refer to the water permeability from the completely moist inner milieu to a completely dry outer atmosphere— standardized circumstances. In such circumstances of constant and maximal pressure gradient they present a value which is indeed reciprocal to the resistance against water loss. Yet, difficulties of two kinds may arise.

The resistance to water vapor loss, representing directly the quality of the barrier, is easily defined in such a way that it is only very slightly dependent upon temperature [9]. This is in accordance with theoretical considerations and has been proved to reflect the reality. The dependency of permeability and water vapor loss measurements upon temperature is on the contrary considerable. This dependency is theoretically known. Scheuplein [10] dealt extensively with the dependence of human skin water vapor loss (WVL) upon temperature. His measurements lead to the following equation:

$$\text{WVL} = 10.5 \ e^{-6.0/RT} + 10^{11} \ e^{-19.7/RT}$$

From this relationship it follows that there are two individual energies of activation for the actual WVL, being 6.0 and 19.7 Kcal/mole. Two different parallel pathways can be visualized in human skin according to these activation energies. Diffusion through "pores", partial openings such as intercellular spaces and appendages which occupy a small fraction ($f = 10^{-5}$), is dominant at low temperatures (below 6°C), but increases only slowly with temperature owing to the small activation energy of 6.0 Kcal/mole. Diffusion through the "bulk" of the horny layer, and especially the "immobilized" water contained in this layer, rapidly becomes dominant at higher temperatures (above 6°C) owing to the larger temperature coefficient of 19.7 Kcal/mole. At room temperatures the flux via both mechanisms is approximately equal according to Scheuplein [10].

Translated into temperature independent barrier terms Scheuplein's results may be described as follows: parallel barriers (parallel pathways) are seen to be present in a direction perpendicular to the surface of the skin. Their barrier qualities differ. The resulting barrier of the skin changes in its location when the temperature decreases below 6°C. This change can be understood as the result of a change in phase, for barrier properties of a material are only constant as long as the material does not change phase (e.g., solid-liquid, etc.) [9].

The barrier of the skin can not only be thought to be split into different barriers perpendicular to the surface of the skin, but also in successive horizontal regions. In the consideration of such different horizontal parts (e.g., after application of substances upon the skin) its quality should preferably be stated in the dimensions of a resistance or barrier, and not in the dimensions of a permeability or water vapor loss. For successive resistances can simply be added together and permeabilities cannot. This complication caused Blank's experiments about the gradual removal of the horny cell layers to be misinterpreted for 13 years [2, 3]. It means that all investigations concerning additional barriers on the skin (application of ointments, petrolatum, wool fat, and so on) should preferably be expressed in the dimensions of resistance [9]. The way in which this can best be done mathematically has been dealt with at length for the reduction of the water vapor loss from lakes after covering with a monomolecular layer of various substances [11], and was extended to the application of ointments on the skin [9].

The renewed construction of a removed horny layer barrier of the skin, and thus the problem of its repair, have not yet been considered in this way but may be so discussed in the future. A necessary condition in such a discussion is a thorough knowledge of the factors involved in the reconstruction of the horny layer.

Summarizing location and quality of the water barrier of the skin together, it has to be considered that although the water barrier is restricted to the skin's horny layer, it is composed of various different layers. A variation exists both parallel to, and perpendicular to, the surface of the skin. At the moment very little, or nothing, is known about the contribution of each of these barrier parts to the overall barrier quality of the skin and its variations.

OTHER PROPERTIES RELATING TO BARRIER FUNCTIONING

"Structure and function are not two sides of a coin; they are the very substance of that coin" [12]. A knowledge of location and quality is necessary to a good understanding of the water barrier, but some other properties relative to the functioning of the barrier must also be considered.

The horny layer cells originate from the granular layer cells, and then gradually move outwards, or are moved outwards, from the body until they are lost as scales [13]. In the meantime, they function as protection for the other parts of the skin from which they originate. This function, however, cannot be accidental. The outgrowth is a programmed sequence, otherwise the thickness of the horny layer could not be so constant. Chalones have been implicated in the regulation of this growth [14].

Constant regulation is a necessity for the ordered maintenance of the outgrowing horny layer, since many environmental variables exert their influence. Varying humidity and varying temperature continuously change the barrier properties of the horny layer because of secondarily exerted hysteresis phenomena [15–17]. Diurnal variation of the barrier has not only been demonstrated in normal

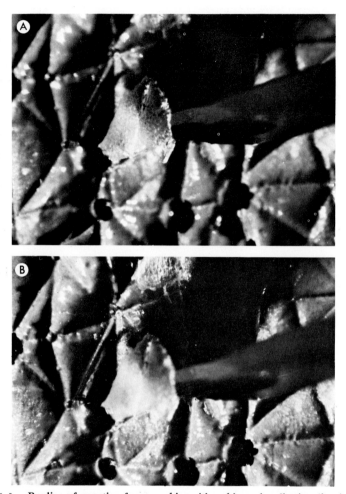

Fig. 7–1.—Replica of sweating forearm skin, with a skin scale adhering (but inverted) to the replica (the injection needle points to it). **A**, focused on the scale, **B**, focused on the replica surface.

healthy skin [18], but also in regenerating irritated skin as a part of the normal process [19]. Skin adapts itself to changed environmental circumstances; in summer the water vapor loss is increased above the water vapor loss in winter [20]. Similar adaptations have been observed following a disease concurrent with high temperature and increased sweating and following exposure to water or physiologic salt solution for one hour a day during a week, which can be considered to be almost harmless, the water vapor loss of forearm skin was also found to be increased [21]. Such influences can be expected to occur in everyday life and in this respect cannot be considered to be "repair". Other characteristics of skin have also been found to be changed; for instance the epidermal turnover time was halved following exposure of the arm to a detergent solution for one hour daily [22]. It has been suggested that the factor which changes the water vapor loss is the extraction of water soluble substances from the skin [23, 24], which influences the composition of the stratum corneum.

The conclusion must be that in fact even healthy skin is permanently in a condition of dynamic equilibrium instead of a stable invariable state. It is, therefore, practically impossible to distinguish sharply between the normal variable steady state of the skin and the repair state following a normal minor infliction occurring in everyday life.

It is obvious that a covering of dry horny layer cells will reduce the water vapor loss compared to the situation in which the scale has been lost from the skin. The loss of scales occurs gradually in healthy skin and is a normal process [10]. Figure 7-1 is a photograph of a replica of forearm skin. A scale which has been turned over from the neighboring replica surface can be seen; an injection needle has been placed between the replica and the scale. The large spherical holes in the replica have been formed by sweat drops from pharmacological stimulation and they appear to be located at the crosspoints of skin folds of this forearm [25]. A similar picture is presented in Figure 7-2. Three different areas have been selected: A, B and C. The black rings represent the rims of capsules applied for sampling the water vapor lost from such skin areas; A″, B″ and C″ referring to 1 mm.² and A′, B′ and C′ referring to 0.125 mm.² skin. The broad black circle is the area underneath the capsule's rim which will not lose water to

Fig. 7–2.—Replica of sweating forearm skin. S′ and S″, impressions of sweat droplets covered by horny layer scales. A″, B″ and C″, areas covered by 1 mm.² water vapor loss measuring capsule. A′, B′ and C′, areas covered by 0.125 mm.² water vapor loss measuring capsule. h, hole in the replica due to a hair. Areas of 1 mm.² like A″, B″ and C″ are relatively representative of an average; areas of 0.125 mm.² like A′, B′ and C′ vary in their aspect and do not represent an average sampled area.

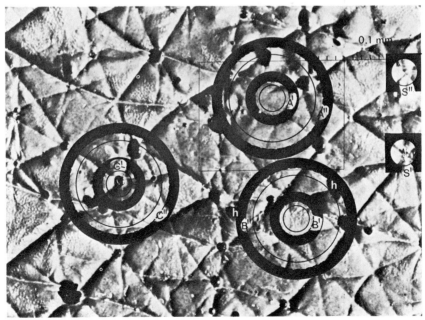

the inside of the capsule. The area between the broad black and the inner black circle is the area underneath the rim which will lose water into the inside of the capsule. The skin areas actually sampled are, therefore, the areas inside the broad black rings. The influence of the rim of the capsule (only relevant in capsules covering small areas) upon the potential lines of water flow through the 15 μ thick stratum corneum [26] is shown in Figure 7-3. This experimental problem, first described in the measurement of the water vapor loss from the thicker human nail, was not considered in measurements on forearm skin. [27].

Measurements of the water vapor loss of the areas shown in Figure 7-2 have been made, though not yet published. The water vapor loss from the larger areas of 1 mm.² could be performed with the same accuracy and reliability as in normally measured areas of 20 mm.² and larger. This implies that the sampled area of 1 mm.² suffices as a sample and presents a good average water vapor loss. The photograph of the skin surface confirms this opinion.

The water vapor loss from the smaller areas of 0.125 mm.² could only be performed with appreciably less accuracy. Obviously areas A′ B′ and C′ are not sufficiently similar in their water vapor loss. This can be confirmed from the photograph. The water vapor loss from B′ may be relatively low when the scale seen in the photograph adheres to the skin and will be relatively high as soon as this scale has been removed from the skin, for instance by rubbing or during the manufacture of the replica. The water vapor loss from C′ may be relatively high because six skin folds come together at the crosspoint in the middle where a sweat duct opening ends. Flexible skin can be supposed to be relatively high in water content and also in water vapor loss from its horny layer. The water vapor loss from A′ may be intermediate between these two values.

From these considerations it is evident that even in healthy skin the water barrier of the skin, located in its horny layer, is dependent on its local structure and function and is formed and renewed continuously. Its properties vary from site to site and from period to period.

Fig. 7–3.—The relative dimensions of a 0.125 mm.² sampling cup are shown in comparison with a semi-diagrammatic representation of the structure of the epidermis of the general body surface. The potential lines of the water flow through the stratum corneum are significantly disturbed by the presence of the impermeable rim of the cup and the effective sampling area is larger than the inside area of the cup. (From Kuno, Yas, Human Perspiration, 1956. Courtesy of Charles C Thomas, Publisher, Springfield, Ill.)

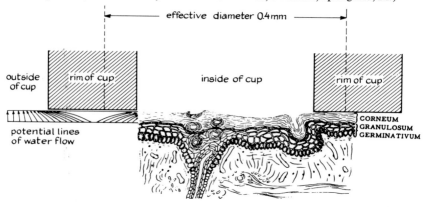

REGENERATION OF THE WATER BARRIER AFTER REMOVAL

The consequences of the removal of parts of the epidermis of the forearm are schematically represented in Figure 7-4 [28]. As a consequence of removal the water vapor loss of the skin is increased above the normal value. This increase has been plotted along the abscissa (IWVL). Removal of a part of the horny layer results in a small increase in the water vapor loss at time 0 (e.g., 0.1 mg. cm.$^{-2}$h^{-1}) which only gradually, and often irregularly, returns to normal. Practically complete removal of the horny layer results in a more appreciable increase in the water vapor loss (e.g., 1 mg. cm.$^{-2}$h^{-1}). Complete removal of the barrier, consisting of stratum corneum and stratum granulosum, results in a highly increased water vapor loss; being more than 20 mg. cm.$^{-2}$h^{-1} at time 0. It is nearly two months before the water vapor loss returns to less than 0.01 mg. cm.$^{-2}$h^{-1} above normal, this being the sensitivity of the method of measurement and about 2% of the average water vapor loss of human forearm skin.

The regeneration to a normal water vapor loss proceeds in two phases. The first phase (T) lasts about a week. During that week the water vapor loss is rapidly reduced (Figs. 7-5 and 7-6). The second phase (TF or F) lasts several weeks. The water vapor loss is only very gradually reduced to normal values. The transition of the first phase into the second phase is clearly coupled with scaling of the (usually parakeratotic) horny layer formed during the first phase. Obviously the rapidly formed parakeratotic horny layer of the first week is only a temporary barrier, which is soon shed. Mechanically, this horny layer is deficient

Fig. 7–4.—Injury and regeneration of forearm skin following the removal of the illustrated parts of the epidermis: *1*, the stratum corneum disjunctum. *2*, the entire stratum corneum—disjunctum and conjunctum. *3*, the stratum corneum and the stratum granulosum. *4*, the entire epidermis. The water vapor loss is very much increased after removal of the entire horny layer, as indicated by the gray area. (From Spruit and Malten [28].)

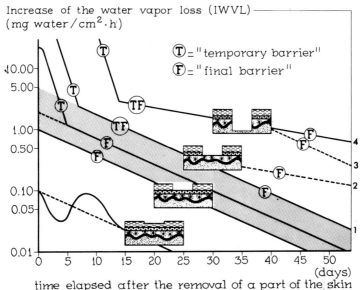

Increase of the water vapor loss (IWVL)
(mg water/cm^2·h)

$\textcircled{T}$ = "temporary barrier"
$\textcircled{F}$ = "final barrier"

time elapsed after the removal of a part of the skin
(days)

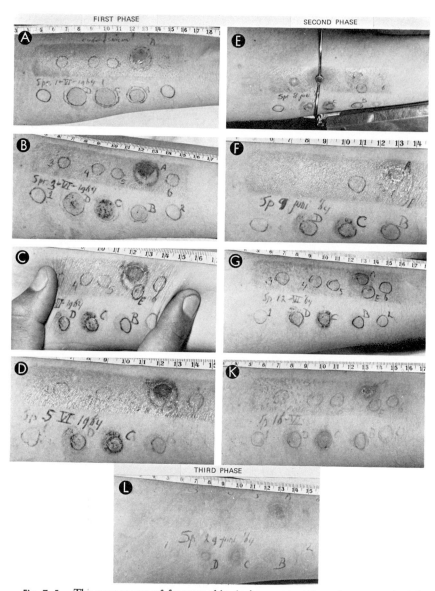

Fig. 7-5.—The appearance of forearm skin during regeneration after removal of the horny layer by stripping and after injury to the skin by exposure to alkali. Sites *1* and *2* are the controls of normal noninjured skin. The horny layer of the skin has been stripped at sites *3, 4, 5, 6, A* and *E*. At site *E*, a plastic cup has been fixed to the stripped skin by nobecutane during the exposure to 0.02 N NaOH at site *A*. At sites *B, C* and *D* the skin has been exposed to 0.02, 0.03 and 0.03 N alkali respectively. Three phases are distinguished: a, 0–5 days after injury (temporary barrier formation); b, 5–15 days after injury (visibly chapping final barrier formation); c, 15–60 days after injury (final barrier formation).

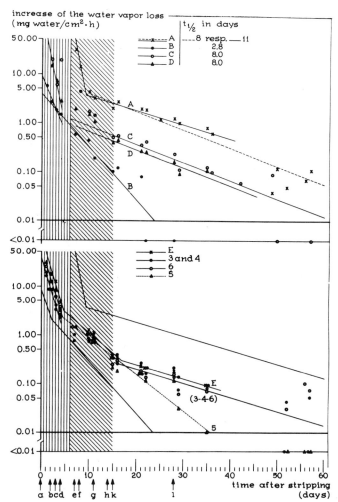

Fig. 7–6.—The increase in the water vapor loss measured at each site of the skin of Figure 7-5 during the regeneration time of about 2 months. (See also the legend of Figure 7-5.)

because of a lack of flexibility. As a barrier to water loss it is very effective, especially when it is composed of dry material just before it is lost as scales. The growth and loss of the material is schematically presented in Figure 7-7. As long as parts of the temporary barrier have not yet been removed the water vapor loss is reduced more effectively than can be achieved by the final barrier which is left after the scaling of the temporary barrier layer.

The formation of the final barrier layer, which will later be removed much more gradually, starts some days after the formation of the temporary barrier layer when this formation has reached a noticeably reduced water vapor loss and the growth (mitosis also) has slowed down [29]. It is believed to be regulated by a feedback mechanism which should be dependent on permeability [14]. A semilogarithmic relationship exists [30], which can be expressed as:

$$t_{1/2} \log \frac{(w_r - w_n)\ t = 0}{(w_r - w_n)\ t = t} = t \log 2$$

t is the time passed since the injury occurred, $(w_r - w_n)$ is the increase in the water vapor loss (IWVL)—being the difference between the water vapor loss of regenerating skin (w_r) and the water vapor loss of nearby normal skin (w_n). It is evident from this formula that the water vapor loss from a normal skin site must always be measured as a control during a series of measurements of the regeneration rate. As an appreciable variability between water vapor loss measurements on different days may occur under normal everyday circumstances in normal skin, the water vapor loss at the control sites is always measured imme-

Fig.7–7.—Scheme of the regeneration of forearm skin after removal of the horny layer by "stripping" with sellotape. **A**, measured course of the regeneration of increased water vapor loss (IWVL) with time. **B**, growth and removal, or wear and tear, of "temporary" and "final" barrier layer: Working hypothesis. (From Spruit [32].)

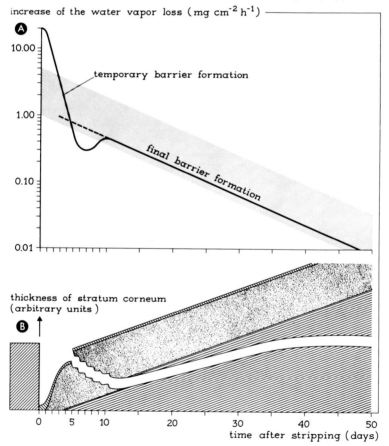

increase of the water vapor loss ($mg\ cm^{-2}\ h^{-1}$)

temporary barrier formation

final barrier formation

thickness of stratum corneum (arbitrary units)

time after stripping (days)

increase of the w.v.l.

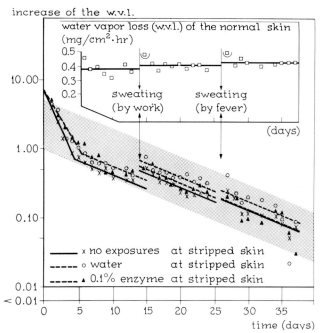

water vapor loss (w.v.l.) of the normal skin (mg/cm²·hr)

sweating (by work)

sweating (by fever)

(days)

_____ x no exposures at stripped skin
------ o water at stripped skin
----- ▲ 0.1% enzyme at stripped skin

time (days)

Fig. 7–8.—The course of the repair of the water barrier at three sites of forearm skin injured equally by stripping with cellophane tape. One of the sites was exposed to water, another to a 0.1% solution of a proteolytic enzyme for one hour on six successive days. The repair was disturbed twice by excessive sweating.

diately following or preceding the measurement of the water vapor loss at the regenerating injured site of the skin. The value $(w_r - w_n)$ has to be calculated from the results of almost simultaneous measurements.

The so-called "half-regeneration-time" $(t_{1/2})$ can easily be found from the slope of the final barrier formation in the graph by reading the time in which the IWVL has been reduced to half its former value. On average it is about 7 days (5–11 days). The limitation of the water vapor loss by the skin starts in a human being about ten days before birth (term). The half-regeneration time during this period has been found to be 3 days [31]. As a result the values of the IWVL during the regeneration period are usually found in the gray area of Figures 7-4 and 7-7.

Basically, the final barrier formation is observed as a straight line semi-logarithmic decrease in the water vapor loss. Attention should be paid to avoiding additional irritation during the regeneration period which lasts for more than a month. Excessive and longlasting sweating increasing the water vapor loss of the skin is one such additional injury. This occurred artificially 14 days after the injury and accidentally 4 weeks after the injury in the experiment shown in Figure 7-8. The measurement of the water vapor loss at two control sites (w_n) is therefore also used as a check that no environmental changes occurred during the experimental period. Skin in repair is more easily attacked than normal skin, and extraction of water soluble components presents a special problem.

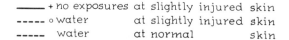

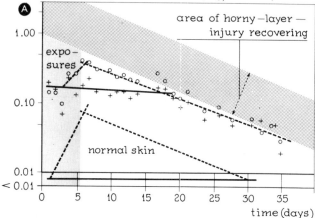

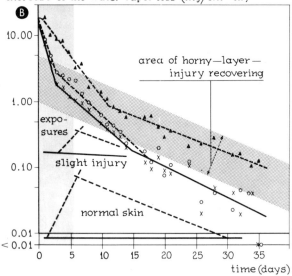

Fig. 7–9.—**A**, course of repair of forearm skin slightly injured at time 0 by a very dilute NaOH solution. Normal skin and injured skin were additionally exposed to water for one hour on six successive days [21]. **B**, course of repair of forearm skin after stripping and supplemental exposure to water or a 0.1% solution of a proteolytic enzyme for one hour during six successive days. The simultaneously conducted experiments of **A** are also indicated.

Sometimes—especially when the injury has been more severe, but also dependent on environmental circumstances—two straight lines are found. The point of inflection between these two straight lines ($TF - F$) is usually accompanied by the occurrence of scaling of the horny layer (second phase (TF), Fig. 7-5); less pronounced than the scaling appearance of the temporary layer (first phase (T), Fig. 7-5), though still obvious. The quality of the final barrier formation can be influenced by many environmental and other factors, just like the qualities of the precursors of the final barrier. In Figure 7-7B, the barrier's "quality" has been depicted as if it were simply the thickness of the horny layer.

The multiplicity of factors, endogenous and exogenous, which govern the regeneration of the skin's water barrier complicate investigation. When, however, several sites of the same skin are investigated at the same time, exogenous factors are largely ruled out as possible causes of differences between simultaneous investigations, since temperature, humidity, etc. are the same in the various investigations. Under these circumstances very reproducible curves have been found [32]. In these investigations it was found that water, physiologic saline and some other substances may influence the regeneration only transitorily or not at all, when applied upon the temporarily formed barrier layer after 24 hours or more following a standardized irritation (Fig. 7-9). Even the scaling of the skin and the dips between temporary and final barrier formation were found to be identical [32]. Thus, the effect of various factors is difficult to predict and each should be controlled.

REPAIR OF THE WATER BARRIER AFTER IRRITATION BY PURE SOLVENTS

The complete removal of the material which composes the water barrier, the horny and granular layers, is a simple but quite radical change. There are many ways in which the water barrier can be modified without removal. The slight variation in the water content of the horny layer brought about by changing the humidity of the environment leaves the layer unimpaired when the change does not last for very long [15]. Longer lasting changes in humidity are thought to cause alterations of the appearance of the skin ("dry skin" in winter) [2, 33].

Some other potential sources of "dry skin" may be slightly more harmful. Housewives who quite often have their hands in dishwater containing household detergents may suffer from "dry skin". Their skin becomes harsh, rough, red and cracked [22, 34]. Skin which is cracked can not be repaired until it regenerates; its water vapor loss and permeability are high. The skin has to recover from this infliction which can be thought of as a disease condition. The suggestion that the injury has been caused, at least partly, by extraction of water soluble substances from the skin [23, 24] is obvious. Liquid water alone may cause the same effect experimentally, but to a lesser degree [21]. The result of the exposure to liquid water apparently involves a change in the composition of the horny layer material. It has been suggested that the water content of the horny layer is reduced by reduction of its content of water binding substances [23].

Similar occupational hazards are encountered by persons who constantly expose their hands and forearms to other solvents, as do painters, service station attendants, etc., and who must subsequently effectively clean the exposed areas.

Again, the result is an extraction of material from their horny layer. The extraction causes the appearance of a dry skin and an increased water vapor loss.

Factors which influence this extraction-irritation of the skin by solvents are twofold. The efficiency of the extraction will be influenced by the character of the solvent, and by the condition of the individual skin, dependent upon several secondary circumstances [35]. After the extraction an altered horny layer is left. The kind and the degree of the alteration of the horny layer will determine the way in which repair will proceed. An example of such a repair following irritation of forearm by exposure to petroleum ether for 20 and 30 minutes has been illustrated in Figure 7-10 [32, 36]. The principal difference from Figure 7-7 is that the horny layer has been extracted but not removed.

Fig. 7–10.—Scheme of repair of forearm skin following irritation by exposure to petroleum ether for 20 or 30 minutes. **A**, measured course of regeneration of the skin's increased water vapor loss with time. **B**, hypothetical scheme of corresponding growth and removal by scaling (see also Fig. 7-7 and [32]).

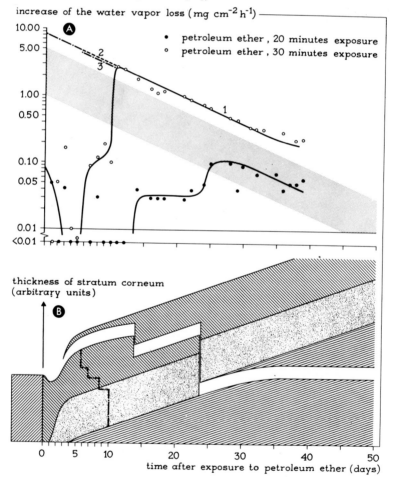

Figure 7-10A presents the measurements of the increased water vapor loss after exposure to petroleum ether, the lower part of the figure (B) presents a schematic suggestion of the development of the repair processes, principally the repair following the 20 minute exposure [32]. Contrary to the former case in which the horny layer was removed, important parts of the horny layer remain covering the underlying skin, and are able to protect the skin to some degree. The petroleum ether extracted horny layer is seen to protect the skin very efficiently from water vapor loss, perhaps not immediately after the exposure when the water vapor loss sometimes appears very moderately increased, but certainly a few days after the exposure until about 14 days after the exposure. The water vapor loss has even been reduced to less than the water vapor loss of the normal unexposed skin during this period. Some scaling occurs thereafter, resulting in a very moderately increased water vapor loss. Only about 24 days after the exposure does some scaling occur again. Nothing of the original temporary horny layer now remains and subsequent repair consists only of the further development of the final barrier layer.

The more severe infliction of a 30 minute exposure causes earlier removal of the temporary barrier layer. Cracking and scaling are more pronounced. The final barrier formation becomes the sole repair process at an earlier stage. Since there is greater extraction of the horny layer a more deficient, more brittle temporary barrier layer is left.

In general, several possibilities occur following extraction of the horny layer by a solvent. As far as the formation of the temporary barrier is concerned three of the obvious possibilities are presented schematically in Figure 7-11. The unbroken lines represent the course of the increased water vapor loss of the skin during the regeneration period. The result of the irritation by exposure to the extracting solvent can be threefold: the increase in the water vapor loss at time 0 (often accidentally) coincides with the increase which is caused by the irritating power of the solvent, as determined by the following final barrier layer formation during the repair period; the horny layer has been more severely damaged so that the water vapor loss is increased more than correlates with the start of a final barrier formation; and the horny layer composition has been changed so that it protects the skin from water vapor loss to a certain amount. These cases will be discussed.

The degree of injury to the water barrier can be seen from the extrapolated course of the repair during the final barrier formation, extrapolated to time 0 (broken lines 2). The repair might continue along a straight line (first along line 2 and then along line 1) like a simple "final barrier formation" (Fig. 7-11A). This only occurs when the water vapor loss is increased very moderately to about 1 mg. cm.$^{-2}$h^{-1}, and even then not so often. More often, the horny layer appears to have been affected by the solvent. At time 0 of the injury, the infliction results in an increase in the water vapor loss. Usually, the resulting horny layer material dries and effectively protects the skin from an excessive water vapor loss, but as a result of the drying it starts scaling and falls off the skin after some four days. Thereafter, skin repair proceeds normally. A parakeratotic horny layer following removal of the horny layer by stripping behaved similarly (Fig. 7-7).

In the above conception the contribution of the "temporary barrier" to the water vapor loss protection at time 0 is nil. The contribution increases with time as the layer dries and alters. The temporary layer and its contribution to the protection are lost some 4 days after the injury. This contribution is determined and graphically represented by curve 3, being the difference between curves 2 and 1 in Figure 7-11A.

A more severe injury may affect the underlying layers and postpone the repair of the final barrier formation (Fig. 7-11B). The final barrier formation has been extended back to time 0 by the broken line 2. The measurement of the increase in the water vapor loss at time 0 reveals that at that time the final barrier formation cannot yet have begun. The earliest date at which the final barrier formation could have started according to Figure 7-11B, is at the crosspoint of curves 1 and 2 three days after the injury. In this figure the temporary barrier formation after three days can be described by line 3 similarly to Figure 7-11A. The real final barrier formation will probably be postponed for more than three days and start shortly before the temporary barrier layer is lost as scales.

The result of an exposure to an irritant can also be that the horny layer becomes less permeable for water (Fig. 7-11C). The increase in the water vapor loss is greatly reduced. An effective temporary water barrier is formed by the extraction of the solvent and the efficiency improves until the barrier layer is lost as scales, see also Figure 7-10.

An important factor of difference between the course of repair along the lines

Fig. 7–11.—Schemes of various courses of repair of the water barrier following injury to the horny layer. Unbroken lines (*1*) = measured course; broken lines (*2*) = extrapolation of "final barrier formation"; broken lines (*3*) = protecting influence of "temporary barrier" calculated from *2 − 1* (not representing an IWVL). A, injury (measured as IWVL) at time 0 coinciding with the IWVL from "final barrier formation" (extrapolated line 2). B, injury at time 0 more severe than obvious from "final barrier formation." C, injury masked from the beginning by the formation of a temporary barrier layer. D, petrolatum applied to the injured skin for 6 successive days.

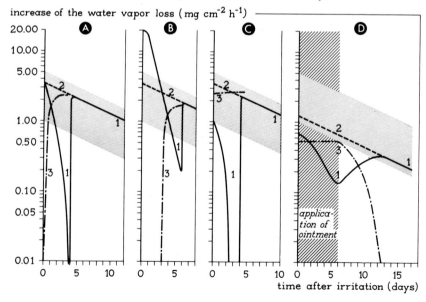

increase of the water vapor loss (mg cm^{-2} h^{-1})

time after irritation (days)

of Fig. 7-11 is the severity of the irritation at time 0. Yet the resulting injury has not been so different that a deviating "final barrier formation" occurred. The ultimate final barrier formation is not only dependent on the degree of the injury at time 0, but also on the course of the temporary barrier formation. The quality of the temporary barrier layer is dependent on the nature of the extracting solvent, the extraction time and on several environmental circumstances and the original condition of the skin. This implies that the quality of the temporary barrier formation can be influenced artificially. The quality of the temporary barrier layer would be improved if it did not "dry out" and crack during the later days of its existence, or would be improved so much that it resembled the quality of the final barrier during its repair. This has been artificially achieved in one experiment by the application of petrolatum to the injured skin (Fig. 7-11D). The application of petrolatum should be repeated daily as it is otherwise removed by the clothes and so on. The layer of petrolatum protects the skin from excessive water loss [9, 36].

During the application of the ointment in this experiment the contribution of the petrolatum temporary barrier was found to be constant (line 3 in Fig. 7-11D). The petrolatum was applied for 6 days; the water vapor loss increased after the application of the ointment was stopped and the residual ointment removed completely. It was obviously gradually lost during the next 7 days. Water vapor loss measurement during the period 15–45 days after the injury revealed the course of the final barrier formation. Extrapolation to time 0 (line 2) and the calculation of the difference between the values of curves 2 and 1 compared with the values of curve 3 showed that in this experiment temporary barrier and final barrier formation coincided. The petrolatum served as a substitute for the temporary barrier; a noncracking one.

Prevention of extraction or improvement of the condition of the skin before injury (for example, the extraction by exposure to petroleum ether) should, in principle, be possible. The natural condition of the original skin appeared to clearly influence the result. When the original skin was relatively easily injured by exposure to petroleum ether, previously applied petrolatum neither increased nor decreased the resistance of the skin to the solvent. When, however, the original skin was initially relatively resistant to the exposure to petroleum ether, the application of petrolatum before the exposure diminished its resistance to the injury and resulted in a more severely injured skin. Such results suggest that petrolatum, for example, can be used to help the repair of an injured skin, but that the application of the petrolatum should be terminated in due course in order to allow the skin to build up its own, usually more effective, protecting qualities.

REPAIR OF THE WATER BARRIER AFTER IRRITATION BY CHEMICALLY REACTIVE SUBSTANCES

Chemically irritating substances applied to the skin will either be in solution or, after application to the skin, at least partly dissolve in water or sweat. The nature of the solvent and its irritating capacity will influence the degree of irritation of the substance. When the solvent is water, the direct influence of the solvent itself will be very small.

In alkaline milieu in which the OH⁻ concentration in the water is greatly raised, the skin is known to be noticeably injured. It is obvious to ask at which concentration the OH⁻ ion will start its irritating influence.

As an example, the same forearm skin was exposed to different OH⁻ concentrations at several sites at the same time during one hour. The increased water vapor loss of these skin sites was measured daily from the day after the exposure until 40 days later; the result is seen in Figure 7-12 [28]. Though the irritation has been very small at pH 11.3, it is already considerable at pH 11.5–11.8 and really severe, accompanied by blister formation, at pH 12.0. Obviously, a critical pH near pH 11.3 exists in this forearm skin. Simultaneously, it has been observed that the amount of OH⁻ ions disappeared very slowly from the solution when the pH was below 11.2. The normal rate of carbon dioxide diffusing from the skin into alkaline solution neutralizes the OH⁻ at alkalinities below pH 11.2. Thereafter another mechanism appeared to exist by which many OH⁻ ions were used at an appreciably faster rate, and the faster as the pH rose more above 11.2. This chemical reaction (proteins are denatured at pH above 11.5 [37, 38]) obviously causes the injury to the skin from which it is repaired according to the curves in Figure 7-12.

After the first exposure, the skin has been irritated and usually a temporary

Fig. 7–12.—Regeneration of forearm skin following exposure to a solution at the indicated pH for one hour, as estimated from the increased water vapor loss of the skin (IWVL). *T*, temporary; *F* and *FF*, final barrier formation. Compare with Figure 7-4. (From Spruit and Malten [28].)

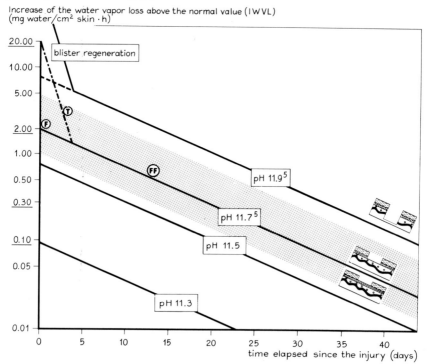

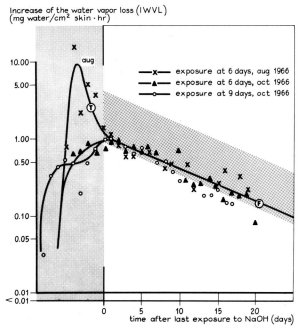

Increase of the water vapor loss (IWVL)
(mg water/cm² skin · hr)

—x— exposure at 6 days, aug 1966
—▲— exposure at 6 days, oct 1966
—o— exposure at 9 days, oct 1966

time after last exposure to NaOH (days)

Fig. 7–13.—Injury to and regeneration of the water barrier of forearm skin after exposure to 0.5 ml. 0.03 N NaOH per cm.² skin for one hour on successive days. Final barrier formation (*F*) was identical in different ambient circumstances; temporary barrier formation (*T*) shows clear adaptation of the skin to subsequent alkali exposures in August. (Derived from Spruit and Malten [28].)

barrier layer has been formed which will stay at the skin for some days and then fall off as scales. This temporary barrier layer proved to have an increased resistance against injury by the repetitive exposure to alkaline solution. The measurements in Figure 7-13 show an example of improved protection [28, 39].

The sensitivity to injury by alkali can vary considerably between skin of various individuals and is very dependent on environmental circumstances. The skin can also adapt itself to the irritating substance very gradually subsequent to repeated exposure to low concentrations. A property of the temporary barrier layer has then, to some degree, been adopted by the final barrier layer.

The phenomenon of protection against exposure to high OH⁻ concentrations by the temporary barrier layer has also been observed in exposures to other chemically reactive substances (Fig. 7-14) [35]. An 18% solution of phenol in resorcinol-formaldehyde resin is more irritating than 13.5% solution of phenol in this resin, because of the increased phenol concentration. This is also evident from single exposures of the skin to the irritant. Repeated exposure for one hour on 6 successive days, however, ultimately caused the same injury with 18% and 13.5% phenol in resin solutions, although in two different individuals (B and dK) to a different degree. The time course of the final barrier formation in these individuals coincides exactly, though not quantitatively. In the case of the less concentrated irritant, the temporary barrier layer formation more gradu-

Increase of the water vapor loss (mg water/cm^2 skin • hr)

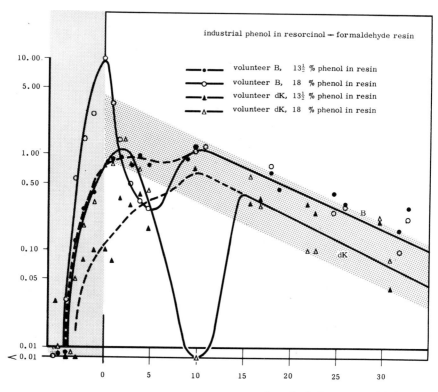

industrial phenol in resorcinol ← formaldehyde resin

——•—— volunteer B,   13½ % phenol in resin
——○—— volunteer B,   18 % phenol in resin
——▲—— volunteer dK, 13½ % phenol in resin
——△—— volunteer dK, 18 % phenol in resin

time after last exposure to phenol (days)

Fig. 7–14.—Injury to and regeneration of forearm skin after exposure to industrial phenol in resorcinol-formaldehyde resin for one hour on 6 successive days.

ally passes into the final barrier layer formation concurrent with less pronounced scaling of the temporary layer, as is evident from the more smoothly decreasing broken curves of the figure. Contrary to experiments after petroleum ether extraction, the temporary layer formed after phenol in resorcinol-formaldehyde resin appeared to be more adhesive to the skin following the more irritating phenol concentration. Differences in hardening of the resin at different phenol concentrations may influence the differences in scaling properties of the temporarily formed barrier layer. Consequently, many factors will influence the processes of protection and repair. For the time being the only way to investigate the process, therefore, seems to be the practical investigation, as the results cannot yet be predicted due to the complexity of the influencing factors.

One exception may be presented to prove the rule. A proteolytic enzyme which will not attack the horny layer of intact normal skin, or slightly injured skin (Fig. 7-8), is able to attack more severely injured skin even during the temporary barrier formation period a day after the injury (see Fig. 7-9B). The injuring capacity succeeded in retarding the final barrier formation. The stratum corneum is not a substrate for this enzyme, although other proteins are.

SUMMARY

The water barrier of the skin is extended over the horny, and mature granular layer, only. Its barrier quality is not constant during the course of time. It varies diurnally and seasonally depending on the humidity and temperature of the environment. It appears easily adaptable to changing conditions. When it meets more severe inflictions from the outside, a temporary barrier layer is formed, which is apparent from the scaling occurring after some 5 days. Although this temporary layer is functionally superior in terms of its water barrier formation and resistance to irritants, its mechanical qualities soon become deficient. It is therefore replaced by the so-called final barrier, whose properties gradually improve semi-logarithmically with a half-value of about 7 days.

Some examples are given of the different courses of repair following an injury to the horny and granular layer or less severe injury. It is indicated how the course of repair might be influenced by the application of petrolatum which is a material with relatively good water barrier properties.

REFERENCES

1. Wolf, J.: Das Oberflächenrelief der menschlichen Haut, Z. mikr.-anat. Forsch. 47: 351, 1940.
2. Blank, I. H.: Factors which influence the water content of the stratum corneum, J. Invest. Dermat. 18:433, 1952.
3. Blank, I. H.: Cutaneous barriers, J. Invest. Dermat. 45:249, 1965.
4. Spearman, R. I. C.: Some light microscopical observations on the stratum corneum of the guinea-pig, man and common seal, Brit. J. Dermat. 83:582, 1970.
5. Rothberg, S., *et al.*: Glycine-C^{14} incorporation into the proteins of normal stratum corneum and the abnormal stratum corneum of psoriasis, J. Invest. Dermat. 37: 497, 1961.
6. Spruit, D.: The water-barrier of stripped and normal skin, Dermatologica 141:54, 1970.
7. Smith, J. G., *et al.*: The epidermal barrier. A comparison between scrotal and abdominal skin, J. Invest. Dermat. 36:337, 1961.
8. Burch, G. E., and Winsor, T.: Diffusion of water through dead plantar, palmar and dorsal human skin and through toe nails, Arch. Dermat. 53:39, 1946.
9. Spruit, D.: The interference of some substances with the water vapour loss of human skin, Dermatologica 142: 89, 1971; Am. Perf. Cosm. 86(8):27, 1971.
10. Scheuplein, J.: Analysis of permeability data for the case of parallel diffusion pathways, Biophys. J. 6:1, 1966.
11. La Mer, V. K.: *Retardation of Evaporation by Monolayers. Transport Processes* (New York: Academic Press, Inc., 1962).
12. Montagna, W.: Something old, J. Invest. Dermat. 55:203, 1970.
13. Goldschmidt, H., and Kligman, A. M.: Desquamation of the human horny layer, Arch. Dermat. 95:583, 1967.
14. Bullough, W. S.: The rejuvenation of the skin, J. Soc. cosm. Chem. 21:503, 1970.
15. Spruit, D., and Malten, K. E.: Humidity of the air and water vapour loss of the skin. The changing permeability, Dermatologica 138:418, 1969.
16. Spruit, D.: Variation of the insensible perspiration of human skin, Am. Perfumer Cosm. 81:25, 1966.
17. Lamke, L. O., and Wedin, B.: Water evaporation from normal skin under different environmental conditions. Acta dermat.-venereol. 51:111, 1971.
18. Shahidullah, M., *et al.*: Diurnal variation in transepidermal water loss, Brit. J. Dermat. 81:866, 1969.
19. Spruit, D.: The diurnal variation of water vapour loss from the skin in relation to temperature, Brit. J. Dermat. 84:66, 1971.

20. Heerd, E., and Oppermann, C.: Untersuchungen über die Wasserdampfabgabe kleiner Hautflächen beim Menschen. III. Der jahreszeitliche Einflusz auf die Perspiratio insensibilis, Pflügers Arch. ges. Physiol. 291:174, 1966.

21. Malten, K. E., and Spruit, D.: The supposed damaging influence of water, physiologic saline, a proteolytic enzyme and pyroglutamic acid on normal and regenerating skin, Ann. Ital. Derm. clin. sper. 23:80, 1969.

22. Baker, H., and Kligman, A. M.: Technique for estimation turnover time for human stratum corneum, Arch. Dermat. 95:408, 1967.

23. Jacobi, O. K.: Nature of cosmetic films on the skin, J. Soc. cosm. Chem. 18:149, 1967.

24. Laden, K., and Spitzer, R.: Identification of a natural moisturizing agent in skin, J. Soc. cosm. Chem. 18:351, 1967.

25. Spruit, D., and Reijnen, A. T. A.: Pattern of sweat gland activity on the forearm after pharmacological stimulation, Acta dermat.-venereol. (In press).

26. Kligman, A. M.: The Biology of the Stratum Corneum, in Montagna, W., and Lobitz, W. C. (eds.): *The Epidermis* (New York: Academic Press, Inc., 1964).

27. Spruit, D.: Measurement of water vapor loss through human nail in vivo, J. Invest. Dermat. 56:359, 1971.

28. Spruit, D., and Malten, K. E.: Estimation of the injury of human skin by alkaline liquids, Berufsdermatosen 16:11, 1968.

29. Brophy, D., and Lobitz, W. C.: Injury and reinjury to the human epidermis. II. Epidermal basal cell response, J. Invest. Dermat. 32:495, 1959.

30. Spruit, D., and Malten, K. E.: Epidermal water-barrier formation after stripping of normal skin, J. Invest. Dermat. 45:6, 1965.

31. Singer, E. J., et al.: Barrier development, ultrastructure, and sulfhydryl content of fetal epidermis, J. Soc. cosm. Chem. 22:119, 1971.

32. Spruit, D., and Malten, K. E.: Water vapour loss and skin barrier: An evaluation and some new findings, Tr. St. John's Hosp. Dermat. Soc. 57:2, 1971.

33. Day, R. L.: Dry skin and chapping aids, J.A.M.A. NS6:650, 1966.

34. Suskind, R.: Cutaneous cleansing in health and disease, J. South. M. A. 55:996, 1962.

35. Malten, K. E., and Spruit, D.: Horny layer injury by solvents, Berufsdermatosen 16:135, 1968.

36. Spruit, D., et al.: Horny layer injury by solvents. II. Can the irritancy of petroleum ether be diminished by pretreatment? Berufsdermatosen 18:269, 1970.

37. Matoltsy, A. G., et al.: Studies of the epidermal water barrier. II. Investigation of the chemical nature of the water barrier, J. Invest. Dermat. 50:19, 1968.

38. Zimmer, C.: Alkaline denaturation of DNA's from various sources, Biochim. et biophys. acta 161:584, 1968.

39. Spruit, D.: Evaluation of skin function by the alkali application technique, Curr. Prob. Dermat. 3:148, 1970.

8

Effect of Local Wound Environment on Epidermal Healing

David T. Rovee, Ph.D.,* Carole A. Kurowsky, R.N.,*
Joan Labun* and Anne Marie Downes, B.A.*

A multiplicity of quantitative methods for measuring the repair of a surgical incision can be found in the literature, but nearly all these methods rely on parameters of dermal healing, e.g., gain in tensile strength, hydroxyproline content to reflect collagen synthesis, hexosamine content, weight of granulation tissue, DNA content to reflect fibroplasia and others [1]. The parameters for measuring the events in epidermal wound healing are fewer and not as well described.

Although epidermal healing may be of relative insignificance to the surgeon [2] who is interested in wound strength, infections, dehiscence and scar formation, it is a prime concern in the repair of partial-thickness graft donor sites, dermabraded areas, "take" in autografting and other partial-thickness defects such as abrasions, blisters and superficial lacerations. The quality of the epidermal healing may also influence subsequent repair in the dermis [3]. The initial wound strength in a surgical incision largely reflects adhesive forces of the fibrin clot and the cohesiveness of the epidermal continuum which can reestablish during the so-called lag phase of healing [4, 5].

The dynamics of epidermal healing can be divided for the purpose of understanding into three phases: epithelial migration to cover the defect, cell division to supply new cells replacing those lost by wounding and differentiation of a new epidermis, a true regenerative process, reestablishing the various strata and functions of this tissue [6]. The exact sequential order or degree of overlap in these processes has not been shown clearly. In fact, the actual or coincidental dependency of one upon the other, for example, migration being accompanied by mitosis, is in dispute [3, 6–10].

Numerous investigators have described the epithelialization of cutaneous wounds by histological examination [11–13]. Only recently, however, have some of the ultrastructural aspects of repairing human skin been reported [14]. By the use of tritiated thymidine or colchicine derivatives some information about the cell kinetics in human wound healing has been reported [15, 16]. The recently

*Department of Skin Biology, Johnson & Johnson Research, New Brunswick, New Jersey.

published technique of using small amounts of topically applied colcemid with occlusion to arrest mitosis in intact or altered epidermis is welcomed by those investigators reluctant to use tritium in vivo, and those familiar with the local toxicity and the difficulty of obtaining volunteers for uncomfortable, multiple, intradermal injections of colchicine [17]. Topical application of the drug also allows for the use of minute quantities for the local stathmokinetic effects with little evidence of toxicity.

The morphological return of a differentiated epidermis following wounding has been described and can be correlated neatly with the return of a physiological parameter, namely water-barrier function, which can be measured precisely by electrical hygrometry [18, 19].

It has been shown that various medicaments or dressings can exert major effects on epithelial migration in cutaneous wounds, either enhancing or retarding epithelialization [20–24]. It is thought that those inert dressings which enhance epithelial migration do so by virtue of maintaining hydration of the exposed wound tissues, or thereby reducing the factors inimicable to wound repair— mechanical trauma, desiccation, etc. [11, 24]. Several investigators have shown that maintaining tissue hydration by the application of plastic film dressings has hastened epithelialization as much as two-fold as compared to air exposed wounds [22]. Even the less occlusive dressings reduce the time required for epithelial migration by reducing dehydration necrosis [25].

Recently, Maibach [26] and Born [27] have shown that inert films or tapes alter the cell kinetics in normal epidermis, reducing the already low base line of cell turnover. Whether these inert films produce this effect by acting as an artificial barrier which may control a part of the kinetic response in an unknown manner, or whether they alter the patterns of normal desquamation and thus the functional demands for new cells is not understood. The fact that topically placed films have any impact at all on the kinetics of normal epidermis raises questions as to their effect on epidermal wounds.

Since cell migration can be altered significantly by changes in the local wound environment brought on by dressings, a study of the environmental effects on epidermal wound healing should also consider the impact of the treatment on cell division and differentiation of a new epidermis.

In our present investigation we have endeavored to gather information on all three phases of epidermal healing since they can be affected by changes in the local wound environment. Attempts have also been made to understand the interrelationship of cell division and cell migration in cutaneous wounds.

MATERIAL AND METHODS

Choice of Wounds in Humans

To study the biological problems of migration, mitosis and differentiation in epidermal wounds, the partial-thickness incision was chosen. The wounds are 15 mm. long, and approximately 0.3 mm. deep. Since the lesion extends completely through the epidermis and into the dermis, epithelial migration must occur to reestablish an epidermal continuum. Also, important in the healing of wounds of this type are a mitotic response and differentiation of a new stratum corneum. Because of the minor discomfort associated with the wound, no anesthetic is required, and subject acceptance of the procedure is good. The slight bleeding can be controlled by mild pressure with a gauze sponge. In this study, all incisions were made on the dorsal aspects of the forearms, perpendicular to the longitudinal axis of that appendage.

For the study of mitotic response or differentiation of epidermis, the tape stripped wound was considered to offer some advantages over the incision since the stripped wound has a larger surface area and mitotic counts could be made over large amounts of wound tissue, rather than being restricted to the wound edges. Also, hygrometric studies of the return of water barrier function could be done readily on the large area strip wounds, thus allowing the measure of the return of this physiological parameter to reflect differentiation.

The stripped wound was inflicted by placing a heavy, industrial grade, pressure sensitive adhesive tape onto the area of skin to be wounded. The tape is removed slowly, and another piece of tape of the same dimensions placed on the site. Sequential strippings are continued until the stratum corneum is completely removed, and the "glistening layer" of skin is reached.

These wounds were made on the upper backs of human subjects. For mitotic studies, the stripped areas were 0.5×2.0 inches. For hygrometric studies, the areas were 2×2 inches.

Dressings Used to Alter Local Wound Environment

To maintain hydration of wound tissues, thus preventing dehydration necrosis, impermeable plastic films (Saran Wrap®) were placed over the wounds and held in place with a pressure sensitive adhesive tape (Dermicel® Tape). Further studies were made with a partially occlusive dressing construction consisting of a polyethylene coated, nonwoven fabric backed by a porous vinyl film (Dermicel® Adhesive Bandage).

Incisions

A series of experimental wounds was made on the dorsal aspect of the forearms of six adult male volunteers. The skin was shaved and swabbed with 70% ethanol. Small incisions, perpendicular to the longitudinal axis of the forearm were made with a sterile scalpel, blade #11. The linear wounds were 15 mm. long and approximately 0.3 mm. deep. Hemostasis, when necessary, was established by firm pressure with a gauze sponge.

Equal numbers of wounds on each subject were air exposed or occluded with a sterile plastic film (Saran Wrap®) held in place by adhesive tape (Dermicel® Tape), according to a randomized procedure. Daily observations and photographs were made. Paired biopsies (i.e., air exposed and occluded wounds) were taken at 12, 18 and 24 hours and 2, 3, 4, 5 and 7 days according to a schedule which provided data from all subjects on the first three days.

In another group of 15 subjects, incisions were made, covered with a partially occlusive dressing, or air exposed. This study was to determine if currently used dressings have an effect on the repair of the wound. Biopsies were obtained at 1, 2 and 3 days post wounding.

Paraffin or frozen sections were made of the biopsy samples after fixation in Bouin's solution or immediately after the tissues were obtained. The fresh sections, cut at $4–8\mu$, were fixed in Wolman's solution and routinely stained with hematoxylin and eosin for histological study. Histological parameters of interest were the degree of inflammatory response, the completion of epithelialization, scab formation, dermal and epidermal dehydration and differentiation of a new epidermis.

In a separate series of air exposed or occluded forearm incisions on six additional subjects, the mitotic response of the epidermis at the wound edges was studied by a modification of the method of Fisher and Maibach [17]. Metaphase figures were accumulated over a six-hour period by topical application of a colcemid cream. An application of approximately 25 mg. 0.5% colcemid in a nonionic base was made to the incision. This treated site was then covered with an occlusive patch containing an additional 40 mg. of the colcemid cream. The applications were made so all biopsies could be taken between 1:00 P.M. and 3:00 P.M. Metaphase figures were counted in at least 10 cross sections, each being 50–75μ apart. Counts were restricted to 3 high dry ($\times$430) fields on both sides of the incision, and including the cut edge. Biopsies were taken at 12 hours, 1, 2, 3, 5 and 7 days. The counts were expressed as metaphase figures per high dry field, referred to as the *mitotic index* in this report.

Procedure for Studying Mitotic Response in Tape Stripped Wounds

Eighteen 2.0 $\times$ 0.5 inch strip wounds were made on the backs of each of six male subjects. The wounds were spaced at least 5 cm. apart, and oriented with a 2 inch dimension parallel to and either side of the vertebral column. In a random fashion, nine wounds were left air exposed and nine others were dressed with an occlusive film (Saran Wrap®).

According to a random schedule, pairs of treated and untreated wounds were biopsied at 12 hours, 1, 2, 3, 5, 7, 10, 12 and 14 days post stripping. Prior to biopsy, colcemid was applied as described earlier in this chapter. Each wound was biopsied only once to avoid effects of the biopsy procedure on mitotic response.

The wound tissues were fixed in Bouin's solution, and routine paraffin cross sections were cut at 6μ and stained with hematoxylin and eosin. Sections were taken serially over a distance of approximately 1 mm. Counts were made across six high dry fields in the center of ten sections, each being 50–75μ apart. Therefore, a total of 60 fields was counted for each treatment and time period studied.

The data for each subject were analyzed separately, comparing the air exposed and occluded wound mitotic indices. The onset, magnitude and duration of the response were noted.

To compare the occluded and air exposed wounds, the areas under both of the plotted curves for each subject were determined in arbitrary units, the variances calculated, and a z-test of significance was run if the variances were equal.

Since there is some subjectivity in recognizing metaphase figures, some slides were counted by two of the authors (DTR, CAK) and interobserver reliability determined by a correlation coefficient.

Hygrometric Study of Strip Wounds

Four 2 $\times$ 2 inch adhesive tape stripped wounds were made on the upper backs of each of four human subjects. The initial transepidermal water loss (TWL) for each stripped area and for an adjacent intact site was determined using the air flow hygrometry system described by Baker and Kligman [28]. Following the initial TWL readings, two of the wounds were covered with Saran film dressings and two were left as untreated controls. TWL readings were taken on all four wounds on days 1, 2, 3, 4, 7, 10 and 15 following stripping. The TWL values were expressed as percent damage according to the formula:

$$\text{percent damage} = \frac{x}{y}\,(100)$$

$$\text{where } x = \text{TWL for day 1, 2, 3, 4, 7, 10 or 15}$$
$$y = \text{TWL for day 0}$$

RESULTS

Epithelial Migration and Differentiation in Partial Thickness Incisions

By 12 hours post incision, air exposed incisions show an intense inflammatory infiltrate composed mainly of polymorphonuclear leukocytes. Epidermal cells at the cut edges are dehydrated and lie at the periphery of the scab. There is no apparent migration of epithelium at this time (Fig. 8-1A).

Fig. 8–1.—A, air exposed incision at 12 hours showing heavy scab formation, dehydration of epidermis at wound edges, intense inflammatory infiltrate and gaping of wound edges. B, occluded incision at 12 hours with few inflammatory cells seen within fibrin network, no discrete "poly band," suppression of scab formation, no tissue loss through dehydration, and no apparent migration. Protrusion of epithelial cells at right cut edge is a sweat duct. C, air exposed incision at 18 hours showing gaping, lack of migration, incorporation of dehydrated epidermis at superficial periphery of scab and delineation of dehydrated mass from viable surface by a "poly band." D, occluded incision at 18 hours (frozen section) showing progression of epithelial migration from stratum basale and stratum spinosum. The tip of the left migrating wedge of cells is only one cell thick.

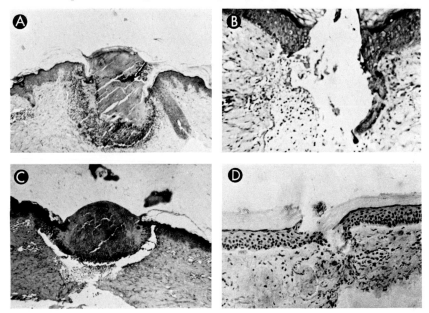

The 12-hour occluded incisions contain only few inflammatory cells. There is no gross dehydration, although cells at the cut edges of epidermis appear somewhat pyknotic. There is no scab formation, and epithelial migration has not yet begun (Fig. 8-1B).

At 18 hours, the air exposed incisions have a well formed scab made up of dried serum, necrotic epidermis from the edges of the wound, lysed red cells and neutrophils, and fibrin. Epithelial migration is not apparent. A fibrin net appears at the wound base infiltrated by a few polymorphonuclear leukocytes (Fig. 8-1C).

The epithelium of 18-hour occluded incisions is actively migrating to close the wound. At the distal tips of the migrating "tongues," the epithelium is only 1–2 cells thick and 3–4 cells thick at the more proximal regions. There is an apparent increase in volume of the epithelial cells at the wound margins. A very slight inflammatory infiltrate is present in and around the fibrin clot at the wound base. Some portions of the incisions have an epithelial continuum reestablished at this time period. The continuum varies from 1–8 cells in thickness. There is no scab formation, but the most superficial epidermal cells are pyknotic (Fig. 8-1D).

Twenty-four hours after incision, the epithelial edges of the air exposed wounds gape apart a distance of 200–700μ. In some of these wounds, it appears that cells from the basal and spinous layers of the epidermis are beginning to migrate beneath the developing scab. The stratum granulosum and the stratum corneum do not participate in the migration. At this time period, many polymorphonuclear leukocytes are incorporated into the eschar along with dried serum and some superficial dermis, characterized by collagenous fibers and fibroblasts. The superficial part of the wounded epidermal edges desiccates in air exposure, the nuclei become pyknotic and these slips of dead epidermis overlie the peripheral, top margins of the scab, thus, regularly forming an "epidermal capping" (*cf.*, Ordman and Gillman [8]). A fibrin network is present in the base of the incision and within it are polymorphs. Mitotic figures can be seen in sections of 24-hour untreated incisions without the aid of colchicine or other inhibitors. The mitoses, normally restricted to the basal layer of epidermis, occur both basally and suprabasally in the wounded samples (*cf.*, Epstein and Sullivan, [15]). Dividing cells have not been observed at the actively migrating tips of epithelium, as most mitoses occur 15–20 or more cell widths proximal to the tips (Fig. 8-2A).

Epithelialization of incisions covered with Saran film is complete at 24 hours. No scab formation or desiccation of superficial tissues is seen. A much smaller cellular infiltrate is present than in the air exposed wounds. The most superficial epithelial cells bridging the wound are pyknotic, and no keratohyalin granules are present. However, some of the wounds do exhibit a parakeratotic surface even at one day. The wound epithelium is equal to or exceeds the thickness of the surrounding uninvolved epidermis (100–200μ thick). A few mitotic figures can be found, but the mitotic response does not appear as marked as in the air exposed incisions. A fibrin network containing polymorphs is seen in the base of the wound (Fig. 8-2B and C).

By two days, the air exposed incisions show considerable dermal loss via dehydration and incorporation into the base of the large scab. Although a few wounds may be epithelialized, most of the incisions still have a defect of 100–150μ to be bridged by epithelium. Some, due to excessive desiccation, show no

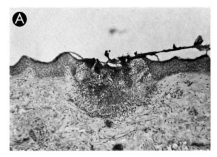
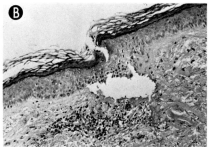
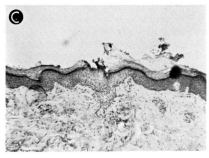

Fig. 8–2.—A, air exposed incision at 24 hours showing gaping edges, beginnings of migration, dehydrated epidermis capping the scab and intense inflammatory infiltrate. Migrating tip of epithelium at right will be lost with further dehydration. B and C, two occluded incisions at 24 hours showing thick epithelial continuum at wound site.

apparent progression of epithelialization, and gape widely (400–700μ). Typically, necrotic epidermis is seen capping the scab. Many polymorphs are incorporated into the eschar. In a few cases, it appears that all the wounded dermis is lost through dehydration, and that the epithelial tongues are migrating over uninvolved dermis. Close examination, however, reveals a small amount of fibrin interposed between dermis and epithelium. When epithelialization has proceeded, a granular layer and subsequent parakeratosis are seen at the most proximal margins of the new epithelial bridge.

Two-day wounds occluded with Saran film are completely epithelialized, and a parakeratotic stratum corneum is present. Keratohyalin granules are present in an apparently normal stratum granulosum. The wound epidermis is slightly hyperplastic. There is no scab formation, no evidence of tissue dehydration, and little inflammatory infiltrate. A fibrin net is seen in the wound base.

Air exposed incisions are reepithelialized by three days. Characteristically, the new epithelial surface is approximately 80μ below the surface of the normal epidermis, due to the sloughing of a large, dry, dermal mass in the scab. Necrotic epidermis can be seen still capping the scab. A few mitotic figures appear at the wound site, and a parakeratotic barrier is present. Most wounds do not have a stratum granulosum at this time period, and fibrin remains in the wound base (Fig. 8-3A and B).

Three-day wounds occluded with Saran film exhibit no signs of dehydration, no scab, no dermal loss and little inflammatory infiltrate. The wounds are epithelialized and invariably have a stratum granulosum and parakeratotic barrier. The surface of the wound epithelium is at the same plane as the surrounding,

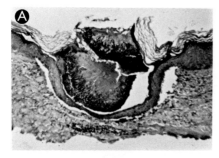

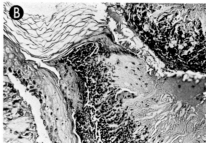

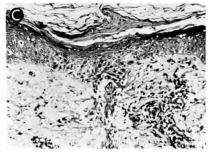

Fig. 8–3.—A, air exposed incision at 3 days showing heavy scab formation capped by dehydrated epidermis. Epithelialization is complete, but the new epidermal surface is approximately 80μ below the surface of the uninvolved epidermis. **B,** higher magnification of 3 day air exposed incision showing an "epidermal cap" over the scab, migration of epithelium deep to the eschar and absence of stratum granulosum. **C,** occluded incision at 3 days. Migration of epithelium was at same plane as uninvolved epidermis. Parakeratotic as well as some normal horn is present. Stratum granulosum has reformed.

uninvolved epidermis (Fig. 8-3C). Occasionally, polymorphs appear around the sweat ducts, presumably due to blockage of the ductal opening know to occur under occlusive therapy.

Air exposed incisions have a well differentiating, parakeratotic epidermis with a stratum granulosum at four days. Otherwise, there is no apparent difference from the three-day wounds.

The four-day incisions occluded with Saran film appear normal with respect to the epidermis, but can be localized by the repairing dermis with the remaining fibrin network.

Both the fifth day air exposed and occluded incisions are differentiating a new barrier. Stratum granulosum is evident in all wounds. The air exposed wounds still have a heavy scab overlying the depressed wound surface.

Healing is complete at seven days with respect to the differentiation of a new epidermis, but the scab is still intact in the air exposed wounds. The epithelium of air exposed incisions remains at a lower plane than the uninvolved epidermis, and grossly, a linear groove ("epidermal scar") may persist for more than six months.

Effects of Clinically Used Dressing on Partial Thickness Incisions

The histological study of air exposed and partially occluded 1-day incisions in 10 subjects revealed that none of the air exposed controls and 60% of the treated wounds were reepithelialized. Inflammatory infiltrate was less pronounced in the treated group than in the air exposed wounds. Although some tissue was lost through dehydration under the partially occlusive cover, scab formation and tissue desiccation were minimal compared to the air exposed group.

For the study of both 2- and 3-day wounds, 6 subjects, some of whom had been observed at 1-day, were available for biopsy. At two days, 66% of the treated incisions had reepithelialized, and a stratum granulosum, indicative of normal differentiation, was apparent in some of the wounds. None of the air exposed wounds were epithelialized.

By three days, 83% of both the treated and air exposed wounds had completed epithelialization. A stratum granulosum was present in 16% of the air exposed and 83% of the covered wounds.

Mitotic Response in Incisions as a Function of Time and Treatment

The MI of the intact, normal, forearm epidermis ranged from 0.498 to 2.233 with a mean of 1.147 in the six subjects studied (Table 8-1).

Both the air exposed and the occluded incisions showed bursts of mitotic response by 2–3 days—the MI, however, remained above the average normal base line (1.147) at seven days in 6 of the 12 incisions studied at that period (Table 8-2).

The magnitude of the mitotic responses was greater in the air exposed than the occluded incisions (Fig. 8-4). The total response (or duration of elevated response) was also higher in the air exposed incisions except in subject JWB (Fig. 8-4) (z-test, $p < 0.05$ for subjects JB, JS, RJK, RK, LC; $p > 0.05$ for subject JWB).

Fig. 8–4.—Composite graph showing mitotic response as a function of wound age and treatment in incisions in six subjects.

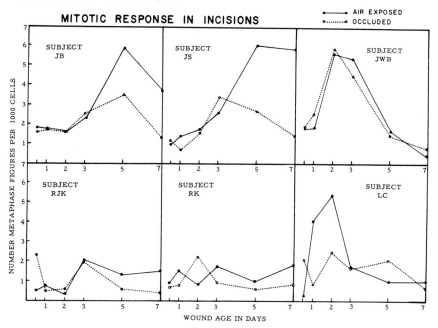

Table 8-1
Mitotic Indices of Epidermis

Subject	Back	Forearm
JWB	.500	.498
EA	.400	—
JS	.383	.867
JB	.500	.533
RK	.450	.517
RJK	.398	2.233
LC	—	2.233

Table 8-2
Incision: Mitotic Index Printout

Subject	Day	Air $\pm$ S.D.	Saran $\pm$ S.D.
JWB	0.5	1.783 $\pm$ 1.303	1.850 $\pm$ 0.777
	1	1.883 $\pm$ 0.993	2.567 $\pm$ 0.963
	2	5.583 $\pm$ 1.862	5.867 $\pm$ 1.096
	3	5.350 $\pm$ 2.040	4.500 $\pm$ 1.112
	5	1.733 $\pm$ 0.756	1.500 $\pm$ 0.725
	7	0.483 $\pm$ 0.567	0.867 $\pm$ 0.747
JB	0.5	1.883 $\pm$ 1.075	1.550 $\pm$ 0.964
	1	1.783 $\pm$ 0.783	1.750 $\pm$ 1.083
	2	1.600 $\pm$ 0.807	1.617 $\pm$ 0.825
	3	2.317 $\pm$ 1.049	2.500 $\pm$ 1.033
	5	5.933 $\pm$ 1.831	3.500 $\pm$ 0.792
	7	3.733 $\pm$ 0.800	1.300 $\pm$ 0.766
JS	0.5	1.000 $\pm$ 0.864	1.233 $\pm$ 0.810
	1	1.417 $\pm$ 0.926	0.700 $\pm$ 0.696
	2	1.800 $\pm$ 1.038	1.567 $\pm$ 1.015
	3	2.700 $\pm$ 0.944	3.433 $\pm$ 1.798
	5	6.067 $\pm$ 1.471	2.683 $\pm$ 0.965
	7	5.850 $\pm$ 2.146	1.483 $\pm$ 0.725
LC	0.5	0.283 $\pm$ 0.555	2.100 $\pm$ 1.674
	1	4.100 $\pm$ 2.290	0.867 $\pm$ 0.853
	2	5.433 $\pm$ 2.860	2.450 $\pm$ 2.190
	3	1.600 $\pm$ 0.906	1.517 $\pm$ 1.097
	5	1.000 $\pm$ 0.759	2.133 $\pm$ 1.268
	7	1.000 $\pm$ 0.759	0.650 $\pm$ 0.685
RJK	0.5	0.517 $\pm$ 0.725	2.350 $\pm$ 1.325
	1	0.683 $\pm$ 0.748	0.450 $\pm$ 0.565
	2	0.367 $\pm$ 0.581	0.567 $\pm$ 0.789
	3	2.000 $\pm$ 1.551	1.950 $\pm$ 1.466
	5	1.300 $\pm$ 1.293	0.550 $\pm$ 0.622
	7	1.467 $\pm$ 0.965	0.417 $\pm$ 0.530
RK	0.5	0.917 $\pm$ 0.787	0.683 $\pm$ 0.833
	1	1.500 $\pm$ 1.214	0.783 $\pm$ 0.865
	2	0.783 $\pm$ 0.846	2.217 $\pm$ 1.606
	3	1.700 $\pm$ 1.183	0.933 $\pm$ 0.899
	5	0.950 $\pm$ 0.769	0.317 $\pm$ 0.469
	7	1.783 $\pm$ 1.530	0.750 $\pm$ 0.968

Table 8-3
Incisions: Areas Under the Mitotic Response Curves

Subject	Treatment	Area (Arbitrary Units)	Variance	Z
RK	A*	4.607	0.031	5.926†
	O*	3.182	0.027	
JWB	A*	7.778	0.014	0.728
	O*	6.893	0.018	
JS	A*	9.357	0.012	14.195†
	O*	6.893	0.018	
JB	A*	9.442	0.013	12.784†
	O*	7.376	0.013	
RJK	A*	4.286	0.037	3.892†
	O*	3.303	0.027	
LC	A*	6.114	0.026	2.776†
	O*	5.435	0.033	

*A = Air Exposed, O = Occluded.
†Significantly different at P < 0.05 by Z-test.

Table 8-4
Average Mitotic Indices of Forearm Incisions

Day	Air ± S.E.	Saran ± S.E.
0.5	1.056 ± 0.261	1.628 ± 0.248
1	1.894 ± 0.474	1.186 ± 0.330
2	2.411 ± 0.842	2.381 ± 0.746
3	2.611 ± 0.572	2.472 ± 0.535
5	2.830 ± 1.009	1.780 ± 0.504
7	2.386 ± 0.828	0.911 ± 0.165

Characteristically, the magnitude and duration of the mitotic response are greater in the air exposed than in the occluded incisions. There occasionally was an elevated MI at 12 hours post incision in the occluded wounds which may represent a difference in onset of the response. The areas under the curves were significantly higher for air exposed wounds than the occluded wounds in all subjects except JWB (z-test, p < 0.05, Table 8-3).

The average responses in incisions appear in Table 8-4 and Figure 8-5.

Mitotic Response in Strip Wounds as a Function of Wound Age and Treatment

The mitotic indices for normal, intact, back epidermis ranged from 0.383 to 0.500 with a mean of 0.439 (Table 8-1).

All peaks of mitotic activity in occluded strip wounds occurred at a wound age of 2 days (Fig. 8-6 and Table 8-5). In the air exposed strip wounds, initial peak activity occurred at 2–3 days with two subjects showing secondary peaks at 5 or 7 days. In the air exposed wounds, the MI peaked at 3 days in three sub-

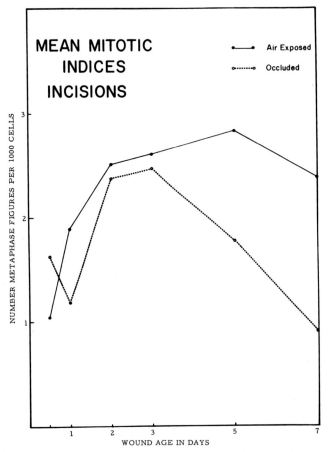

Fig. 8–5.—Average mitotic response to incision in six subjects as a function of wound age and treatment.

jects, at 2 days in two subjects and was equal at 2 and 3 days in one subject (Fig. 8-6 and Table 8-5).

In all subjects except JB, the magnitude of peak MI was greater in the air exposed than in the occluded wounds. The total mitotic activity estimated by areas under the response curves was significantly higher in the air exposed wounds (Table 8-6 and Fig. 8-6).

Strip wounds which were occluded approached base-line values (<1.0) of MI at wound ages of 5 to 10 days (Table 8-5). Air exposed wounds returned to base-line values between 7 and 14 days. Three wounds in the exposed group remained above base line (>1.0) at 12 days.

The average mitotic responses for the two treatment groups are seen in Table 8-7 and Figure 8-7. From these averages, it can also be seen that the occluded wounds peak at 2 days, one day before the exposed wounds. The duration of the response is shorter in the occluded group, and the MI values are lower throughout the period of kinetic response.

Table 8-5
Strip Wound: Mitotic Index

Subject	Day	Air ± S.D.	Saran ± S.D.
EA	0.5	0.700 ± 0.646	0.750 ± 0.654
	1	0.733 ± 0.634	3.783 ± 1.728
	2	19.067 ± 2.928	7.683 ± 1.672
	3	8.700 ± 1.587	3.500 ± 0.930
	5	13.833 ± 4.633	2.550 ± 0.872
	7	7.950 ± 3.311	1.367 ± 0.712
	10	1.900 ± 0.656	0.900 ± 0.602
	12	1.517 ± 0.701	0.817 ± 0.624
	14	0.850 ± 0.547	0.517 ± 0.504
RJK	0.5	2.283 ± 1.106	1.433 ± 0.909
	1	4.283 ± 0.761	3.983 ± 1.017
	2	6.917 ± 2.102	7.833 ± 1.815
	3	8.417 ± 1.629	5.333 ± 1.174
	5	7.817 ± 1.600	6.000 ± 1.402
	7	13.350 ± 2.910	5.533 ± 1.443
	10	3.100 ± 1.053	0.583 ± 0.671
	12	1.350 ± 0.860	0.733 ± 0.778
	14	0.550 ± 0.723	0.450 ± 0.561
RK	0.5	0.450 ± 0.565	0.467 ± 0.623
	1	0.867 ± 0.676	0.767 ± 0.745
	2	7.133 ± 2.920	10.600 ± 3.562
	3	17.517 ± 3.685	3.383 ± 1.195
	5	3.750 ± 1.480	1.167 ± 0.717
	7	1.433 ± 0.998	0.650 ± 0.633
	10	1.933 ± 1.087	0.433 ± 0.621
	12	1.417 ± 0.926	0.567 ± 0.593
	14	0.400 ± 0.494	0.433 ± 0.563
JB	0.5	0.367 ± 0.520	0.483 ± 0.596
	1	0.650 ± 0.659	0.350 ± 0.481
	2	12.717 ± 3.979	14.450 ± 5.153
	3	11.183 ± 3.789	3.267 ± 2.162
	5	6.817 ± 4.192	2.133 ± 1.589
	7	2.067 ± 1.039	1.133 ± 0.892
	10	1.000 ± 1.042	0.700 ± 0.743
	12	0.633 ± 0.637	0.417 ± 0.591
	14	0.417 ± 0.591	0.317 ± 0.537
JS	0.5	0.683 ± 0.748	1.433 ± 0.945
	1	1.317 ± 1.049	0.583 ± 0.619
	2	11.900 ± 3.935	11.417 ± 3.016
	3	11.917 ± 4.492	2.600 ± 1.786
	5	6.167 ± 3.421	1.200 ± 0.935
	7	2.883 ± 2.116	1.033 ± 1.025
	10	0.733 ± 0.733	0.550 ± 0.565
	12	0.467 ± 0.566	0.333 ± 0.510
	14	0.450 ± 0.622	0.383 ± 0.524
JWB	0.5	1.217 ± 1.415	2.083 ± 1.225
	1	0.717 ± 0.739	0.400 ± 0.558
	2	12.250 ± 4.700	13.850 ± 4.062
	3	18.050 ± 5.060	3.200 ± 1.482
	5	5.867 ± 6.492	0.983 ± 0.725
	7	3.150 ± 2.680	0.883 ± 1.075
	10	0.600 ± 0.887	0.350 ± 0.547
	12	0.883 ± 0.715	0.383 ± 0.555
	14	0.500 ± 0.651	0.417 ± 0.591

Table 8-6
Strip Wounds: Areas Under the Mitotic Response Curves

Subject	Treatment	Area (Arbitrary Units)	Variance	Z*
RK	A†	16.474	0.067	
	O†	9.243	0.059	20.440
JWB	A†	15.909	0.131	
	O†	9.010	0.069	15.397
JS	A†	15.655	0.097	
	O†	9.193	0.078	15.422
JB	A†	15.673	0.075	
	O†	10.514	0.080	13.106
RJK	A†	23.167	0.032	
	O†	16.933	0.042	22.943
EA	A†	22.400	0.036	
	O†	13.013	0.042	33.467

*All are significant at $P < 0.05$.
†A = Air Exposed, O = Occluded.

Fig. 8–6.—Composite graph showing six subjects' mitotic response to tape stripping of the epidermis as a function of wound age and treatment.

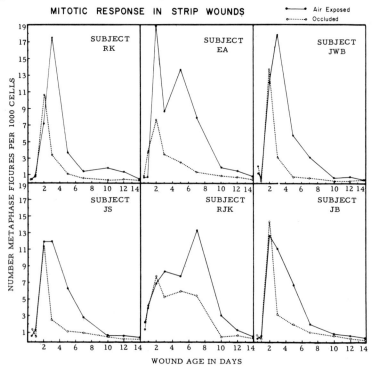

Table 8-7
Average Mitotic Indices of Strip Wounds

Day	Air ± S.E.	Saran ± S.E.
0.5	0.950 ± 0.293	1.108 ± 0.264
1	1.428 ± 0.579	1.644 ± 0.711
2	11.680 ± 1.834	10.972 ± 1.175
3	12.630 ± 1.723	3.553 ± 0.378
5	7.384 ± 1.411	2.339 ± 0.778
7	5.139 ± 1.893	1.767 ± 0.760
10	1.544 ± 0.389	0.586 ± 0.080
12	1.028 ± 0.180	0.542 ± 0.081
14	0.528 ± 0.683	0.420 ± 0.027

Fig. 8–7.—Average mitotic response to stripping as a function of wound age and treatment.

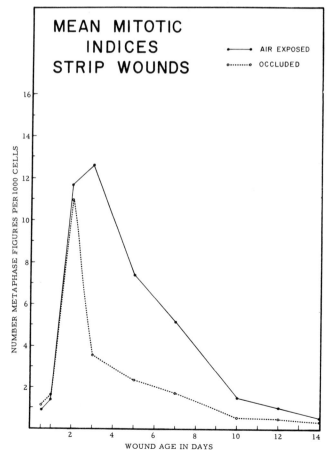

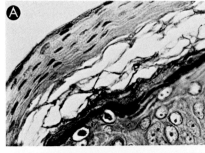

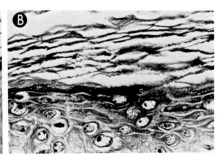

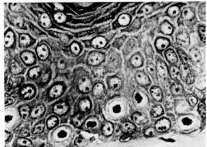

Fig. 8—8 (above).—A, seven-day, air
exposed strip wound showing parakeratotic crust covering surface. Note the
regeneration of normal horn beneath
crust. B, seven-day, occluded strip wound
with apparently normal stratum corneum
and no loss of cells in a crust.

Fig. 8—9 (left).—Typical colcemid
metaphase figures seen in all phases of
this study.

The interobserver reliability of the mitotic counts for the study is reflected by
a correlation coefficient (r) of 0.966 obtained by a comparison of microscopic
counts of two of the authors.

Throughout the first 7 days of forced regeneration, the air exposed strip
wounds could be distinguished histologically by the presence of a thick, parakeratotic crust, whereas the occluded wounds showed only a developing stratum
corneum (Fig. 8-8). Typical colcemid figures are seen in Figure 8-9.

Table 8-8
Transepidermal Water Loss and Percent Damage in Strip Wounds
as a Function of Wound Age and Treatment

Subject	Treatment	Average % Damage at Day							Avg. TWL at 0 Time (mg./cm.^{2}/hr.)	Normal Skin TWL (mg./cm.^{2}/hr.)
		1	2	3	4	7	10	15		
WV	A*	59	14	8	4	2	1	1	25.94	0.20
	O*	28	4	3	2	1	0	1		
AD	A*	30	10	7	3	2	2	1	31.59	0.15
	O*	33	6	6	2	2	2	1		
HL	A*	38	8	8	2	2	1	1	33.60	0.19
	O*	19	4	4	1	1	1	1		
BS	A*	51	10	6	3	1	1	0	40.10	0.17
	O*	48	7	4	1	1	1	0		
Average	A*	44	10	7	3	2	1	1	32.81	0.18
Values	O*	32	5	4	1	1	1	1		

*A = Air Exposed, O = Occluded.

Water Loss Through Stripped Skin as a Function of Wound Age and Treatment

Water loss (TWL) through intact skin averaged 0.18 mg./cm.²/hr. for the four subjects. At 0 time after stripping, the average TWL was 32.81 mg./cm.²/hr. Over the first 4 days of forced regeneration, it is seen that the occluded wounds have regained significantly better barrier function than the exposed wounds. By 7 days, the differences in TWL in the two treatment groups were not significant, the average values being approximately 1% (percent damage) at 7, 10 and 15 days.

The data are summarized in Table 8-8.

DISCUSSION

Maintenance of wound tissue hydration overtly alters the course of all phases of epidermal healing. Migration of epidermal cells, the single most important factor in reestablishing a continuum of epidermis, occurs within 18–24 hours post incision, if dehydration is prevented by placing an occlusive film over the wound. With air exposure, 2–3 days are required for completion of epithelialization. The differences in migratory patterns of epithelial cells in the air exposed and covered wounds have also been reported in experimentally produced blisters [10] and excisions in pigs [21, 22, 24] and humans [23]. It has been interpreted that air exposure of denuded dermis with subsequent dehydration and incorporation into the scab presents a mechanical barrier to epithelial migration, since the epithelial cell must move deep to the crust migrating only on a viable wound surface [24]. In the present study, it was seen that not only the superficial wound dermis, but also the epidermis at the wound periphery is incorporated into the scab. It may be that the presence of this dead, dry tissue in the wound has a quantitative influence on the early inflammatory infiltrate as the occluded wounds exhibited significantly fewer inflammatory cells.

Because the epithelial migration occurred deep to the scab in air exposed incisions, a new epidermal surface resulted at a plane below the uninvolved epidermis. This depressed new surface remains as a linear groove or "epidermal scar" for as long as six months in some subjects (summarized in Fig. 8-10). It is interesting to speculate how the development of this type of scar relates to the similarly appearing scar (pock marks) in acne or chicken pox. When hydration was maintained with occlusion, migration of epithelial cells occurred at the same plane as the uninvolved epidermis, thereby leaving no "epidermal scar."

Recent ultrastructural studies have shown that the migrating epidermal cells in air exposed blister beds contain more inclusions resembling extracellular fibrin than do the epidermal cells in intact blisters; it was suggested, as a possibility, that this phagocytic activity of epidermal cells consumed energy needed for migration, and resulted in a slower repair in the de-roofed than in the intact blisters [10]. It follows that the same differences in phagocytosis exist in the air exposed and occluded incisions studied in the present report. Other interpretations can be made, for example, the dry mass may simply present a mechanical barrier to migration [10].

Study of the kinetic response to incision showed that a burst in mitosis oc-

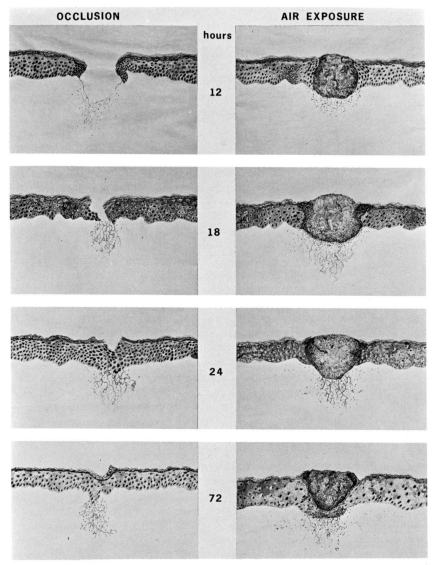

Fig. 8–10.—Diagrammatic summary of epithelialization in air exposed or occluded incisions. Note that completion of epithelialization occurs at 18–24 hours under occlusion and at 2–3 days in air exposure. There is no scab formation in occluded incisions and no apparent tissue loss through dehydration. Note the plane of new epidermis in air exposed incisions at 72 hours. See text for complete description.

curred at 2 to 3 days irrespective of air exposure or occlusion. It was interesting that the increase in mitotic activity had not returned to normal base-line values at the end of the 7 day period of study. It is not known what need there may be for new cells at that point in repair.

Since few epidermal cells are lost through dehydration in the occluded incisions, there is not a great demand for new cells, and in fact, the mitotic response was lower in this treatment group. Many epidermal cells are incorporated in the scab in air exposed incisions and this loss might be important in triggering the greater mitotic activity seen in this group of incisions.

The intact epidermis of the forearm was noted to vary considerably in baseline mitotic activity (Table 8-1); this range has been reported by other investigators [17]. The mitotic activity in normal back epidermis was found to be much more consistent with a very small range (Table 8-1). This may be explained by the fact that back skin is probably traumatized much less in everyday activities than forearm skin which is scraped, scratched, bumped and irradiated by sunlight. Because of the uniformity in normal back epidermis, this site is more suitable for our study of cell kinetics in healing strip wounds.

The relationship, coincidental or dependent, of migration and mitosis has been discussed by other investigators, most concluding that migration occurs independently of cell division [29]. When studying air exposed incisions, epithelialization is completed at the same time there is a burst in mitotic activity at the wound site. Does this burst in mitosis necessarily follow reestablishment of an epithelial continuum, or is the timing coincidental? The pattern of mitotic response was qualitatively the same in occluded incisions where epithelialization was completed at 18–24 hours, so it would seem that these data argue against a causal relationship between the two events.

The epithelial continuum seen in occluded incisions at 24 hours is 4–8 cells thick. Because this stratification occurs prior to a burst in mitosis, it is suggested that the epithelial cells move over one another, thus forming a multilayered epithelium. Ultrastructural studies also suggest an early layering of epithelial cells by migration, not mitosis [10].

Mitotic response to wounding was studied with somewhat more clarity in stripped skin than in incisions, since large areas of responding wound tissue could be harvested. Cell division was not restricted to an edge, and the insult itself was uniform. This type of forced regeneration has been reported in the past [15, 19], but the investigators have not carried the results to a return to base-line levels. As previously published, air exposed strip wounds show a peak in mitotic activity at 2–3 days post stripping [15]. All the occluded wounds peaked at 2 days. The total response (area under curves) and duration of response were greater in the air exposed than in the occluded strip wounds. The magnitude of the peaks was also greater in the air exposed wounds. Two subjects showed secondary bursts of mitosis in air exposed wounds at 5 and 7 days, possibly due to excessive drying and cracking of the tissue, since these were studied during the winter when ambient humidities were extremely low (Relative Humidity = 5–15%). The occluded wounds returned to base-line levels of mitosis between 5 and 10 days, varying with the subject. Air exposed wounds reached base line between 7 and 14 days with three subjects showing elevated mitotic activity at 12 days (>1.3, base line = 0.4).

Our data do not reflect a highly cyclical response as reported by some investigators [15], possibly because of the duration of the colcemid application (six hours) or because all biopsies were obtained at the same time of day.

The lower mitotic activity seen in occluded strip wounds might be explained on the basis of less tissue loss (through dehydration) than in air exposed wounds. If an inhibitor of mitosis (chalone) [30] is contained in the epidermal cells, the parakeratotic slough seen in air exposed wounds (Fig. 8-8A) would be important in the kinetic response reported. A mitotic response in stripped skin might better be thought of as a two-fold response based on our findings. There is a response to stripping away the stratum corneum possibly mediated by the mechanical trauma or loss of an inhibitor as well as a secondary mitotic response to the cell loss through dehydration. This secondary cumulative response was eliminated by maintaining hydration with occlusion. A similar interpretation of reduced DNA synthesis in normal human skin covered with occlusive dressings was made by Born, who explained his findings on the basis of an enrichment of a physiological regeneration inhibiting substance in the epidermis due to decreasing peripheral loss by surface drying and desquamation [27, 31].

The return of barrier function as measured hygrometrically was altered by the occlusive dressings. The young wounds had a slightly, but significantly better barrier than the air exposed wounds, indicating earlier onset of stratum corneum differentiation. Thus, it has been shown that all phases of epidermal wound healing can be altered by changes in the local wound environment.

Further study of the kinetic findings reported are underway since several questions arise concerning the effect, and also methodological error. For example, do differences in barrier reformation in the two treatment groups alter the penetration of colcemid or the duration of mitotic arrest? Other investigators have seen the same type of result as we report in different systems (intact normal or psoriatic skin) using intradermal tritiated thymidine [27]. The technique of using topical colcemid yields reproducible results in normal skin where the stratum corneum is intact, and the mitotic indices obtained agree with reported indices obtained by other methods. The value for air exposed strip wounds also resemble values reported by other investigators [15]. There was no clear cut correlation between barrier properties and mitotic response measured in the present study. Therefore, it is suggested that the differences in mitotic response seen in air exposed and occluded wounds are real, rather than artifact. Nonetheless, animal studies using tritiated thymidine and systemic colchicine are underway to further elucidate the effects of dehydration on the mitotic response to wounding.

It has been shown that all phases of epidermal repair are altered under occlusive films. Migration of epidermal cells and differentiation occur earlier when hydration is maintained and the mitotic response is reduced. The earlier migration seen in incisions covered by more conventional dressings can also be explained on the basis of hydration. Although the present studies dealt with extremes of wound environment, it would be of interest to study effects of more subtle changes in environment, variables which may account for diverse literature reports of wound healing.

Although occlusion enhances epidermal wound healing, it is not suggested as a clinical practice since increased bacterial populations also occur under occlusive dressings. Still, occlusion has, with careful scrutiny, been usefully employed clinically in the treatment of donor sites [32], mesh grafts [33] and dermabraded skin [34]. The lack of major infections seen under occlusion in the presence of increased bacteria may be due to the absence of large amounts of necrotic tissue since viability is maintained with hydration. It is through maintaining hydration, more or less, that dressings exert their more or less beneficial action on epidermal wound healing [11].

SUMMARY

In humans, the three phases of epidermal wound healing (migration, mitosis and differentiation) are altered by changes in the local wound environment brought about by placing occlusive films over the wound site.

In partial thickness incisions, 2 to 3 days are required for reestablishing an epithelial continuum by migration in air exposed wounds, but maintaining tissue hydration by occlusion shortens this time requirement to 18 to 24 hours. The qualitative pattern of mitotic response is not altered, however, the mitotic indices are lower in occluded than air exposed incisions. Bursts in mitosis occur at 2 to 3 days post incision, but counts have not returned to normal by 7 days. With occlusion, not only is epithelialization complete at 24 hours, but there is a stratification of epithelial cells (4–8 cells thick) before the major mitotic responses. This suggests the independence of migration and mitosis in the healing incision.

Mitosis during forced regeneration was studied in tape stripped skin. The magnitude and duration of mitotic response were greater in air exposed than occluded strip wounds. From these data, it appears that the kinetic response to stripping is mediated in a two-fold fashion: Mitosis in response to removing the stratum corneum, and a second, cumulative mitotic response to cells lost through dehydration.

Based on these findings, it is seen that the local wound environment should be considered in interpreting patterns of epidermal healing.

ACKNOWLEDGMENTS

The authors thank Miss C. Finegan and Mrs. E. Church for their technical assistance in the preparation of histological samples, Miss J. Labun for preparing the graphs and diagrams, Miss E. Hahn for typing the manuscript, and Mr. K. Young for illustrations. Thanks are also due to Drs. J. W. Bothwell and C. B. Linsky for suggestions in the preparation of the manuscript.

We extend special thanks to those volunteers who, because of their interest in this research, participated as volunteers in the study.

REFERENCES

1. Van Winkle, W.: The tensile strength of wounds and factors that influence it, Surg. Gynec. & Obst. 129:819, 1969.
2. Viljanto, J., and Niinikoski, J.: Haavan optimaalinen ja supernormaali paraneminen, Duodecim 85:1170, 1969.
3. Van Winkle, W.: The epithelium in wound healing, Surg. Gynec. & Obst. 127:1089, 1968.
4. Ordman, L. J., and Gillman, T.: Studies in the healing of cutaneous wounds III.

A critical comparison in the pig of the healing of surgical incisions closed with sutures or adhesive tape based on tensile strength and clinical and histological criteria, Arch. Surg. 93:911, 1966.

5. Rovee, D. T., and Miller, C. A.: Epidermal role in the breaking strength of wounds, Arch. Surg. 96:43, 1968.

6. Johnson, F. R.: The reaction of epithelium to injury, Scient. Basis Med. Ann. Rev. 276, 1964.

7. Viziam, C. F., Matoltsy, A. G., and Mescon, H.: Epithelialization of small wounds, J. Invest. Dermat. 43:499, 1964.

8. Ordman, L. J., and Gillman, T.: Studies in the healing of cutaneous wounds I. The healing of incisions through the skin of pigs, Arch. Surg. 93:857, 1966.

9. Matoltsy, A. G., and Viziam, C. B.: Further observations on epithelialization of small wounds, J. Invest. Dermat. 55:20, 1970.

10. Krawczyk, W.: A pattern of epidermal cell migration during wound healing, J. Cell Biol. 49:247, 1971.

11. Hartwell, S. W.: Surgical wounds in human beings. A histological study of healing with practical applications: I. Epithelial healing, Arch. Surg. 19:835, 1929.

12. Gillman, T., Penn, J., Bronks, D., and Roux, M.: A re-examination of certain aspects of the histogenesis of the healing of cutaneous wounds, Brit. J. Surg. 43:141, 1955.

13. Gillman, T., and Penn, J.: Studies in the repair of cutaneous wounds, Med. Proc. 2 (suppl.):121, 1956.

14. Odland, G., and Ross, R.: Human wound repair. I. Epidermal regeneration, J. Cell Biol. 39:135, 1968.

15. Epstein, W. L., and Sullivan, D. J.: Epidermal Mitotic Activity in Wounded Human Skin, in Montagna, W., and Billingham, R. E. (eds.): *Advances in Biology of Skin*, Vol. 5 (New York: Pergamon Press, 1964).

16. Epstein, W. L., and Maibach, H. I.: Cell renewal in human epidermis, Arch. Derm. 92:462, 1965.

17. Fisher, L. B., and Maibach, H. I.: The effect of corticosteroids on human epidermal mitotic activity, Arch. Derm. 103:39, 1971.

18. Matoltsy, A. G., Schragger, A., and Matoltsy, M. N.: Observations on regeneration of the skin barrier, J. Invest. Dermat. 38:251, 1962.

19. Pinkus, H.: Tape stripping in dermatological research. A review with emphasis on epidermal biology, J. Ital. Derm. 107:1115, 1966.

20. Scapicchio, A. P., Constable, J. D., and Opitz: Comparative effects of silver nitrate and sulfamylon acetate on epidermal regeneration, J. Plast. & Reconstr. Surg. 41:319, 1968.

21. Winter, G. D.: Formation of the scab and the rate of epithelization of superficial wounds in the skin of the young domestic pig, Nature 193:293, 1962.

22. Winter, G. D., and Scales, J. T.: Effect of air drying and dressings on the surface of a wound, Nature 197:91, 1963.

23. Hinman, C. D., and Maibach, H. I.: Effect of air exposure and occlusion on experimental human skin wounds, Nature 200:377, 1963.

24. Harris, D. R., and Keefe, R. L.: A histologic study of gold leaf treated experimental wounds, J. Invest. Dermat. 52:487, 1969.

25. Bothwell, J. W., and Rovee, D. T.: The effect of dressings on the repair of cutaneous wounds in humans, in Harkiss, K. J. (ed.): *Surgical Dressings and Wound Healing* (London: Bradford University Press, 1971).

26. Maibach, H. I.: Personal communication.

27. Born, W.: Epidermale DNA-Synthese unter Occlusiv-Verbänden im Tritium-Thymidin-Autoradiogramm, Ztschr. Haut.-Geschl. 44:305, 1969.

28. Baker, H., and Kligman, A. M.: Measurement of transepidermal water loss by electrical hygrometry, Arch. Derm. 96:441, 1967.

29. Kischer, C. W.: Epithelization, Excerpta Medica Internat. Congress Ser. 229:197, 1970.

30. Bullough, W. S.: Epithelial Repair, in Dunphy, J. E., and Van Winkle, W. (eds.): *Repair and Regeneration* (New York: McGraw-Hill Book Co., Inc., 1968).

31. Born, W., and Bickhardt, R.: Zur Regelung des Zellnachschubs in der Epidermis, Klin. Wchnschr. 46:1312, 1968.
32. Harris, D. N.: Personal communication.
33. Hagstrom, W. J., Nassos, T. P., Boswick, J. A., and Stuterville, O. H.: The importance of occlusive dressings in the treatment of mesh skin grafts, J. Plast. & Reconstruct. Surg. 38:137, 1966.
34. Orentreich, N.: Personal communication.

Part IV

Interactions and Regeneration

Introduction

Rupert E. Billingham, D.Sc. *

Despite the tremendous investment of effort in the study of wound healing the clinical benefits to date have been disappointingly small. Our knowledge still doesn't extend very far beyond descriptive accounts, at the levels of the light and electron microscopes, of the principal morphologic events involved in the natural repair of different types of tissues. Unfortunately, better understanding of the profound effects of nutritional deficiency states and adverse hormonal influences on wound healing has not led to the development of means to promote supernormal rates of healing, or even hinted that this may be a feasible goal. No topical agents have yet been found that accelerate the healing process very markedly. One would like to believe that long-overdue breakthroughs may occur and that one day wound healing research will accomplish much more than rationalize empirically evolved surgical practices and define and realize the optimal conditions that allow Nature to function at maximal efficiency. Have mammals lost, irretrievably the dramatic regenerative powers of some of their distant ancestors? Are there any alternatives to the current, rapidly developing practice of replacing damaged or diseased tissues and organs by grafting?

Although it is most unlikely that any of the work which forms the subject matter of the contributions in the present section was carried out specifically to study wound healing, it is germane to this subject. It deals with the analysis of various kinds of tissue interactions for both the genesis and maintenance of various epithelia of the body, with the chemical definition and biological properties of an agent that has a truly remarkable influence on the growth of epidermal cells, and finally with an extension of an important experiment of Nature which hints that to procure *de novo* neogenesis of skin is a feasible objective.

*Department of Cell Biology, The University of Texas Southwestern Medical School at Dallas, Dallas, Texas.

9

In Vivo Approaches to the Analysis of the Conservation of Epidermal Specificities

*Alan E. Beer, M.D. and R. E. Billingham, D.Sc.**

Ideally, wound healing has as its end result the complete restoration of the status quo ante with respect to both structure and function of affected tissues and organs. Consequently, any systematic study of wound healing as it relates to those epithelia of the body, notably that of skin, which are continually undergoing self renewal through proliferative and differentiative activity of cells in the basal layer, must include definition of the mechanism(s) responsible for the faithful conservation of their characteristic properties—structural and other—throughout the life span of the individual.

There are many qualitatively different kinds of superficial epidermis, including the generalized form that covers the trunk of most mammals, the thick, tough and mitotically active epidermis of the sole of foot, and foot pads and the exquisitely transparent epidermis of the cornea. In addition, there is a great range of structurally and functionally disparate epidermal appendages including hairs, nails, claws, hard superficial scales and glands of many types [1]. All of these are potential sources of new epithelium to resurface superficial lesions.

It is well documented experimentally that, in embryonic development, the differentia of the skin result from heterotypic or inductive interactions between ectodermal and mesenchymal precursors of epidermis and dermis [2–4]. However, we still know very little about the nature and modus operandi of the postulated mediators of these interactions, apart from the fact that they are capable of diffusing across cell-impermeable Millipore filters in tissue culture systems [5].

So far relatively little attention has been devoted to analysis of the factors responsible for the faithful conservation of the specificities of the qualitatively distinct epidermal differentia throughout life. The connective tissue or dermal substrates upon which the various types of epidermis rest, and which intimately invest its appendages, are properly credited with providing essential mechanical support and facilitating metabolic exchanges between the avascular epidermis

---

*Department of Cell Biology, The University of Texas Southwestern Medical School at Dallas, Dallas, Texas.

and the vascular plexus in the papillary layer. There is uncertainty, however, whether the dermis is also the continuing source of morphogenetic "instructions" committing those epidermal cells which leave the germinal layer to one or other of a wide diversity of pathways of differentiation. In other words, do epidermal specificities reflect subtle, qualitative regional differences in the dermis acting upon an equipotential basal layer? The alternative possibility, by no means mutually exclusive, is that there are inherited differences of developmental origin between the germinal layer cells in qualitatively different components of the epidermal system which enable them to breed true of their own accord.

Another related question, which has intrigued many investigators, is whether the germinal cells of other types of epithelium of nonectodermal origin, e.g., those of the transitional epithelium of the bladder, or the epithelium that lines the ileum, are intrinsically and irreversibly different from those of the epidermis [6, 7].

The purpose of this contribution is to present in outline the results of previous work that bears upon the conservation of epidermal specificities in the adult, and to describe a new approach to the analysis of epithelial specificities and interrelationships.

THE BEHAVIOR OF FITTED SPLIT THICKNESS GRAFTS OF VARIOUS TYPES OF SKIN TRANSPLANTED HETEROTOPICALLY

In a variety of rodent and other species it has been established that relatively thin, split thickness grafts of skin having regionally distinctive properties of its superficial epidermis, transplanted to anatomically unnatural sites prepared in trunk skin or elsewhere on the body, faithfully maintain their original specificity of epidermal type [8–10]. If a thin graft of guinea pig's sole of foot skin, which is closely similar to that of human sole, is transplanted to a site on its chest where it is protected by hair and no longer subjected to wear and tear, its epidermis maintains a high rate of proliferation and continues to produce a thick, tough and functionally redundant cuticle. Likewise, grafts of the highly vascular semi-transparent "skin" that constitutes the wall of the hamster's cheek pouch rigidly conserve their original properties following transplantation to the trunk, as do grafts of tongue "skin". Histological study of long established heterotopic transplants of these various types of skin revealed that the boundary between the graft and host skin types of epithelia is always distinguishable almost to a cellular interface. Such findings indicate that all the information required to determine the characteristic structure of a particular type of epidermis must be contained within even the thinnest split thickness skin graft. However, they do not discriminate between the roles of the epidermis and dermis in the maintenance of epidermal specificities.

An unfortunate restriction is imposed upon this particular experimental approach by the fact that although skin grafts can be separated cleanly into their epidermal and dermal moieties by means of trypsin or other enzymes, fitted grafts of pure epidermis transplanted to host sites devoid of all native dermis fail to prevent rapid contracture of the epithelialized wound, prematurely obliterating the tissue under study. In even the thinnest of split thickness grafts the presence of dermal tissue inhibits this process.

THE BEHAVIOR OF SPLIT THICKNESS GRAFTS
TRANSPLANTED IN OPEN STYLE

In adult rabbits, because of their size, it is easy to prepare extensive wounds or graft beds, up to 7 × 6 cm., by surgical excision of the full thickness of the skin down to the surface of the vascular plane overlying the panniculus carnosus [11]. When such wounds are maintained under dressings, granulation tissue soon develops and not until 25–30 days are they reduced to insignificant dimensions by the process of wound contracture [12, 13]. If small, split-thickness grafts of various types of skin are transplanted to the centers of such freshly prepared wounds, epithelium unaccompanied by connective tissue elements grows out centrifugally from their margins over the extremely hospitable ad hoc mesenchymal substrate, producing hyperplastic epidermis. This enables one to compare both macroscopically and microscopically the annuli of epidermal outgrowth generated by different types of skin on a common, anatomically unnatural substitute for dermis. This approach has yielded highly suggestive evidence that the germinal layers of lingual, corneal, ear and vaginal epidermis differ intrinsically from one another with respect to the properties of the epidermis they can generate. On this type of wound bed newly generated corneal epidermis retains its transparency, that of tongue produces a thick, tough compact cuticle and the overall staining and other properties of its more proximal cells closely resemble those of normal lingual epithelium. The epithelial outgrowth from ear skin has a thick, opaque waxy looking flaking cuticle, and that of vagina is devoid of a cuticle [14]. There are other more subtle differences at the microscopic level.

Unfortunately wound contracture and the migratory ingrowth of native epithelium from the wound margins restricts the informative duration of this type of experiment to 20–25 days. This observation period is insufficient to exclude the possibility that the observed conservation of specificities by the outgrowing epithelia is due to the continued presence of inductive stimuli of dermal origin not yet completely "diluted out" by the migratory and proliferative activity of the cells with which they are associated. Although ingenious means of preventing wound contracture have been developed [15, 16], they have not proved satisfactory for facilitating the analysis of the regional specificities of either pure epidermal grafts or of epidermal outgrowth from split-thickness grafts. Another shortcoming of this approach is that the epidermis available for study is always hyperplastic.

Despite its deficiencies this experimental approach has also yielded evidence bearing upon the interrelationship between mammary gland epithelium and that of trunk skin in adult rabbits [17]. Coarse suspensions of autologous mammary tissue in Hanks' solution, distributed over the surfaces of extensive full thickness beds on adult female hosts gave rise to multiple foci of epithelial outgrowth by the tenth postoperative day. Within 18–20 days the entire wounds were resurfaced by heavily keratinized hyperplastic epidermis, indistinguishable from that which is produced by suspensions of epidermal cells produced from ear or trunk skin [16, 18]. Of course these observations do not reveal whether the resultant superficial epidermis reflected the activity of ductal or secretory alveolar cells, or both.

STUDIES ON FITTED DERMOEPIDERMAL RECOMBINANT GRAFTS

A much more satisfactory and more critical means of analyzing epidermal specificities entailed the production of heterotypic recombinant grafts in guinea pigs and hamsters [19]. This involved the enzymic cleavage of thin shavings of skin into their dermal and epidermal moieties and then replacing one type of epidermis upon a sheet of dermis naturally associated with a different kind of epidermis. The resultant recombinant grafts were then transplanted to full thickness beds of appropriate size prepared in the skin of the side of the chest of genetically compatible adult hosts and maintained under observation for periods up to 100 days. This allowed the epidermis ample time for several cycles of complete self renewal before histological study.

Needless to say, an essential prerequisite for this approach was the demonstration that recombination of the separated dermal and epidermal components from the *same* type of skin (i.e., homotypic recombination) produced grafts that faithfully regenerated the specificity of the epidermal type concerned. In particular, recombined dermis and epidermis from sole of foot, or from ear skin, produced grafts that, after subsidence of the hyperplastic and other changes associated with the healing-in phase, were indistinguishable from grafts of intact skin of similar origin and temporal standing.

In the guinea pig it was found that heterotypic recombinant grafts from ear, trunk and sole skin components, in various combinations, always expressed the epidermal specificity naturally associated with the dermal component. This suggests that the germinal layer cells of these particular forms of epidermis are potentially equivalent or equipotential.

However, when epithelia from tongue or esophagus were recombined with sole or ear dermal substrates they consistently retained their distinctive histological characteristics indefinitely. In hamsters, too, lingual and esophageal epithelia retained their specificities when caused to grow upon ear skin dermis. In addition the distinctive epidermis that lines the cheek pouch in this species was similarly found to retain its specificity when recombined with ear skin dermis.

These various findings indicate that the specificities of trunk epidermis (including those of ear and sole) behave as if they were determined by the continuous influence of regionally distinctive morphogenetic stimuli from the dermis— i.e., their basal layer cells are equipotential within certain limits. In addition, there are other aberrant types of epidermis, including those of tongue, esophagus and hamster's cheek pouch (and probably cornea and vagina too, see page 189) whose specificities seem to be intrinsically determined.

Although, because of technical difficulties, the outcome of recombining ear skin epidermis with tongue or cheek pouch dermis has not yet been tested, it seems unlikely that the range of its equipotentiality would be sufficient to enable it to generate the specificities normally associated with these types of connective tissue.

It is pertinent at this juncture to mention some interesting findings of Briggaman and Wheeler [20]. They showed that whereas grafts of pure epidermis, from human skin, degenerated rapidly on transplantation to the chorioallantoic membranes (CAM) of chick embryos, such grafts consistently survived, displaying normal mitotic and differentiative activity when recombined with dermis prior to grafting irrespective of whether the latter was of autologous, homologous or heterologous origin, inverted or otherwise, or whether it had been devitalized by freezing and thawing.

However, the inability of the pure epidermal grafts to survive on the CAM almost certainly does not reflect a rigid dermal dependency on their part, since Briggaman and Wheeler [21] have recently reported that epidermis is well maintained on the CAM following recombination with tendon, tendon sheath or fascia. To study the influence of various nondermal mesenchymal environments on the differentiative potentiality of epidermis, Billingham and Silvers [17] injected suspensions of rat tail skin epidermal cells into the hamstring or lingual muscles, the spleen, and beneath the renal capsule. In all of these sites the cellular grafts produced multiple, small epidermal cysts with cuticular debris on the inside and viable Malpighian cells on the outside, separated from host tissue by a thin layer of dermis like fibrous connective tissue. In most instances biopsy specimens taken 90 days postoperatively revealed that hair follicles complete with dermal papilla were associated with these cysts in addition to well differentiated sebaceous glands. When hamster cheek pouch epidermal cell suspensions were transplanted to similar sites they, too, produced epithelialized cysts but these were totally devoid of appendages. Barker and Billingham (unpublished) have found that small grafts of pure rat tail skin epidermis survive and maintain the general appearance of epidermis when transplanted beneath the renal capsule. In this environment the epithelium displayed no tendency to migrate over the renal tissue bed or to produce appendages. Likewise, the present authors have found that split thickness grafts of rat tail skin remain perfectly healthy following transplantation to this site, but, again, the epidermis does not grow beyond the limits of its native dermis.

STUDIES ON THE TRANSPLANTATION OF VARIOUS TYPES CF SKIN TO THE UTERUS

Recently we have been studying the fate of free skin grafts and of suspensions of viable epidermal cells, prepared from tail skin, introduced into the uterine lumen of genetically compatible virgin adult female rat hosts (Fig. 9-1) [22]. The purpose of these grafts was to simulate Nature's transplants, i.e., blastocysts which implant naturally onto the endometrial surface and develop into embryos.

In the initial experiment the skin grafts, short cylinders of everted tail skin, were inserted via a short longitudinal incision made near the utero-tubal junction of the uterine horns of virgin rats which immediately received a single intramuscular injection of 50 micrograms of estradiol benzoate in sesame oil. This was to simulate the surge of endogenous estrogen believed to be essential for the successful implantation of blastocysts. Histological studies on sequentially removed biopsy specimens revealed that, by the fifth postoperative day, the grafts had become well attached to the untraumatized endometrial surface and had acquired a blood supply. Indeed, skin grafts in this ectopic site closely resembled similar grafts transplanted orthotopically to beds prepared in the integument of the trunk on other rats. Once they had implanted successfully, and in the absence of any further exogenous estrogen, intrauterine skin grafts were able to survive indefinitely as evidenced by the histological appearance of grafts of 100 or more

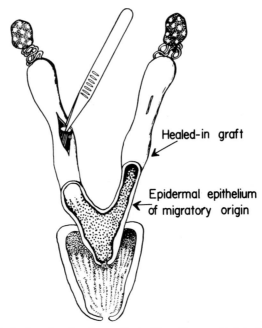

Healed-in graft

Epidermal epithelium
of migratory origin

Fig. 9–1.—Illustration showing the method of inserting a cylindrical tail skin graft into the lumen of a rat's right uterine horn. The resurfacing of the endometrium by migrating epidermal epithelium from an established skin graft in the left uterine horn is shown. Epithelium is beginning to migrate into the contralateral uterine horn.

days' standing. They regenerated sparse crops of hair characteristic of tail skin within two weeks of transplantation and retained all the structural features normally associated with this type of skin. The only abnormality was the gross enlargement and hypersecretory activity of the sebaceous glands, associated with intense mitotic activity of their peripheral cells (Fig. 9-2). In no case did histological examination reveal any tendency on the part of the skin epidermis to migrate outward beyond its own native dermal margins, the interface between endometrial and skin epithelia remaining incisively distinct.

It is pertinent to mention that in the absence of the exogenous estrogen only a very small proportion (about 8%) of the skin grafts implanted on the endometrial surface of virgin female rats. However, complete success did attend the transplantation of skin into the uteri of rats grafted 4 or 5 days after what subsequently proved to have been a successful mating, and which did not receive estrogen.

When the influence of maintaining the hosts of intrauterine skin grafts in a state of chronic physiologic estrogen dominance was investigated (these animals were given an intramuscular injection of 50 micrograms of estradiol benzoate at operation and weekly thereafter), the graft epidermis behaved in a remarkable and totally unexpected manner. From the twelfth postoperative day on it began to migrate centrifugally from the graft margins over the surrounding endometrial surface. In most instances the leading edge of the skin epidermis appeared to

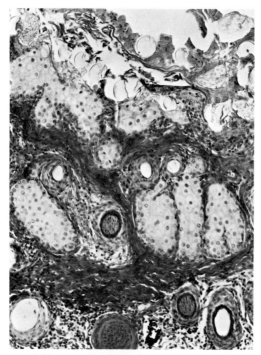

Fig. 9–2.—Striking hyperplasia of the sebaceous glands in a skin graft growing in the uterus of a rat maintained in estrus. ($\times$ 75).

advance by undermining the tall columnar cells comprising the native epithelium of the endometrium, maintaining contact with and becoming firmly adherent to the superficial mesenchymal stroma of the uterine mucosa (Fig. 9-3A). In some cases, however, the skin epithelium grew over the endometrial epithelium, which subsequently became attenuated and disappeared, again leaving a typical Malpighian or basal layer of the epidermis bonded to uterine mesenchymal tissue as before.

Cephalad, this estrogen-facilitated migration of epidermis never transgressed the uterotubal junction (Fig. 9-3B). Ectopic skin epidermis was never observed in either the fallopian tube or in the ovarian bursa. In the caudal direction, however, the field of migratory activity of the graft epidermis was much less constricted. Within 3–4 weeks postoperatively most animals evidenced the forthcoming of the growth of tongues of stratified, well keratinized skin epithelium down to and passage through the cervical os into the ungrafted uterine horn. Indeed, when sufficient time was allowed to elapse, the native epithelium of this organ, too, suffered partial replacement by skin epidermis.

Once skin grafts had become established on the endometrium of normal rats under the influence of a single injection of estrogen, oophorectomy performed 14 days postoperatively had no adverse effect on their well being. In the absence of further estrogen treatment no epidermal migration took place in the uteri of

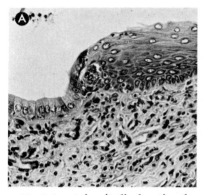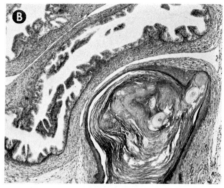

Fig. 9–3.—**A**, longitudinal section through a rat's uterus grafted with skin 14 days previously, showing an advancing tongue of stratified epidermal epithelium of graft origin which is firmly attached to the endometrial mesenchymal substrate and is also undermining the "native" endometrial epithelium. ($\times$ 120). **B**, longitudinal section through the utero-tubal junction in a rat which received a skin graft in its right uterine horn 100 days before and which has been maintained in chronic estrus. Note the complete failure of epidermis to migrate into the fallopian tube. ($\times$ 30).

castrated hosts, even from grafts of long standing in this milieu. However, epidermal migration from such grafts could be initiated at will and caused to replace neighboring endometrial epithelium simply by commencement of chronic estrogen inoculation (50μg. weekly) at any time after the grafting operation. This consideration also applied to intrauterine skin grafts in normal female rats which had received a single injection of exogenous estrogen at the time of operation.

STUDIES ON THE MODUS OPERANDI OF ESTROGEN IN FACILITATING EPIDERMAL MIGRATION IN THE UTERUS

Where two entirely different types of epithelium naturally abut onto one another at various sites in the body, as for example at the mucocutaneous borders, the location of the frontier is rigidly conserved. Indeed, if through any change of the *milieu intérieur,* one type of epithelium suddenly began to replace its neighbor, the consequences for the individual might be serious. Think how disastrous it would be for us if, as a consequence of some hormonal or vitamin status, epidermal epithelium were able to transgress these natural and biologically important frontiers replacing, for example, the native epithelium of the cornea or the small intestine with one having entirely different structural and physiological properties.

The estrogen dependent capacity of skin epithelium to replace the indigenous endometrial epithelium was an unexpected finding, with possible clinical implications. The obvious question that arose was whether the hormone acted upon receptors in the uterine substrate, affecting the behavior of the epidermis indirectly, or whether it acted upon receptors associated with the epidermal cells.

Failure of estrogen treatment to alter the migratory properties of epidermis from open fit skin grafts transplanted orthotopically in rats, or transplanted to other ectopic sites in the body cavity sustains the provisional conclusion that the estrogen dependent migration of epidermis within the uterus results from the action of the hormone upon the host organ, rather than upon the cells of graft origin.

FATE OF EPIDERMAL CELLULAR GRAFTS IN THE UTERUS

In the light of previous observations that autologous epidermal cell suspensions in rabbits, seeded over the surfaces of extensive, full thickness cutaneous wounds, give rise to foci of epidermal outgrowth which eventually coalesce and resurface the entire graft bed, the fate of introducing cellular grafts of epidermis into the uterine lumen was investigated.

When suspensions of epidermal cells were introduced into the uteri of normal, nonestrogen treated virgin female rat hosts no evidence was obtained of the successful implantation of these cells. However, if the host was treated with estrogen at the time of inoculation of the epidermal cell suspension, small foci of epidermal proliferation were demonstrable histologically in all recipients killed on the twelfth postoperative day (Fig. 9-4A). Once established, and provided that the host received chronic estrogen treatment, these epidermal bridge heads rapidly expanded through the mitotic and migratory behavior of the cells. What is so remarkable here is that monodisperse or at least small clumps of basal layer epidermal cells were able to gain a permanent foothold on the intact, completely epithelialized endometrial surface.

Irrespective of whether it originated from a suspension of epidermal cells or from a free skin graft implanted in the uterus of a rat subsequently maintained on chronic estrogen, the epidermis that replaced endometrial epithelium, and which represented a naturally produced heterotypic recombinant on a completely untraumatized uterine mesenchymal bed, displayed no tendency to interact with the latter to generate any of the appendages characteristic of the integument, such as hair or sebaceous glands. Apart from its invasive displacement of

Fig. 9–4.—**A**, section through uterine horn injected with a suspension of epidermal cells 12 days previously. Note the small, concave plaque of epidermis which has begun to invade a superficial uterine gland ($\times$ 75). **B**, transverse section through a rat's uterus in which epidermis from a skin graft has migrated into and relined a uterine gland. Note the squamous cell debris in the lumen of the gland. ($\times$ 190).

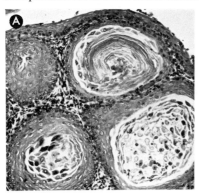
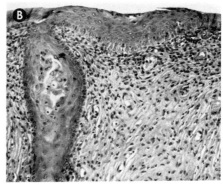

the superficial endometrial epithelium, skin epidermis readily grew down into the crypts of the uterine glands, completely replacing the native epithelial cells by an epithelium of stratified, nonsecretory structure (Fig. 9-4B).

TRANSPLANTATION OF OTHER TYPES OF "SKIN" TO THE UTERUS OF ESTROGEN TREATED RATS

The findings described above suggested that transplantation of various regionally distinctive types of skin to the uteri of rats maintained under chronic estrogen might afford a convenient and critical test of the equipotentiality or otherwise of the cells of their germinal epithelial layers. In other words, would the epithelium from a given type of graft maintain its specificity when caused to grow over and become united to endometrial mesenchymal tissue?

Vaginal and cervical epidermis are closely similar to that of the integument and juxtaposed to endometrial epithelium at the level of the cervix. To elucidate the interrelation of these two phenotypically distinct types of epithelia, small grafts of vaginal tissue, in practice short cylinders of vagina, were inserted into the hosts' uteri according to our standard procedure. Under conditions of chronic estrogen dominance, vaginal epithelium displayed vigorous migratory activity, replacing endometrial epithelium and faithfully conserving its distinctive histological features (Fig. 9-5).

Lingual epidermis differs incisively from skin or vaginal epidermis with respect to its cytostructure and the highly distinctive three-dimensional pattern of the interface between its basal layer and its connective tissue substrate. When small rectangular grafts of lingual mucosa, freed as far as possible from muscle, were placed in the uterus they implanted readily and their epidermis displayed a capacity for migration that was strikingly superior to that of tail skin. This finding is consonant with the rapidity with which small lesions in the intact tongue become reepithelialized. More important, the specificity of the epithelium which grew out from the tongue grafts over the endometrium was unmistakably that of

Fig. 9–5.—Section through uterus grafted with vaginal "skin" 21 days previously to show the advancing edge of migrating vaginal epithelium which is in contact with and displacing columnar endometrial epithelium. ($\times$ 75).

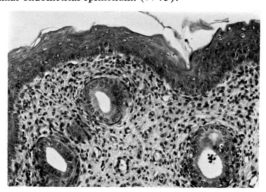

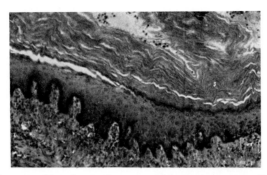

Fig. 9–6.—Lingual epidermis of migratory origin from a tongue "skin" graft of 14 days' standing in a rat's uterus. Note the typical re-entrant pattern presented by the superficial endometrial stroma in contact with the basal layer cells of the epithelium, and the compact laminated structure characteristic of the cuticle of the tongue. (× 30).

tongue (Fig. 9-6), corroborating previous evidence that this is an epithelium *sui generis*.

Hamster cheek pouch epidermis had previously been shown to retain its specificity when recombined with ear skin dermis. When small, rectangular grafts of this type of "skin" were inserted into the uteri of hormonally treated hamsters they healed in rapidly and the epithelium also replaced neighboring native endometrial epithelium, retaining its specificity (Fig. 9-7A).

Fig. 9–7.—**A,** photomicrograph showing epithelium which originated from a graft of hamster cheek pouch mucosa placed in the uterus 60 days before which is slowly replacing the endometrial epithelium. Note the incisive difference between the two types of epithelia where their cells abut one another. (× 600). **B,** photomicrograph showing endometrial epithelium which has overgrown the dermis of a graft of hamster cheek pouch "skin" placed in the uterus 60 days previously. (× 260).

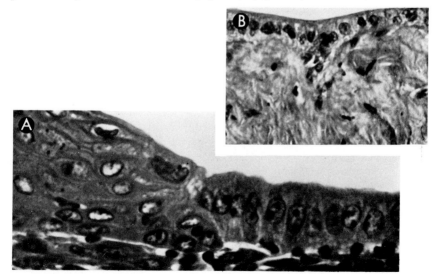

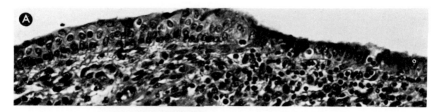

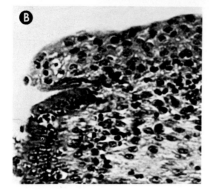

Fig. 9–8.—Transitional epithelium of
bladder which is invasively replacing native
endometrial epithelium in a rat's uterus. The
graft of bladder mucosa was placed in the
uterus 45 days previously. ($\times$ 190).

It has also been noted that whenever there was denuded cheek pouch connective tissue in this type of graft, it became resurfaced by a layer of tall, columnar
endometrial cells, rather than by its own type of epithelium (Fig. 9-7B). This
hints that endometrial epithelial cells can form a stable tissue when caused to
recombine with pouch skin dermis.

Corneal epidermis appears, on the basis of several lines of indirect evidence,
to be another type of epidermis whose cells will breed true to type when caused
to grow upon an alien mesenchymal substrate. A variety of attempts were therefore made to get it established in the uterine milieu in an effort to obtain more
critical evidence bearing upon this premise. Unfortunately, the introduction of
fragments of cornea, corneal epidermis isolated from its stroma by means of
trypsin, and cultured corneal cells into the uterus has consistently failed to result
in the establishment of the grafts.

Transitional epithelium of bladder, is of nonectodermal origin, and has its
own distinctive histological features including the absence of a cuticle. Small
grafts of bladder mucosa were freed as far as possible from muscle and deeper
tissue and inserted into the uteri of estrogen treated rats. They healed in readily
and the epithelium displayed a migratory potential that was superior to that of
tail skin but significantly inferior to that of lingual epidermis. The bladder epithelium which displaced endometrial epithelium proved to be perfectly stable,
even after cessation of the estrogen treatment of the host (Fig. 9-8).

Experiments are currently in progress to study the outcome of causing sheets
of lingual and tail skin epithelia of migratory origin to meet one another as a
consequence of growing over the uterine stroma. In practice this simply involved
transplantation of small grafts of tongue mucosa and tail skin to separate locations in the uteri of rats maintained in chronic estrus and allowing migratory epi-

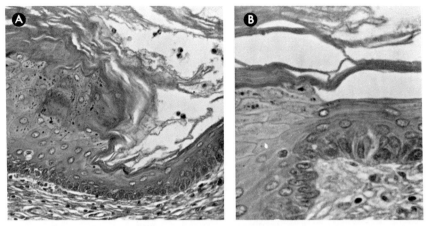

Fig. 9–9.—**A,** junction between outgrowing epithelial sheets originating from grafts of lingual mucosa and tail skin which were implanted 60 days before at remote sites in the same uterine horn of a rat. Both types of epithelia have invasively replaced the native endometrial epithelium and have probably formed a stable artificial "mucocutaneous" border. Each epithelium has conserved its own characteristic structural specificity. (× 260). **B,** high power view of junction between lingual and tail skin epithelia of migratory origin on uterine mesenchymal substrate. (× 600).

thelial outgrowths to make contact. Preliminary observations indicate that these two types of epithelia form a stable interface, a sort of artificial mucocutaneous border at their point of abutment, which is incisively distinct in histological sections as illustrated in Figure 9-9.

CONCLUSIONS

The observations that, under the conditions of chronic estrogen stimulation of the host, the epithelia from grafts of tail skin, hamster cheek pouch, vagina and bladder enjoy a strong selective advantage over the native endometrial epithelium of the uterus which they replace with an epithelium of their own particular structural specificity has a number of interesting implications:

1. They lend strong support to the previous conclusion that intrinsic, inheritable differences do exist between the germinal layer cells of certain types of epidermal and other epithelia of the body.

2. The marked structural differences between uterine epithelium and that of the squamous epithelium of the vagina and cervix are not due to the influence of different kinds of mesenchymal stromata acting upon a common, equipotential lineage of germinal cells.

3. They raise and leave unresolved the question of the nature of the estrogen dependent process that enables various kinds of alien epithelia to trespass upon and actually "take over" the stroma of the endometrium.

4. Finally, they suggest that some reported instances of "epidermidization" of the uterine epithelium, in both man and certain laboratory animals, may in fact be the result of migratory displacements of squamous epithelium from the

cervix or vagina into the uterus, facilitated by abnormalities of hormonal status or vitamin deficiency states. Relevant to this premise are observations that in perinatal human females the squamocolumnar junction of the uterine cervical epithelium advances to the level of the internal os of the uterus during the height of the estrogenic stimulus that reaches the fetus from its mother during gestation [23] and inward migration of cervical squamous epithelium toward the uterus takes place in adult mice maintained in estrous [24].

The experiments reviewed represent only a very crude, superficial approach to analysis of the origin and continued maintenance of epidermal and other epithelial specificities throughout life. The results indicate that certain epidermal differentia differ from one and other only with respect to the morphogenetic or regulatory influences that impinge upon their germinal layers from subjacent localized mesodermal or dermal cell populations, and canalize the differentiation of the cells along one of a variety of alternative pathways. Other epithelia, notably those of tongue, esophagus, hamsters' cheek pouch and bladder behave as if their developmental repertoire is much more restricted, being intrinsically determined and much less susceptible to extraneous regulatory influences.

Wessels [4] has presented the attractive thesis that the alternative forms or somatic phenotypes which the epidermis, and presumably certain other types of epithelia, may assume may be due to the differential activity of the members of a general class or series of epithelial genes, in response to hormone like influences emanating from qualitatively different mesenchymal or dermal cell populations. As a result of inductive type processes that take place in ontogeny, the determinative status of some epithelia may be more restricted than that of others, depending upon which particular (and how many) epithelial genes have been permanently repressed (and are not therefore easily derepressible) and which particular epithelial genes are still susceptible to derepression by appropriate factors or instructions of mesenchymal origin.

It is an unfortunate fact that most students of epidermal wound repair have totally neglected the considerable body of knowledge available concerning the natural, cyclical self destructive and self renewal activity of the primate endometrial epithelium which McMinn [13] aptly described as a special type of recurring "acute ulceration". Although the function of this self inflicted wounding of the uterine surface still awaits a satisfactory answer, it affords a striking model of the complex way in which hormones can affect the well being and activity of epithelia in general. Surely the time has come for gynecologists to adopt a less parochial attitude to the stratified epithelia in their domain and for dermatologists to pay more attention to the fascinating epithelialized territories that lie hidden beneath the surface of the body.

SUMMARY

Various heterotopic and other kinds of grafting experiments carried out on adult rodents are reviewed which bear upon the problem of the rigid conservation of the structural and functional specificities of epidermal and other types of epithelia throughout life. These indicate that the germinal layer cells in many structurally and functionally distinctive types of epidermis are equipotential, and that their characteristic mode of differentiation is determined by interaction with the particular type of dermis, or dermal cell population that forms their normal substrate.

However there are exceptions, including the epidermis of tongue, cornea, esophagus, hamster's cheek pouch and the transitional epithelium of bladder whose specificities are maintained even when they are caused to grow upon anatomically unnatural types of mesenchymal bed.

A new approach to the analysis of epithelial specificities is described. This entails transplantation of various types of skin, or other epithelialized tissue to the uteri of rats maintained in chronic estrus. Under these conditions various types of epithelia tested migrate centrifugally beyond the limits of their native mesenchymal substrate invasively replacing the endometrial epithelium of the uterus on a massive scale, and in so doing, producing natural epithelial/mesenchymal heterotypic recombinants.

BIBLIOGRAPHY

1. Billingham, R. E., and Silvers, W. K.: Some Unsolved Problems in the Biology of Skin, in Lyne, A. G., and Short, B. F. (eds.): *Biology of the Skin and Hair Growth* (Sydney: Angus and Robertson, 1965).
2. Billingham, R. E., and Silvers, W. K.: Origin and conservation of epidermal specificities, New England J. Med. 268:677, 1963.
3. Wessels, N. K.: Differentiation of epidermis and epidermal derivatives, New England J. Med. 277:21, 1967.
4. Wessels, N. K.: Some thoughts on embryonic inductions in relation to determination, J. Invest. Dermat. 55:221, 1970.
5. Wessels, N. K.: Tissue interactions during skin histodifferentiations. Developmental Biol. 4:87, 1962.
6. Joseph, J., and Thomas, G. A.: The behaviour of autografts of ileum transplanted into the urinary bladder in rabbits, J. Anat. 92:551, 1958.
7. Joseph, J.: Autografts of ileum and lining of urinary bladder to the ears of rabbits, J. Anat. 25:27, 1960.
8. Billingham, R. E., and Medawar, P. B.: Pigment spread and cell heredity in guinea pigs' skin, Heredity 2:29, 1948.
9. Billingham, R. E., and Medawar, P. B.: A note on the specificity of the corneal epithelium, J. Anat. 84:50, 1950.
10. Billingham, R. E., and Silvers, W. K.: Studies on Cheek Pouch Skin Homografts in the Syrian Hamster, in Wolstenholme, G. E. W., and Cameron, M. P. (eds.): *Ciba Foundation Symposium on Transplantation* (London: J. & A. Churchill, Ltd., 1962).
11. Billingham, R. E., and Medawar, P. B.: The technique of free skin grafting in mammals, J. Exper. Biol. 28:385, 1951.
12. Russell, P. S., and Billingham, R. E.: Some aspects of the repair process in mammals, Prog. Surg. 2:1, 1962.
13. McMinn, R. M. H.: *Tissue Repair* (New York: Academic Press, Inc., 1969).
14. Krohn, P. L.: The behaviour of autografts and homografts of vaginal tissue in rabbits, J. Anat. 89:269, 1955.
15. Breedis, C.: Differentiation and redifferentiation in skin, Nat. Cancer Inst. Monograph 10:21, 1962.
16. Karasek, M. A.: Growth and differentiation of transplanted epithelial cell cultures, J. Invest. Dermat. 51:247, 1968.
17. Billingham, R. E., and Silvers, W. K.: Dermoepidermal Interactions and Epithelial Specificity, in Fleischmajer, R., and Billingham, R. E. (eds.): *Epithelial-Mesenchymal Interactions* (Baltimore: Williams and Wilkins Co., 1968).
18. Billingham, R. E., and Reynolds, J.: Transplantation studies on sheets of pure epi-

dermal epithelium and on epidermal cell suspensions, Brit. J. Plast. Surg. 5:25, 1952.

19. Billingham, R. E., and Silvers, W. K.: Studies on the conservation of epidermal specificities of skin and certain mucosas in adult mammals, J. Exper. Med. 125: 429, 1967.

20. Briggaman, R. A., and Wheeler, C. E.: Epidermal-dermal interactions in adult human skin: role of dermis in epidermal maintenance, J. Invest. Dermat. 51:454, 1968.

21. Briggaman, R. A., and Wheeler, C. E.: Epidermal-dermal interactions in adult human skin. II. The nature of the dermal influence, J. Invest. Dermat. 56:18, 1971.

22. Beer, A. E., and Billingham, R. E.: Implantation, transplantation, and epithelial-mesenchymal relationships in the rat uterus, J. Exper. Med. 132:721, 1970.

23. Schneppenheim, P., Hampert, H., Kaufmann, C., and Ober, K. G.: Die Beziehungen des Schleimepithals zum Plattenepithel an der Cervix Uteri in Lebenslauf der Frau, Arch. Gynäk. 190:303, 1957-58.

24. Baggish, M. S., and Woodruff, D. J.: The occurrence of squamous epithelium in the endometrium, Obst. & Gynec. Surv. 22:69, 1967.

The expenses of some of the work described in this article were supported in part by U.S. Public Health Service Grant AI 07001 and The Lalor Foundation.

10

Epidermal Growth Factor:
Chemical and Biological Characterization*

Stanley Cohen, Ph.D.† and John M. Taylor, Ph.D.†

During the course of the studies on the nerve growth promoting protein of the submaxillary gland of the male mouse [1], it was observed that partially purified extracts of these glands caused gross anatomical changes when injected daily into newborn mice. Among the specific tissue changes observed were the precocious opening of the eyelids (6–7 days instead of the normal 12–14 days), and the precocious eruption of the incisors (6–7 days instead of the normal 9–10 days). By means of a biological assay based on the precocious opening of the eyelids of the newborn mouse, a polypeptide responsible for this effect was isolated [2]. The biological activity was subsequently found to be due to a direct stimulation of the proliferation and keratinization of epidermal tissue; therefore, the polypeptide has been termed epidermal growth factor (EGF). The chemical and physical properties of EGF will be described, followed by a discussion of its biological activity.

CHEMISTRY OF THE EPIDERMAL GROWTH FACTOR

Early Characterization

The isolation procedure for EGF involved standard methods of protein purification. In a typical preparation, the submaxillary glands of 150 adult male mice, having a wet weight of approximately 22–25 Gm., yielded from 5–7 mg. of pure EGF, with a recovery of approximately 20% of the original activity. EGF was estimated to be approximately 0.5% of the dry weight of the submaxillary gland protein.

The isolated material appeared to be relatively pure and homogeneous by several different criteria. EGF showed only a single component when it was exam-

---

*This manuscript will be included in The Thirtieth Symposium of the Society for Developmental Biology, 1971.

†Department of Biochemistry, Vanderbilt University School of Medicine, Nashville, Tennessee.

ined in the analytical ultracentrifuge, having a sedimentation coefficient ($s_{20, w}$) of 1.25 S. Paper electrophoresis in buffers of different pH, and paper chromatography in a variety of solvents showed only one spot after staining with protein dyes. The material was antigenic; and cellulose acetate immunoelectrophoresis of the factor against its antiserum revealed only one precipitin band.

The ultraviolet absorption spectrum of the purified factor was observed to be typical for proteins, with a 280 to 260 optical density ratio of 1.6. EGF was found to be heat stable and nondialyzable. Its biological activity was stable to boiling in water but was destroyed by heating in dilute alkali or dilute acid. Biological activity was also destroyed by incubation with chymotrypsin or a bacterial protease, but was only partially lost after incubation with trypsin. These data strongly suggested that the factor was polypeptide-like in nature [2].

Chemical and Physical Properties

A more detailed study of the chemical and physical properties of EGF has been undertaken [3, 4]. Studies of the amino acid composition, summarized in Table 10-1, indicate the absence of three specific amino acid residues: lysine, alanine and phenylalanine. The calculated number of residues was based on one histidine residue per mole of polypeptide. The presence of six half-cystine residues has been confirmed by amino acid analysis of the S-aminoethylated derivative of EGF. No free sulfhydryl groups were detected, indicating the probable existence of three disulfide bridges within the molecule. In addition, no detectable hexosamines have been found.

A minimum molecular weight of 6,166 to 6,554 was calculated from the amino acid composition. This molecular size is supported by low speed sedimentation equilibrium studies, which indicate a molecular weight of 6,400, and by gel filtration studies on columns of BioGel P-10, which suggest an approximate molecular weight of 7,000.

Table 10-1
Amino Acid Composition of Low Molecular Weight EGF*

Amino Acid	Residues/Mole	Amino Acid	Residues/Mole
Lysine	0	Alanine	0
Histidine	1	Half-cystine	6
Arginine	4	Valine	2
Aspartic Acid	8–9	Methionine	1
Threonine	2	Isoleucine	2
Serine	6–7	Leucine	4
Glutamic Acid	3–4	Tyrosine	5
Proline	2	Phenylalanine	0
Glycine	6–7	Tryptophan	2
Total residues			54–58
Minimum Molecular Weight			6,166–6,554

*Samples of 100 μg were hydrolyzed in 6 N HCl under vacuum for 24 hours. The average value from two hydrolyses is presented. The calculated number of residues was based on one histidine and four arginine residues per mole of polypeptide. The results were uncorrected for hydrolytic losses. The recovered amino acids amounted to 85% by weight of the starting material. Tryptophan was measured spectrophotometrically. (From Taylor *et al.* [3].)

Table 10-2

Physical and Chemical Properties of Epidermal Growth Factor

Property	Value
Molecular weight in daltons	
sedimentation equilibrium	6,400
gel filtration (BioGel P-10)	7,000
amino acid composition	6,166–6,554
Sedimentation coefficient ($s_{20, w}$)	1.25 S
Partial specific volume ($\bar{v}$) in cm.³/Gm.	0.69
Extinction coefficient ($E_{1\ cm., \ 280\ m\mu}^{1\%}$)	30.9
Isoelectric point	pH 4.60
Tertiary structure	Nonhelical
Number of polypeptide chains	One
Amino-terminus	Asparagine
Carboxyl-terminus	Arginine
Disulfide bonds	Three
Missing amino acids	Lys, Ala, Phe
Hexosamine content	None detected

The values for the molecular weight of EGF reported here differ from the original estimate of 15,000 [2]. The earlier estimate, however, was calculated from the amino acid composition on the basis of one alanine and ten leucine residues per mole. The recent amino acid analyses of EGF, prepared under improved conditions which reduce contamination, do not reveal the presence of a significant amount of alanine.

Studies with chemically modified derivatives of EGF indicate that it is a single chain polypeptide. This conclusion is supported by the finding of only one amino-terminal residue (asparagine) and only one carboxyl-terminal residue (arginine).

The results of these and other investigations on the chemical and physical properties of EGF are summarized in Table 10-2.

High Molecular Weight Form of Epidermal Growth Factor

In crude homogenates of the submaxillary glands of adult male mice, EGF was found to be a component of a high molecular weight complex [3]. The isolation and characterization of this biologically active complex, termed high molecular weight epidermal growth factor (HMW-EGF), will be described below.

The existence of HMW-EGF was first detected by the gel filtration of aqueous extracts of the submaxillary glands on calibrated columns of Sephadex G-75. The result of a gel filtration experiment is shown in Figure 10-1. The eluate fractions were examined by an immunoprecipitation reaction with an antibody to the low molecular weight EGF. The major EGF-antibody precipitating material was observed with the pigmented hemoglobin peak in the 50,000 to 70,000 molecular weight fraction of the eluate. This fraction was also found to be biologically active by means of the eyelid-opening assay in the newborn mouse.

The HMW-EGF was isolated by means of standard methods of protein purification. Based on purification yields, HMW-EGF was estimated to be approxi-

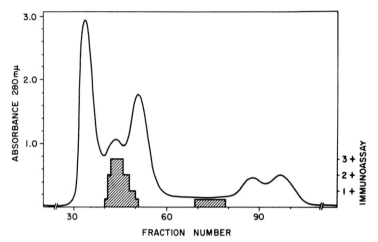

Fig. 10–1.—Gel filtration of a crude extract of male mouse submaxillary glands on Sephadex G-75. A 4.0 ml. extract containing 0.3 Gm. of protein was applied to a Sephadex G-75 column (2.5 × 90 cm.) equilibrated with the elution buffer (0.01 M sodium acetate, pH 5.9, and 0.1 M sodium chloride). The flow rate was 3.8 ml./cm.^{2}/hr. and 5.0 ml. fractions were collected. The hatched areas indicate the immunoprecipitation reaction of the eluate fractions with the antibody to low molecular weight epidermal growth factor. The immunoassay was carried out by layering 25 μl. from each eluate fraction over 25 μl. of antiserum and qualitatively observing the precipitate that formed at the interface after 30 minutes. (From Taylor [38].)

mately 2 to 3% of the dry weight of the submaxillary gland protein, with a recovery of approximately two-thirds of the original material.

High speed sedimentation equilibrium studies indicate that HMW-EGF has a molecular weight of approximately 74,000. It can be reversibly dissociated, under a variety of conditions, into two molecules of the low molecular weight EGF (6,400), and two molecules of an EGF-binding protein (30,000). Conditions for dissociation include adsorption to ion exchange columns, gel filtration in buffers below pH 5.0 and above pH 8.0, and by isoelectric focusing with low pH range ampholyte solutions. The result of an isoelectric focusing experiment is shown in Figure 10-2. Only two major protein peaks are observed above the background absorbance. The peak at pH 4.60 corresponds to low molecular weight EGF, and the peak at pH 5.60 corresponds to the EGF-binding protein. The low molecular weight EGF obtained from the dissociation of HMW-EGF is identical to the EGF as originally isolated by [2]. Criteria of identity include isoelectric point determinations, amino acid composition, carboxyl-terminal residue analysis, gel filtration studies and antigenic identity with an antibody prepared against EGF as originally isolated.

The low molecular weight EGF and the EGF-binding protein can be recombined to form a high molecular weight complex, having approximately the same molecular weight as the native HMW-EGF when examined by sedimentation equilibrium and gel filtration studies. In a typical experiment, equal weights of

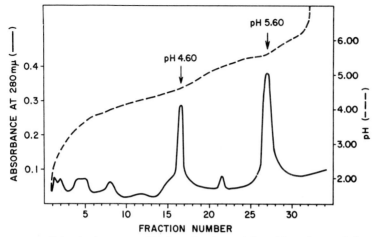

Fig. 10–2.—Subunit character of high molecular weight epidermal growth factor by isoelectric focusing under dissociation conditions. The pH range of the ampholyte solution was from pH 4 to 6. The solid line shows the absorbance at 280 mμ of the fractions (3 ml.) obtained from the isoelectric focusing column. The dashed line represents the pH gradient developed during the experiment. The experiment was performed with 8 mg. of HMW-EGF. (From Taylor *et al.* [3].)

EGF and EGF-binding protein are mixed together in a neutral buffer, allowed to stand for a few hours, then applied to a calibrated column of Sephadex G-100. The results of this experiment are shown in Figure 10-3. The EGF-binding protein alone did not form a precipitate with the EGF antibody, whereas the recombined HMW-EGF did form a precipitate. In addition, the elution volume of the recombined HMW-EGF was similar to that of the native HMW-EGF, and distinctly different from the elution volumes of its two components.

After the HMW-EGF had been isolated, the observation was made that the EGF-binding protein was an arginine esterase, and various enzymatic parameters were measured. The esterase showed a hydrolytic specificity for arginine esters, and for lysine esters to a lesser degree. Significant catalytic hydrolysis was not observed for a variety of other amino acid esters, with no detectable hydrolysis of arginine amide substrates. The rate of hydrolysis of benzoyl-arginine ethyl ester at 25° C was approximately 390 μmoles/min./mg. of enzyme at pH 8.0. The additional observation that EGF possesses a carboxyl-terminal arginine residue suggests that EGF may be generated from a precursor protein by the possible proteolytic action of the EGF-binding esterase.

In a broad context, the observations that certain other polypeptide hormones such as bradykinin [5] and insulin [6] arise from precursors by the proteolytic action of arginine esterases, suggest that the formation of active polypeptide hormones from inactive precursors, by the proteolytic action of a family of arginine esterases, may be a general phenomenon.

It may be noted that the nerve growth factor of the male mouse submaxillary gland, originally isolated by Cohen [1], has been found to be a component of a

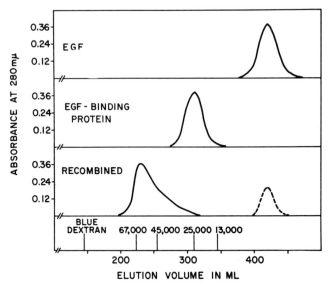

Fig. 10–3.—Recombination of epidermal growth factor binding protein and low molecular weight epidermal growth factor. Samples containing from 8 to 16 mg. of protein in 4 ml. of elution buffer (0.01 *M* sodium acetate, pH 5.9, and 0.1 *M* sodium chloride) were applied to a Sephadex G-100 column (2.5 × 90 cm.) equilibrated with the same buffer. The flow rate was 4.3 ml./cm.^{2}/hr. and 5 ml. fractions were collected. The top curve shows the elution profile of pure low molecular weight EGF. The middle curve shows the elution profile of pure EGF-binding protein. The bottom curve shows the elution profile of the recombined HMW-EGF (the dotted line indicates excess unreacted low molecular weight EGF). At the bottom of the figure the elution volumes and molecular weights of various protein standards: bovine serum albumin (67,000), ovalbumin (45,000), chymotrypsinogen A (25,000), and horse heart cytochrome c (13,000) are shown. (From Taylor *et al.* [3].)

high molecular weight complex, with an approximate molecular weight of 140,-000 [7]. One of the subunits of this complex has been found to be an arginine esterase [8]. The physical and enzymatic properties of this enzyme bear a close resemblance to the EGF-binding esterase. Preliminary immunological evidence indicates that these two enzymes may be nearly identical, raising the possibility that the biosynthesis and activation of the epidermal growth factor and the nerve growth factor may be quite similar, perhaps under the control of the same genetic locus. This possibility is also suggested by their similar sexually dimorphic character and sensitivity to hormonal induction by testosterone.

BIOLOGY OF THE EPIDERMAL GROWTH FACTOR

Effects of EGF In Vivo

The precocious opening of the eyelids and incisor eruption following the daily subcutaneous injection of microgram quantities of EGF is ascribed mainly to an enhancement of epidermal growth and keratinization. A histological examination

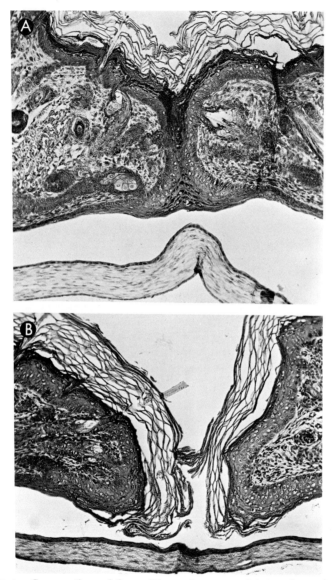

Fig. 10–4.—Cross sections of the eyelid area from control (**A**) and experimental (**B**) 8-day-old rats. The experimental animal had received daily injections (1 μg./Gm. body weight) of EGF. (From Cohen and Elliott [9].)

of these animals revealed enhanced keratinization and an increase in the thickness of the epidermis not only in the eyelid area (Fig. 10-4) but also in the back skin and epithelium lining the mouth [9]. This histological picture has been confirmed by making a number of chemical measurements (protein, RNA, DNA) of pure epidermis obtained by trypsinization of standard areas of skin from 5-day-old control and EGF-treated rats [10, 11]. Farebrother and Mann [12] have extended these histological observations. The most noticeable effects again were seen in the skin. Changes were also noted in the pericardium, kidney capsule and bile duct. A diminution of the thickness and fat content of the dermis was reported. An enhancement of the carcinogenicity of topically applied 3-methylcholanthrene on mouse skin has also been noted [13] in EGF-treated animals.

The eyelid opening effect in newborn rats is demonstrable at a dosage level of 0.1 μg./Gm./day. At higher dosage levels, 1 to 2 μg./Gm./day, there is a distinct growth inhibition of the animals, and after 10 days of treatment, clear morphological changes are visible in the liver, where large accumulations of fat are present. This fatty liver appears to be, almost exclusively, the result of the net accumulation of triglycerides [14].

Effects of EGF on Cells in Culture

EGF has been shown to stimulate epithelial cell proliferation in a number of organ culture systems. The initial observations were made with fragments of skin from the trunk of seven-day chick embryos, cultured in synthetic medium. The number of layers of epidermal cells of control cultures remained almost unchanged during a 48-hour incubation period whereas a marked increase in the number of layers of epidermal cells occurred in the experimental cultures (Fig. 10-5). In the constant presence of H^3-thymidine, almost every basal cell of the EGF-treated cultures became labeled, while in control cultures only very few basal cells contained radioactivity [15].

This proliferative effect of EGF has also been reported for epithelial cells of mouse mammary glands and mammary carcinomas in organ culture [16, 17].

Fig. 10-5.—Cross sections of control (A) and experimental (B) explants of back skin from 7-day chick embryos after 3 days of incubation. The experimental cultures contained 5 μg./ml. of EGF. (From Cohen [15].)

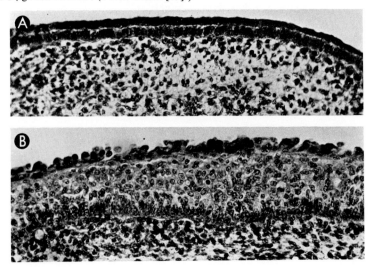

One of the initial morphological effects of the factor is a stimulation of cell migration, demonstrated by experiments in which aggregates of chick embryo epidermal cells were incubated in collagen coated culture dishes for 18 hours. Control cells consistently formed compact flattened colony-like areas while, in contrast, in the presence as little as 0.02 μg./ml. of the factor, the cells spread into a fibroblast-like network [18]. Under these conditions EGF did not enhance thymidine incorporation, indicating that DNA synthesis had not been stimulated.

Biochemical Studies on the Mechanism of Action of EGF

The stimulation of epidermal proliferation in culture is dependent upon a number of conditions, among which are the age of the embryo from which the skin is explanted and whether or not dermal cells are present.

In the following experiments, sheets of pure epidermis derived from the back skin of 9-day embryos were cultured on Millipore filters in a variety of media with or without microgram quantities of EGF. This system was chosen, rather than epidermis or whole skin from younger embryos, to obtain sufficient amounts of tissue for biochemical work and permit studies on the early effects of EGF on a single cell type. The observations and conclusions from a number of studies [19–21] are summarized below:

1. In the control tissues no significant changes occurred in the total amounts of protein, RNA or DNA during the 3-day period of incubation. However, total net protein and RNA in the experimental cultures increased twofold over their initial values during the first 48 hours of incubation. No significant increase in the content of DNA in epidermis cultured in the medium containing EGF was observed (Fig. 10-6). The failure of EGF to stimulate DNA synthesis under these conditions, as well as the clear stimulation of protein and RNA synthesis, has been confirmed in experiments in which the appropriate radioactive precursors (thymidine, orotic acid, uridine and lysine) were added to the medium in the presence and absence of EGF and their incorporation into the tissues studied.

2. EGF appears to rapidly stimulate the transport of certain metabolites. Within 15 minutes following the addition of EGF there is an approximately twofold stimulation of the uptake of radioactive aminoisobutyric acid and uridine into the trichloroacetic acid soluble fraction of the cells. This uptake is not prevented by inhibitors of protein synthesis such as cycloheximide, indicating that the synthesis of new proteins was not required for these permeability changes.

3. During the first 90 minutes following the addition of EGF there is an approximately threefold stimulation of the incorporation of labeled uridine into total RNA. This stimulation is not inhibited by puromycin or cycloheximide.

4. A number of experiments have been performed to partially characterize the nature of the newly formed RNA which appears in the cytoplasm after EGF addition. After a 90-minute incubation period with labeled uridine in the presence and absence of EGF, sucrose sedimentation analysis of the mitochondrial supernatants revealed that the synthesis of all types of RNA discernible on the gradient (4-S, 16-S, 28-S and heterogeneous RNA) were stimulated (approximately four to eight times).

5. In the presence of EGF there is a conversion of preexisting ribosomal monomers into functional polysomal structures. (Controls contained approximately 30% of the total ribosomes as polysomes whereas EGF-treated cells contain

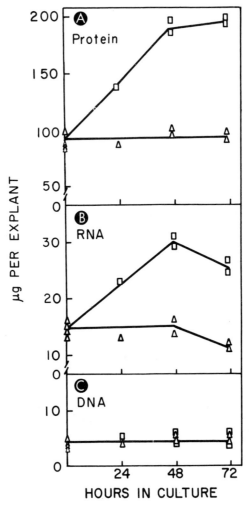

Fig. 10–6.—Changes in total protein (A), RNA (B) and DNA (C) of 8.5-day chick embryo epidermis during culture with 5 μg./ml. of EGF (□) and without EGF (△). (From Hoober and Cohen [20].)

about 60% as polysomes.) This ribosomal monomer-polysome conversion is detectable on sucrose gradients 30 minutes after the addition of EGF to the culture medium, and is observable even in the presence of cycloheximide or in a simple salt medium. It appears, therefore, that the initial transfer of monosomes to polysomes does not *require* the synthesis of new protein or an increased transport of amino acids and glucose. EGF also stimulates the synthesis of new ribosomal subunits.

6. The increase in the ratio of polysomes to monosomes in the epidermal cells under the influence of EGF would suggest that the isolated total ribosomal popu-

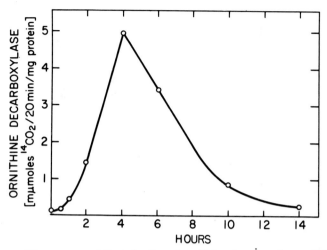

Fig. 10–7.—Time course of the induction of ornithine decarboxylase activity in chick embryo epidermis by EGF. The reaction mixture contained 3.0 μmoles of sodium-potassium phosphate buffer (pH 6.6), 0.1 μmole EDTA, 12 mμmole pyridoxal phosphate, 0.12 μmole of DL-[1-^{14}C] ornithine, and approximately 0.3 mg. tissue protein, in a total final volume of 60 μl. (From Stastny and Cohen [22].)

lation of the EGF-treated cells should be more active in cell-free protein synthesis than in that of control cells. To examine this question, a cell-free protein synthesizing system from cultured chick embryo epidermis was devised. Extracts prepared from epidermis cultured with EGF were over twice as active as extracts of tissue cultured without EGF in incorporating labeled amino acids (using endogenous messenger RNA). This difference was accounted for in the ribosomal fraction of the cells, with no differences detected in the soluble fraction. In addition, the total ribosomal population from treated cells was more active in protein synthesis, even in the presence of polyuridylic acid, than were control ribosomes. This suggested that ribosomes from treated cells had a greater ability to bind messenger RNA in a functional manner than those of control cells. These differences were detectable 30 minutes following the addition of EGF.

We were led to the next series of experiments [22] by the similarities between the response of epidermal cells to EGF and the response of many other cell types to hormonal growth stimulation, and to the results of several groups on the induction of ornithine decarboxylase in liver by partial hepatectomy or growth hormone administration [23–25].

Briefly, EGF induces a marked (40-fold), but transient, increase of ornithine decarboxylase activity in cultures of chick embryo epidermis (Fig. 10-7). The induction of the enzyme is prevented by inhibitors of protein synthesis (cycloheximide, puromycin and fluorophenylalanine), suggesting that de novo synthesis of the enzyme had occurred. However, until the enzyme is isolated or measured in some absolute manner, this conclusion can only be a tentative one.

The induced ornithine decarboxylase activity was reflected in the intracellular accumulation of labeled putrescine in the presence of EGF when labeled orni-

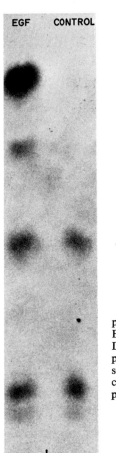

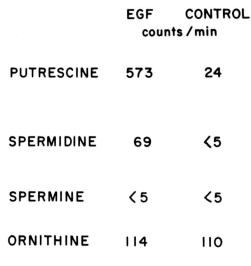

	EGF	CONTROL
	counts /min	
PUTRESCINE	573	24
SPERMIDINE	69	⟨5
SPERMINE	⟨ 5	⟨5
ORNITHINE	114	110

Fig. 10–8.—Intracellular accumulation of polyamines in the presence and absence of EGF. Epidermis was cultured in medium containing DL-[2-14C] ornithine for a four hour period. The polyamines were extracted from the tissue, separated by paper electrophoresis, and the labeled components detected by autoradiographic procedures. (From Stastny and Cohen [22].)

thine (Fig. 10-8) or arginine was present in the medium. EGF also induces lysine decarboxylase activity with a concomitant increase in intracellular cadaverine in the presence of labeled lysine.

The possible biological significance of the transient induction of ornithine decarboxylase activity for growth regulation in cultures of chick epidermis is supported by the finding that EGF induces this enzyme in skin when injected into neonatal mice. The additional observation that the enzyme is induced in the testes of these animals suggests that this polypeptide may also affect epithelia in other organs.

Whereas the induction of the enzyme is prevented by a number of inhibitors of protein synthesis, several other metabolic events (discussed previously), which are stimulated by EGF, are not prevented by inhibition of protein synthesis. These results suggest that the induction of ornithine decarboxylase is an early but secondary event in the action of EGF.

Polyamines have been implicated in a large and diverse number of biological processes [26]. For example, they have been shown to stabilize ribosomes and membranes, and to stimulate the synthesis of protein, DNA, RNA and aminoacyl-transfer RNA. In many of these reactions the polyamines may replace, at least partially, a Mg^{++} requirement and it has been suggested that polyamines may be more important for protein synthesis in vivo than is Mg^{++} [27].

The fact that both steroid [28, 29] and polypeptide hormones may act as inducers of ornithine decarboxylase again suggests that the induction of the decarboxylase is an early, but not necessarily primary, event in the action of these hormones. It is conceivable that the rapid induction of ornithine decarboxylase and the subsequent accumulation of putrescine or polyamines provide a mechanism by which the cell may rapidly alter its internal environment to optimize conditions for a variety of biosynthetic reactions.

Thus, we have described a series of metabolic alterations which accompany the growth stimulating effects of EGF on epidermal cells. Many of these changes appear to take place in a variety of cells when a growth stimulus is applied. Neither the initial binding site nor the "primary" metabolic effect of EGF has been clearly identified.

Synthesis and Storage of EGF

The tubular cells of the submaxillary gland of rodents exhibit sexual dimorphism. The morphology and granule content of these cells are dependent upon the hormonal status of the animal. The cells are developed fully in the male only after puberty, castration results in the atrophy of the tubular portion of the gland and the injection of testosterone into female mice results in a hypertrophy and hyperplasia of these cells [30].

The quantity of EGF present in the submaxillary gland closely parallels this development of the tubular system [18]. A number of other proteins of the submaxillary gland also show this sexually dimorphic character, including nerve growth factor [1, 31], renin [32] and certain arginine esterases [33, 34].

Turkington *et al.* [35] have demonstrated by immunofluorescent staining that EGF is present in specific tubular cells of the submaxillary gland, but it was not detected in any other mouse tissue examined. Moreover, organ cultures of mouse submaxillary gland incorporated labeled amino acids into a protein that was shown to be identical to authentic EGF by polyacrylamide gel electrophoresis after purification by specific immunoabsorption. These results indicate that EGF is synthesized in the mouse submaxillary gland and suggest that the elaboration of EGF may be a specific function of tubular cells.

Radioimmunoassay of EGF

The development of a very sensitive radioimmunoassay for EGF using a rabbit antiserum and iodinated EGF [36, 37] permits further studies on the physiology of this growth promoting polypeptide. The assay is sensitive to as little as 30 ng. of EGF and is not affected by cross reactivity to a variety of polypeptide hormones (ACTH, growth hormone, FSH, LH, TSH or insulin). Using this assay it was possible to quantitatively monitor the accumulation of EGF in the submaxillary gland in male mice of varying age (Fig. 10-9). The EGF content

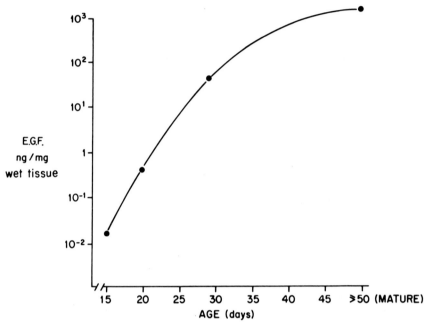

Fig. 10–9.—The content of EGF in the submaxillary glands of male mice during maturation.

of the gland was very low in 15-day-old mice, about 0.016 ng./mg. wet tissue, and increased to levels of about 1000 ng./mg. in glands of mature male mice.

EGF has been found to be present in mouse serum at a level of approximately 1 ng./ml. The stimulation of α-adrenergic receptors (intravenous injection of phenylephrine at 1.5 μg./Gm.) in normal adult male mice leads to a marked increase in the serum levels of EGF, reaching 150 ng./ml. in 60 minutes. These findings support the view that EGF serves a continuing physiological function in the animal, and that its secretion may be regulated by feedback mechanisms.

Considerable amounts of EGF have been detected in normal mouse milk (approximately 200 ng./ml.). In preliminary experiments it has been possible to elicit precocious eyelid opening and incisor eruption by oral administration of EGF to newborn mice. This suggests the possibility that an EGF-like molecule may be present in milk and exert its effects on the neonatal animal.

Although there is at present no direct evidence for the role of the growth factor in normal development and cell control, the following indirect evidence indicates that an important function does exist: EGF was isolated from a mammalian organ; the concentration of the factor in the submaxillary gland is dependent on the hormonal status of the animal; the secretion of EGF into the serum is stimulated by α-adrenergic compounds; and finally, EGF has specific morphological and biochemical effects on epidermis and certain epithelial tissues.

REFERENCES

1. Cohen, S.: Purification of a nerve growth promoting protein from the mouse salivary gland and its neurocytotoxic antiserum. Proc. Nat. Acad. Sc. (U.S.) 46:302, 1960.
2. Cohen, S.: Isolation of a mouse submaxillary gland protein accelerating incisor eruption and eyelid opening in the newborn animal. J. Biol. Chem. 237:1555, 1962.
3. Taylor, J. M., Cohen, S., and Mitchell, W. M.: Epidermal growth factor: High and low molecular weight forms, Proc. Nat. Acad. Sc. (U.S.) 67:64, 1970.
4. Taylor, J. M., Cohen, S., and Mitchell, W. M.: Unpublished data.
5. Schachter, M.: Kallikreins and kinins, Physiol. Rev. 49:509, 1969.
6. Chance, R. E., Ellis, R. M., and Bromer, W. W.: Porcine proinsulin: Characterization and amino acid sequence, Science 161:165, 1968.
7. Varon, S., Nomura, J., and Shooter, E. M.: The isolation of the mouse nerve growth factor protein in a high molecular weight form, Biochemistry 6:2202, 1967.
8. Greene, L. A., Shooter, E. M., and Varon, S.: Subunit interaction and enzymatic activity of mouse 7S nerve growth factor, Biochemistry 8:3735, 1969.
9. Cohen, S., and Elliott, G. A.: The stimulation of epidermal keratinization by a protein isolated from the submaxillary gland of the mouse, J. Invest. Dermat. 40:1, 1963.
10. Angeletti, P. U., Salvi, M. L., Chesanow, R. L., and Cohen, S.: Azione dell' "epidermal growth factor" sulla sintesi di acici nucleici e protine dell'epitelio cutaneo, Experientia 20:146, 1964.
11. Mann, C. B., and Fenton, E. L.: Biological effects of epithelial growth factor and its antiserum in neonatal rats, Biochem. J. 118:33P, 1970.
12. Farebrother, D. A., and Mann, C. B.: The histological effects of epithelial growth factor and its antiserum in the neonatal rat, Biochem. J. 118:33P, 1970.
13. Reynolds, V. H., Boehm, F. H., and Cohen, S.: Enhancement of chemical carcinogenesis by an epidermal growth factor, Surg. Forum 16:108, 1965.
14. Heimberg, M., Weinstein, I., LeQuire, V. S., and Cohen, S.: The induction of fatty liver in neonatal animals by a purified protein (EGF) from mouse submaxillary gland, Life Sc. 4:1625, 1965.
15. Cohen, S.: The stimulation of epidermal proliferation by a specific protein (EGF), Developmental Biol. 12:394, 1965.
16. Turkington, R. W.: The role of epithelial growth factor in mammary gland development in vitro, Exper. Cell Res. 57:79, 1969.
17. Turkington, R. W.: Stimulation of mammary carcinoma cell proliferation by epithelial growth factor in vitro, Cancer Res. 29:1457, 1969.
18. Cohen, S.: Growth Factors and Morphogenic Induction, in M. D. Anderson Tumor Institute: *Developmental and Metabolic Control Mechanisms and Neoplasia* (Baltimore: Williams and Wilkins Co., 1965).
19. Hoober, J. K., and Cohen, S.: Epidermal growth factor. I. The stimulation of protein and nucleic acid synthesis in chick embryo epidermis, Biochim. et biophys. acta 138:347, 1967.
20. Hoober, J. K., and Cohen, S.: Epidermal growth factor. II. Increased activity of ribosomes from chick embryo epidermis for cell-free protein synthesis, Biochim. et biophys. acta 138:357, 1967.
21. Cohen, S., and Stastny, M.: Epidermal growth factor. III. The stimulation of polysome formation in chick embryo epidermis, Biochim. et biophys. acta 166:427, 1968.
22. Stastny, M., and Cohen, S.: Epidermal growth factor. IV. The induction of ornithine decarboxylase, Biochim. et biophys. acta 204:578, 1970.
23. Jänne, J., Raina, A., and Siimes, M.: Mechanism of stimulation of polyamine synthesis by growth hormone in rat liver, Biochim. et biophys. acta 166:419, 1968.
24. Russell, D., and Snyder, S. H.: Amine synthesis in rapidly growing tissues: Ornithine decarboxylase activity in regenerating rat liver, chick embryo, and various tumors. Proc. Nat. Acad. Sc. (U.S.) 60:1420, 1968.

25. Jänne, J., and Raina, A.: On the stimulation of ornithine decarboxylase and RNA polymerase activity in rat liver after treatment with growth hormone, Biochim. et biophys. acta 174:769, 1969.
26. Herbst, E. J., and Bachrach, U. (eds.): Metabolism and biological functions of polyamines, Ann. New York Acad. Sc. 171:691, 1970.
27. Hurwitz, C., and Rosano, C. L.: The intracellular concentration of bound and unbound magnesium ions in *Escherichia coli,* J. Biol. Chem. 242:3719, 1967.
28. Cohen, S., O'Malley, B. W., and Stastny, M.: Estrogenic induction of ornithine decarboxylase in vivo and in vitro, Science 170:336, 1970.
29. Pegg, A. E., Lockwood, D. H., and Williams-Ashman, H. G.: Concentrations of putrescine and polyamines and their enzymic synthesis during androgen-induced prostatic growth, Biochem. J. 117:17, 1970.
30. Sreebny, L. M., and Meyer, J. (eds.): *Salivary Glands and Their Secretions* (New York: The Macmillan Company, 1964).
31. Levi-Montalcini, R., and Angeletti, P. U.: Hormonal Control of the NGF Content in the Submaxillary Salivary Glands of the Mouse, in Sreebny, L. M., and Meyer, J. (eds.): *Salivary Glands and Their Secretions* (New York: The Macmillan Company, 1964).
32. Oliver, W. J., and Gross, F.: Effect of testosterone and duct ligation on submaxillary renin-like principle, Am. J. Physiol. 213:341, 1967.
33. Angeletti, R. A., Angeletti, P. U., and Calissano, P.: Testosterone induction of estero-proteolytic activity in the mouse submaxillary gland, Biochim. et biophys. acta 139:372, 1967.
34. Calissano, P., and Angeletti, P. U.: Testosterone effect on the synthetic rate of two esteropeptidases in the mouse submaxillary gland, Biochim. et biophys. acta 156:51, 1968.
35. Turkington, R. W., Males, J. L., and Cohen, S.: Synthesis and storage of epithelial-epidermal growth factor in submaxillary gland, Cancer Res. 31:253, 1971.
36. Bynny, R. L., Orth, D. N., Cohen, S., Doyne, E. S., and Island, D. P.: Epidermal growth factor radioimmunoassay: Effects of age, androgen, and adrenergic agents on EGF storage and release, J. Clin. Endocrinology 32:A45, 1971.
37. Bynny, R. L., Orth, D. N., Cohen, S., and Island, D. P.: Solid phase radioimmunoassay (RIA) for epidermal growth factor (EGF), Clin. Res. 19:29, 1971.
38. Taylor, J. M.: Epidermal growth factor: High and low molecular weight forms. Doctoral dissertation, Department of Biochemistry, Vanderbilt University, Nashville, Tennessee, 1970.

Much of this work was supported by USPHS grants HD 00700 and FR 06067.

11

Wound Healing and Antler Regeneration

Richard J. Goss, Ph.D. *

Contrary to popular belief, not all mammalian appendages are without the capacity for regeneration. The fact that the vast majority of them do not regenerate testifies to the operation of inhibitory influences, influences which may involve the mechanism of wound healing.

An appendage, by definition, is a protuberance from the body which is covered by skin. Among the lower vertebrates, many of whom are able to replace missing structures, the presence of the skin is essential for regeneration. Skinless limbs in amphibians, for example, if prevented from becoming recovered with epidermis by inserting them into the abdominal cavity, remain incapable of regenerating amputated portions for indefinite periods of time [1]. Only when such limbs are again exteriorized and allowed to heal over with skin is their regenerative ability finally restored. Clearly, the skin is making some indispensable contribution to the regenerative process. This contribution may involve wound healing.

THE ROLE OF WOUND HEALING IN REGENERATION

Two lines of indirect evidence support the contention that wound healing is indispensable for regeneration. The first is that regeneration seldom, if ever, occurs in the absence of wound healing. There are, to be sure, a few kinds of restorative growth which are independent of integumentary wound healing. Lens regeneration in salamanders, for example, is triggered by the removal of the old lens in the absence of any wound to the iris epithelium from which the new lens develops. Similarly, various kinds of compensatory growth in internal organs of the body occur in response to stimuli that do not necessarily require direct traumatization to the reacting tissues. Since none of these tissues is normally enveloped by the integument, it is not surprising that their restoration should be independent of wounds in the skin. During normal ontogeny, of course, the embryo sprouts its appendages without the intervention of an integumentary

---

*Division of Biological and Medical Sciences, Brown University, Providence, Rhode Island.

219

wound. Although the relationship between generation and regeneration is admittedly obscure in these cases, whatever condition may prevail in wound healing may also be shared by the developing limb bud. It is conceivable that the common attribute here could involve an intimate association between epidermis and the underlying mesodermal tissues.

Another line of evidence supporting the hypothesis that wound healing is necessary for regeneration is the results of experiments in which wound healing is precluded. If an amputated stump is sealed off with old skin, then regeneration fails to take place [2]. This suggests that it is not the skin per se which is required for appendage regeneration, but the healing of this skin over the amputated stump. What is it about wound healing over the end of a stump which sets the stage for subsequent regeneration?

Experiments with regenerating newt limbs have emphasized the importance of the apical epidermal cap of cells which is formed in the wound epidermis over the end of an amputated limb [3]. This apical epidermal cap, which becomes heavily innervated, lies in intimate contact with the underlying mesodermal tissues cut through in the process of amputation. It is beneath this cap that a mass of undifferentiated cells accumulates to give rise to the blastema from which the regenerate is ultimately formed. Various experiments indicate that the apical epidermal cap induces the formation of a blastema beneath it, and that it is therefore indispensable for initiating the process of regeneration. Indeed, at any location within a regeneration territory where an adequate nerve supply and a source of competent mesodermal cells are present beneath a wound in the epidermis, there will be established a site of renewed growth. Thus, it is possible to produce accessory limbs by deviating nerves beneath wounds in the skin [4, 5] and also by implanting some kind of irritating material beneath a wound [6]. One is drawn inescapably to the conclusion that a major function of the dermis must be to separate the underlying mesoderm from the overlying epidermis in order to suppress the potential for regeneration that exists everywhere on the surfaces of those appendages which are capable of replacing themselves.

REGENERATION IN MAMMALS

Theories abound as to why birds and mammals are unable to regenerate their appendages, but they are all purely academic in view of our present state of ignorance. Over the years many investigators have attempted with little or no success to induce regeneration in mammalian appendages. It is of some historical interest that Thomas [7], Klintz [8] and von Haffner [9] claimed, with varying degrees of credibility, that the tails of some rodents (especially the dormouse) can regenerate. The nipples of guinea pig and rabbit mammary glands have also been found to undergo limited regeneration [10, 11]. In 1926, Nicholas [12] noted the absence of regeneration in fetal rat digits amputated in utero. Rogal [13], however, unconvincingly claimed that the amputated digits of infant rats would regenerate if their mother had been maintained on diets deficient in vitamins A and D. Equally incredible was the report by Umansky and Kudokotzev [14] that parathyroid hormone, by virtue of its ability to provoke excessive bone destruction, could promote regeneration in the lower arm stumps of 4- to 15-day-old rats. Scharf [15, 16] attempted to delay scar formation in amputated digits of 2-day-old rats (and thereby stimulate regeneration) by the application of trypsin and $CaCl_2$. This approach, however, was no more encouraging than previous ones had been. Schotté and Smith [17, 18] inhibited dermal scar formation in amputated mouse digits by ACTH and cortisone, but their treatments likewise failed to bring about regeneration.

More recently, experiments by Mizell [19, 20] on newborn opossums have met with limited success. Limb amputation of pouch young does not result in regeneration, despite the immaturity of their extremities. However, when central nervous tissue was transplanted to such stumps, outgrowths were produced in some cases. These contained new skeletal elements separate from those in the stump, and possessed short finger-like protuberances. These results are consistent with Singer's theory [21–23] that the loss of regenerative ability may be due to insufficient innervation, a possibility supported by the induction of partial regeneration in the arms of frogs [24] and lizards [25], but not rats [26], following augmentation of their nerve supplies.

In 1965–66, Joseph and Dyson [27, 28] reported that holes 1 cm. square cut through the external ears of rabbits eventually filled in to the point where the aperture was almost completely obliterated. Following initial wound healing around the edges, the surrounding tissues became conspicuously swollen, and during the third week they began to grow in from all sides. This ingrowth continued for the next month or two until the original hole had been reduced in area by averages of 67% and 85% in female and male rabbits, respectively. In two cases, the holes disappeared altogether. This reaction was not attributable to contraction, but was accomplished by the centripetal regeneration of new tissues, including the differentiation of additional cartilage and the development of hair follicles de novo. It has also been found that the regeneration of ear holes is accelerated in rabbits previously subjected to abdominal wounds [29] and that it takes place faster in males than in females [27, 30].

Actually, this phenomenon had been discovered in Moscow in 1953 by Markelova, who described it in her doctoral dissertation. Although Voronzova and Liosner [31] alluded to this work, it seems to have gone either unnoticed or unappreciated by students of regeneration ever since. Preliminary experiments by Grimes and Goss [32] have confirmed that rabbits do indeed regenerate new tissue to fill in holes (up to 1.75 cm. in diameter) punched in their ears. Experience has also shown, however, that mice, rats, guinea pigs, sheep and deer do not regenerate ear tissue.

These studies are reminiscent of the earlier investigations by Clark and Clark [33] on the development of various tissues inside chambers made in rabbit ears fitted with windows. Under these conditions, all tissues except the skin grow in from around the edges of the chamber, and in some cases give rise to cartilage. Similarly, Joseph et al. [34] and Stoll and Furnas [35] have reported the proliferation of new cartilage in the ears of rabbits and guinea pigs at sites from which some of the original cartilage had been removed.

Apropos of hole regeneration in mammals, it is noteworthy that Church and Warren [36] have discovered that full thickness holes 2 cm. in diameter cut in the wing membranes of fruit bats are capable of filling in after only 1 month. This is achieved by a combination of contraction of the surrounding webbing and the production of new tissues at the converging margins of the apertures.

A somewhat similar example has been studied by Taylor and McMinn [37] and Taylor [38] in the case of perforated guinea pig tympanic membranes. These holes may be completely closed in 10 days, although remodeling may go on for 2 months.

ANTLER REGENERATION

Notwithstanding the discouraging prospects for regeneration in mammals in general, the well known annual replacement of antlers in deer justifies a measure of optimism. Here is an example of a histologically complex appendage composed of bone, blood vessels, nerves and skin which regenerates each spring and summer on the frontal pedicles from which the previous year's antlers have been shed. Following closure of the wound over the end of the pedicle, the healing skin rounds up into a bud which rapidly elongates during the succeeding months into a rack of antlers sometimes reaching the length of a meter or more in larger species of deer [39]. These remarkable headpieces grow by the apical proliferation of fibroblasts which subsequently chondrify and ossify as elongation of the shaft progresses. Toward the end of the summer, due to rising levels of testosterone, the bone solidifies, the vascular channels become constricted and the desiccated skin (velvet) peels off. The males are thus provided with dead, bony antlers in time for the autumn mating season, but with the coming of spring the entire process is repeated. During the past few decades this phenomenon has been investigated intensively from the point of view of antler morphogenesis [40], histogenesis [41–44], endocrinology [45–48] and environmental control [49–51].

Skin plays a very important role in antler formation according to the histological investigation of Wislocki [41]. The cells of the dermis may constitute a major source of antler tissues. After the old antlers have been shed, the skin around the upper margin of the pedicle thickens and gives rise to cells which heal over the exposed pedicle bone. Fibroblasts move in beneath the scab, followed by the migration of epidermal tissue from around the edges. Proliferation in the newly healed wound builds up a mass of cells from which the substance of the antler will ultimately differentiate as it grows in length.

Although the histological picture strongly suggests that the dermis may be the source of antler cells, experiments are needed to prove the point one way or the other. It has been shown [40, 52, 53] that if the bone of the pedicle is removed antler regeneration nevertheless takes place. This does not prove that the pedicle bone could not be the source of antler cells, however, because a new pedicle bone may be produced prior to the regeneration of antlers. Similarly, if the skin is removed from the pedicle, it too is replaced, and antler formation still occurs. In fact, one can amputate the entire pedicle without destroying potential sources of antler forming tissues.

The role of epidermis in antler formation has been investigated by Goss [43]. In these experiments, the distal centimeter of pedicle skin was removed, and a hole in the external ear was pulled over the antlers to fit snugly around the circumcised pedicle. The rationale of this experiment was to exclude the epidermis of the pedicle from participating in antler formation. This was achieved by inducing the remaining pedicle epidermis to heal to the inner ear epidermis. Thus, the outer surface of the ear was prevented from healing until such time as the old antler was shed. When this happened, the outer ear epidermis healed over the end of the pedicle. Nevertheless, from such pedicles antlers were produced which were enveloped in epidermis derived originally from the outer surface of the ear. This epidermis shared all the characteristics normally encountered in antler epidermis, including the ability to form new hair follicles and sebaceous glands. One must conclude, therefore, that the specificity of the epidermis is dictated by the nature of the underlying mesodermal tissues.

These mesodermal tissues are particularly important as a potential source of antler cells. To test this possibility, pieces of skin from pedicles and from growing antlers "in velvet" have been grafted to other parts of the body in order to explore the possibility that they might be endowed with the capacity to give rise to antler tissue. Most of these grafts consisted of round "buttons" of skin 1 cm. in diameter punched out with a cork borer. Some, however, were larger pieces, as much as 2 or 3 cm. in diameter. The graft sites were either the surface of the external ear or the front or back of the scalp. The latter locations were less desirable because the deer were more successful in their efforts to dislodge the dressings from such locations. Owing to the flexibility of the ear, it was more difficult for the deer to interfere with the healing of grafts there.

All experiments were carried out on young adult male sika deer *(Cervus nippon)*, except for one fallow deer *(Dama dama)* which was used. Animals were immobilized with succinylcholine chloride (Anectine®) administered intramuscularly with a Cap-chur gun. Supplemental doses were given subcutaneously by hypodermic needle as required during the course of the operations. Regions of the body subjected to surgery were generously injected with xylocaine. Since operations were performed in the field, no attempts were made to be sterile, nor were any required judging from the lack of postoperative infections. To reduce bleeding from pedicles, antlers and ears, rubber tubing was tied tightly around their bases during surgery.

The technique of grafting antler and pedicle skin was as shown in Figure 11-1. The graft site was thoroughly shaved, and a piece of skin the size of the graft was removed. Skin to be transplanted was placed in the previously prepared site after having removed all blood clots. Usually it was unnecessary to suture the edge of the graft to the surrounding skin of the graft site, since neither tended to contract. Using 3-0 silk thread, sutures were placed around the graft site in the intact skin 0.5 to 1.0 cm. from the edge of the graft. Six or eight such sutures were usually sufficient, and the thread was not cut once they were tied in place. Then the graft was smeared with Vaseline, and a wadding of cotton wrapped in gauze was placed over the graft and surrounding skin. The sutures on opposite sides of the graft site were then tied over the cotton so as to exert gentle pressure. This kind of dressing served to press the graft onto the graft bed and to immobilize it with respect to the adjacent tissues. This is important if revascularization is to be achieved. Dressings were left on for two or more weeks, and although not all grafts took, a substantial proportion of successful cases sufficed to yield results.

It was easier to graft skin to the surface of the ear because the tie-over sutures could be passed directly through the full thickness of the ear and around cotton wadding placed over the graft itself and on the opposite side of the ear.

Some grafts appeared to heal in place more successfully than others. In a few

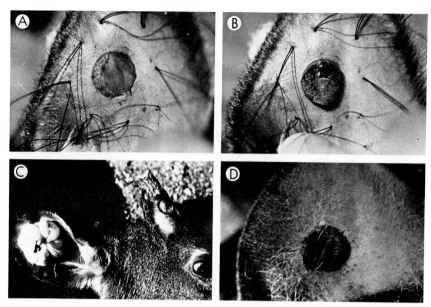

Fig. 11–1.—Stages in the grafting of pedicle skin to inside of external ear. **A,** a circular piece of skin has been removed from the inner surface of the ear in preparation of the graft site (October, 1970). Eight sutures, penetrating the full thickness of the ear, encircle the area. **B,** round piece of pedicle skin, thicker than that on the surrounding ear, in place on graft bed. **C,** completed operation, showing gauze-wrapped cotton dressing held in place over graft by tie-over sutures. Source of graft can be seen on pedicle to the right. **D,** surviving graft the following summer (June, 1971) has grown typical pedicle pelage but shows no signs of developing antler tissue.

cases a desiccated crust of skin on the surface of the graft suggested that the transplant had not survived. Later on, however, such grafts often sprouted hairs and exhibited the texture and pigmentation of the original graft skin. Presumably, enough of the tissue survived to reconstitute the full thickness of the graft in these cases. In all, a total of 8 grafts of antler skin were made during the summer of 1970, of which 6 survived. Of the 12 grafts of skin from the side of the pedicle transplanted during the fall of 1970, 9 survived.

It was anticipated that such grafts might be stimulated to develop into antlers during the spring and summer of 1971 when antler growth was triggered on the ends of the pedicles. However, none of these grafts—neither antler velvet nor pedicle skin, showed signs of developing into antler tissue during the course of the 1971 growing reason (Figs. 11-1D, 11-2A and B). Such negative results might have been expected, however, in view of the fact that the skin that was grafted was derived from the side of the pedicle or shaft of the antler, sites which normally do not sprout antlers. Therefore, it could be argued that the polarity of the skin graft was not conducive to the regeneration of antlers. If this were the case, then it should be possible to bring about heterotopic antler regeneration by grafting skin in such a configuration that it would have a free edge, as in the case of the distal pedicle skin at the time the old antlers are shed. Still another

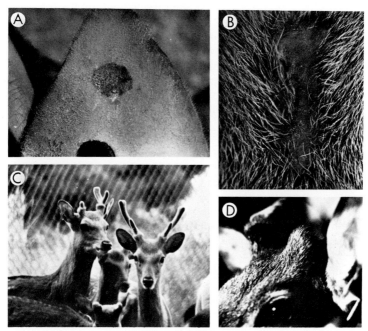

Fig. 11–2.—**A**, graft of antler "velvet" skin on inside of ear, as it appeared in the summer of 1971, one year after transplantation. It can be distinguished by the retention of its original pigmentation, but has failed to grow out as an antler. **B**, a rectangular piece of skin taken from the side of the shaft of an antler was grafted onto the forehead. The following summer, as seen here, it remained unchanged. **C**, the deer on the left is growing an abortive antler from his right pedicle because a flap of pedicle skin was sutured over its end prior to the antler-growing season. **D**, this deer's left pedicle has grown no antler at all as a result of its having been sealed over with a skin flap.

reason why the grafts did not give rise to antlers may have been the absence of a wound. With the exception of the initial antler bud produced by a yearling fawn, antlers originate from the wound which is healed over the ends of the pedicles. It would seem, therefore, that future experiments along these lines will have to take into account the configuration and polarity of the skin graft and must also make provision for the existence of a free edge at the margin of a wound.

In order to determine if an antler can grow in the absence of a wound on the end of its pedicle, 5 deer were subjected to the following operations on their pedicles. In each animal one of the pedicles was shaved and the skin slit longitudinally about halfway down one side. The rest of the skin was carefully separated from the underlying bone around its entire circumference and peeled back out of the way. The bone was then sawed through at a level approximately halfway from the base to the tip of the pedicle, being careful not to mutilate the skin any more than was necessary. This done, the distal skin, which had previously been separated from the bone, was folded over the stump of the pedicle. Excess flaps of skin were trimmed off and the part that fitted over the amputated stump of the pedicle was then sutured in place. These operations were done on different deer at various times from late autumn through the spring, but in all cases well before the antlers were due to be shed. The opposite unoperated pedicles in each case served as controls. Previous experiments have shown that pedicles amputated below the base are nevertheless capable of regenerating antlers [40].

With the advent of the antler growing season, these pedicles failed to produce normal antlers. The full thickness pedicle skin which was sutured over the end of the pedicle did not become involved in the production of antlers. At best, only small abortive antlers sprouted from the corners of these pedicles where the flap of skin had not healed completely to the opposite side (Fig. 11-2C). In one deer, antler growth was completely inhibited (Fig. 11-2D). The 4 others produced antlers measuring from 1.5 to 13 cm. in length, none of which was branched. The difficulty in suppressing antler growth altogether in these experiments testifies to the strong tendency for their regeneration to take place wherever even a small interruption exists in the skin covering the end of the pedicle. In all cases in which antler regeneration was not completely suppressed, the outgrowth formed on the sutured side of the pedicle. Thus, as in other regenerating systems, the existence of a healing wound seems to be a prerequisite for antler development. These results, therefore, indicate that it is not so much the skin itself as it is the healing of an integumentary wound which is so essential for the onset of antler regeneration. It is as significant as it is gratifying that what holds true for the antler is consistent with what is known of most other vertebrate regenerating systems.

SUMMARY

Regeneration can occur in selected mammalian structures, not the least of which are deer antlers. To explore their histogenesis, pieces of skin from antlers "in velvet", or from their pedicles, were grafted to the scalp or ears. Although 75% of these transplants survived through the following summer, none gave rise to new antler tissue. Even the pedicles themselves, from which new antlers normally grow each year, can be prevented from producing antlers if their distal ends are closed over with full thickness skin. Only where a wound is allowed to heal on the pedicle can an antler develop. It is concluded that, as in other vertebrate appendages, regeneration must be initiated in the healing of an integumentary wound.

ACKNOWLEDGMENTS

I am indebted to Mr. Dion Albach, Director of the Roger Williams Park Zoo in Providence, for his generous cooperation in caring for the deer during the course of these experiments. My thanks also to Miss Angela Masso for technical assistance, and to a number of my students who, from time to time, were good enough to lend a hand when the deer were more than one man could handle. This research has been supported by NSF research grant GB-20166.

REFERENCES

1. Goss, R. J.: Regenerative inhibition following limb amputation and immediate insertion into the body cavity, Anat. Rec. 126:15, 1956.

2. Godlewski, E.: Untersuchungen über Auslösung und Hemmung der Regeneration beim Axolotl, Arch. Entw.-Mech. 114:108, 1928.
3. Thornton, C. S.: The effect of apical cap removal on limb regeneration in *Amblystoma* larvae, J. Exper. Zool. 134:357, 1957.
4. Guyénot, E., Dinichert-Favarger, J., and Galland, M.: L'exploration du territoire de la patte anterieure du *Triton,* Rev. Suisse Zool. 55:1, 1948.
5. Kiortsis, V.: Potentialités du territoire patte chez le Triton (adultes, larves, embryons), Rev. Suisse Zool. 60:301, 1953.
6. Ruben, L. N., and Stevens, J. M.: Post-embryonic induction into urodele limbs, J. Morph. 112:279, 1963.
7. Thomas, O.: Regeneration of the tail of mice, Proc. Zool. Soc. London 1905:491, 1905.
8. Klintz, J. H.: Experimentelle Schwanzregeneration bei Bilchen (Myoxidae) und einigen anderen Säugern, Arch. Entw.-Mech. 40:343, 1914.
9. von Haffner, K.: Ergebnisse der histologischen Untersuchung der von E. Mohr beschriebenen Schwanzregenerate von Myoxiden (Bilchen), Zool. Anz. 135:66, 1941.
10. Markelova, I. V.: Regeneration of amputated nipples in guinea pigs, Doklady Akad. Nauk SSSR 72(1):221, 1950.
11. Markelova, I. V.: Regeneration of nipples in rabbits, Biull. Eksp. Biol., Med. 33(6):58, 1952.
12. Nicholas, J. S.: Extirpation experiments upon the embryonic rat, Proc. Soc. Exper. Biol. & Med. 23:436, 1926.
13. Rogal, I. G.: The possibility of regeneration of extremities in rats, Doklady Akad. Nauk SSSR 78:161, 1951.
14. Umanski, E. E., and Kudokotzev, V. P.: Stimulation of the process of regeneration in the mammalian extremity under the action of the parathyroid hormone, Doklady Akad. Nauk SSSR 86:437, 1952.
15. Scharf, A.: Experiments on regenerating rat digits, Growth 25:7, 1961.
16. Scharf, A.: Reorganization of cornified nail-like outgrowths related with the wound healing process of the amputation sites of young rat digits, Growth 27:255, 1963.
17. Schotté, O. E., and Smith, C. B.: Wound healing processes in amputated mouse digits, Biol. Bull. 117:546, 1959.
18. Schotté, O. E., and Smith, C. B.: Effects of ACTH aud of cortisone upon amputational wound healing processes in mice digits, J. Exper. Zool. 146:209, 1961.
19. Mizell, M.: Limb regeneration: Induction in the newborn opossum, Science 161:283, 1968.
20. Mizell, M., and Isaacs, J. J.: Induced regeneration of hindlimbs in the newborn opossum, Am. Zool. 10:141, 1970.
21. Singer, M.: Nervous mechanisms in the regeneration of body parts in vertebrates, in Rudnick, D. (ed.): *Developing Cell Systems and Their Control* (New York: Ronald Press Co., 1960).
22. Singer, M.: The Trophic Quality of the Neuron: Some Theoretical Considerations, in Singer, M., and Schadé, J. P. (eds.): *Progress in Brain Research: Mechanisms of Neural Regeneration* (Amsterdam: Elsevier Press, Inc., 1964).
23. Singer, M.: Some Quantitative Aspects Concerning the Trophic Role of the Nerve Cell, in Mesarovíc, M. D. (ed.): *Systems Theory and Biology* (New York: Springer-Verlag, 1968).
24. Singer, M.: Induction of regeneration of forelimb of the frog by augmentation of the nerve supply, Proc. Soc. Exper. Biol. & Med. 76:413, 1951.
25. Simpson, S. B.: Induction of limb regeneration in the lizard, *Lygosoma laterale,* by augmentation of the nerve supply, Proc. Soc. Exper. Biol. & Med. 107:108, 1961.
26. Bar-Maor, J. A., and Gitlin, G.: Attempted induction of forelimb regeneration by augmentation of nerve supply in young rats, Transpl. Bull. 27:460, 1961.
27. Joseph, J., and Dyson, M.: Sex differences in the rate of tissue regeneration in the rabbit's ear, Nature 208:599, 1965.

28. Joseph, J., and Dyson, M.: Tissue replacement in the rabbit's ear, Brit. J. Surg. 53:372, 1966.
29. Joseph, J., and Dyson, M.: The effect of abdominal wounding on the rate of tissue regeneration, Experientia 26:66, 1970.
30. Dyson, M., and Joseph, J.: The effect of androgens on tissue regeneration, J. Anat. 103:491, 1968.
31. Vorontsova, M. A., and Liosner, L. D.: *Asexual Propagation and Regeneration* (Oxford: Pergamon Press, 1960).
32. Grimes, L. N., and Goss, R. J.: Regeneration of holes in rabbit ears, Am. Zool. 10:537, 1970.
33. Clark, E. R., and Clark, E. L.: Microscopic observations on new formations of cartilage and bone in the living mammal, Am. J. Anat. 70:167, 1942.
34. Joseph, J., Thomas, G. A., and Tynen, J.: The reaction of the ear cartilage of the rabbit and guinea-pig to trauma, J. Anat. 95:564, 1961.
35. Stoll, D. A., and Furnas, D. W.: The growth of cartilage transplants in baby rabbits, Plast. & Reconstruct. Surg. 45:356, 1970.
36. Church, J. C. T., and Warren, D. J.: Wound healing in the web membrane of the fruit bat, Brit. J. Surg. 55:26, 1968.
37. Taylor, M., and McMinn, R. M. H.: Healing of experimental perforations of the tympanic membrane, J. Laryng. & Otol. 79:148, 1965.
38. McMinn, R. M. H., and Taylor, M.: The cytology of repair in experimental perforations of the tympanic membrane, Brit. J. Surg. 53:222, 1966.
39. Goss, R. J.: Problems of antlerogenesis, Clin. Orthop. 69:227, 1970.
40. Goss, R. J.: Experimental investigations of morphogenesis in the growing antler, J. Embryol. & Exper. Morph. 9:342, 1961.
41. Wislocki, G. B.: Studies on the growth of deer antlers. I. On the structure and histogenesis of the antlers of the Virginia deer (Odocoileus virginianus borealis), Am. J. Anat. 71:371, 1942.
42. Wislocki, G. B., and Waldo, C. M.: Further observations on the histological changes associated with the shedding of the antlers of the white-tailed deer (Odocoileus virginianus borealis), Anat. Rec. 117:353, 1953.
43. Goss, R. J.: The Role of Skin in Antler Regeneration, in Montagna, W., and Billingham, R. E. (eds.): *Advances in Biology of Skin,* Vol. 5, *Wound Healing* (Oxford: Pergamon Press, 1964).
44. Goss, R. J., Severinghaus, C. W., and Free, S.: Tissue relationships in the development of pedicles and antlers in the Virginia deer, J. Mammal. 45:61, 1964.
45. Wislocki, G. B., Aub, J. C., and Waldo, C. M.: The effects of gonadectomy and the administration of testosterone propionate on the growth of antlers in male and female deer, Endocrinol. 40:202, 1947.
46. Tachezy, R.: Über den Einfluss der Sexualhormone auf das Geweihwachstum der Cerviden, Säugetierkundliche Mitteilungen 4:103, 1956.
47. Goss, R. J.: The Deciduous Nature of Deer Antlers, in Sognnaes, R. (ed.): *Mechanisms of Hard Tissue Destruction* (Washington: AAAS Publication No. 75, 1963).
48. Goss, R. J.: Inhibition of growth and shedding of antlers by sex hormones, Nature 220:83, 1968.
49. Jaczewski, Z.: The effect of changes in length of daylight on the growth of antlers in the deer (*Cervus elaphus* L.), Folia Biol. 2:133, 1954.
50. Goss, R. J.: Photoperiodic control of antler cycles in deer. I. Phase shift and frequency changes, J. Exper. Zool. 170:311, 1969.
51. Goss, R. J.: Photoperiodic control of antler cycles in deer. II. Alterations in amplitude, J. Exper. Zool. 171:223, 1969.
52. Bubenik, A., and Pavlansky, R.: Von Welchem Gewebe geht der eigentliche Reiz zur Geweihentwicklung aus? III. Mitteilung: Operative Eingriffe am Bastgeweih, Saugetierkundliche Mitteilungen 7:157, 1959.
53. Bubenik, A. B., and Pavlansky, R.: Trophic responses to trauma in growing antlers, J. Exper. Zool. 159:289, 1965.

Part V

Physical and Chemical Factors Affecting Repair

Introduction

Thomas K. Hunt, M.D. *

Part V of this volume continues the emphasis on environmental conditions affecting wound healing and wound infection.

Silver's contribution on oxygen tensions in epithelium before and after injury dramatically emphasized the wide varieties of microclimates found across inert films, eschars and in wounded tissues. Obviously, epithelium exposed to air and liable to drying must proliferate and migrate under hostile conditions. Discussants commented that epithelium prepares for hypoxia by enhancing enzymes of glycolytic metabolism in the initial response to injury and that glycogen stored at the wound edge is used for energy during the migratory process. Oxygen, however, is only one of many potentially important environmental components.

Bothwell reported faster healing in humid climates. This relates well to studies reported earlier in this volume which show that epithelization is faster under water impermeable films.

Bhaskar's enthusiastic report on the use of hemostatic adhesives in oral surgery implies that hemostasis, fixation and coverage by the n-butyl isomer of cyanoacrylate glues provides an ideal environment for healing in the oral cavity. The oral cavity with its constant contamination and its extremely good blood supply may be relatively unique, however, and he cautioned specifically against the use of adhesives in deep wounds where the agent would form a barrier to fibrous union.

Obviously, one hesitates before generalizing on the clinical applicability of environmental control. Plastic films seem to benefit superficial wounds. Yet, even there, further qualification seems necessary. Marple's report on enhancing dermal infectability by stripping injury followed by an inert film occlusion demonstrates that an environment favorable for epidermal cells is also favorable for bacteria.

Waterman's report documented that prophylactic antibiotic irrigation of closed wounds has not been effective. His summary of the literature disclosed a wide variety of results from a variety of experimental designs. His analysis of

---

*Associate Professor of Surgery, University of California School of Medicine, San Francisco, California.

231

experimental conditions facing investigators in this field again emphasized the importance of environmental factors.

Garcia-Velasco reported his studies on keloids and hypertrophic scars. He reported favorable results from intralesional injection of anti-inflammatory steroids.

12

The Effect of Tissue Adhesives on Buccal Wounds

S. N. Bhaskar, D.D.S., Ph.D.*

A family of chemical adhesives with the formula of $CH = C (CN) - COOR$ has the ability to cement moist living tissues and act as hemostatic agents [1, 2]. When embedded in deep tissues they become phagocytosed but are not completely removed from the site of implantation [3, 4]. These materials applied on the surface of wounded skin or mucous membrane act as protective layers and become exfoliated when the underlying tissues heal [5–9]. In a series of studies by the author it was found that of all the cyanoacrylates available, the butyl and the isobutyl were the most acceptable [2–12] because of their physical as well as their biological properties. It has also been shown that an application of the drug can be completed in an average only of 3/10 of a second [8]. When these drugs are used in the oral cavity, it was found that they do not become aspirated and cause no undesirable effects [13]. Administration of butyl and isobutyl cyanoacrylates in animals in dosages which were 36 and almost 1000 times those used in man produced no systemic effects [8] and when applied to the surface of experimentally infected wounds they do not encourage the growth of organisms [14]. Applications of butyl cyanoacrylate and isobutyl cyanoacrylate in the human oral cavity in more than 1000 instances has not produced any evidence of immediate or delayed sensitivity [15]. In addition to the use of these drugs in the management of oral soft tissue wounds they have been found to be effective in providing temporary coverage of wounds which require delayed closure [16]. Their effectiveness has also been successfully demonstrated in the protection of exposed and unexposed dental pulp tissue [17–20].

Therefore, the isobutyl and butyl cyanoacrylates are excellent surface dressings for oral wounds for the following reasons:

1. Quick application uneffected by the presence of saliva or blood in the wound.

2. Bacteriostatic properties.

3. Secondary applications can be made without removing the old dressing.

4. When the tissues heal the dressings are spontaneously desquamated.

---
*Col., DC, Director, United States Army Institute of Dental Research, Walter Reed Army Medical Center, Washington, D.C.

5. Clinically, patients have less postoperative pain, edema or swelling. Postoperative biopsies taken in more than 300 patients do not reveal any implantation of the material in deep tissues.

6. Compared to other methods of dressing oral wounds, these drugs are much easier to apply.

Because of the reasons given above, the butyl and isobutyl cyanoacrylate are used routinely in a number of oral surgical procedures.

Fig. 12–1.—Low **(A)** and high **(B)** power photomicrographs of a bisected rat tongue. Note the marked edema and neutrofil infiltration.

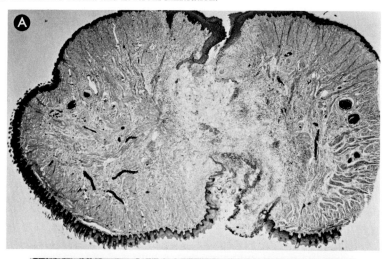

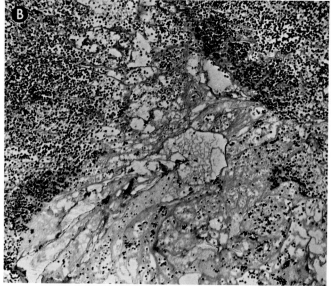

HISTOLOGIC CHANGES ASSOCIATED WITH CHEMICAL ADHESIVES

Animal studies have been conducted on the tissue response to the methyl, ethyl, propyl, butyl, isobutyl, hexyl, heptyl and octyl cyanoacrylates. These show that with the exception of the methyl cyanoacrylate all of these materials are within the acceptable range biologically. The relative incompatibility of methyl cyanoacrylate, in comparison to other materials tested, may be due to the fact that it rapidly degrades to formaldehyde which in turn produces the severe tissue response seen in the area. Of the other cyanoacrylates tested, the butyl and the isobutyl cyanoacrylate were found to be most acceptable based on the fact that they appeared to produce the minimal amount of edema, neutrophil infiltration, necrosis and granulation tissue.

When the methyl cyanoacrylate is used as an adhesive agent the implant site shows severe edema, neutrophil infiltration and necrosis (Fig. 12-1). The interface between the tissue and the drug is ill-defined and the healing is delayed. With higher homologues, such as the isobutyl and butyl cyanoacrylate, the interface at the wound site does not evidence necrosis or severe edema. Inflammatory infiltrate is minimal and connective tissue ingrowth into the incision line occurs rapidly (Fig. 12-2). When these materials are experimentally or accidentally inplanted in deep tissues they undergo partial phagocytosis and in part may be sequestrated from the mucosal surface (Fig. 12-3). Since there is no certainty that a deep implant of this material would be completely eliminated, the recommended use of these adhesives is limited to the surface application.

On skin wounds, the cyanoacrylate dressing reduces the degree and duration of inflammatory response [12]. The reduction of inflammatory exudate is apparently due to the fact that cyanoacrylate forms an adhesive covering on the wound and protects it from secondary infection. It appears most likely that the improved clinical reaction (reduced pain, swelling, edema) seen following use of these adhesives is related to the reduction of the inflammatory response.

APPLICATIONS IN HUMAN ORAL WOUNDS

These drugs have been successfully employed in a number of oral surgical procedures.

Gingivectomy. The usual periodontal dressings applied after a gingivectomy are bulky and difficult to retain. They retract on hardening and thus lead to the collection of saliva and food debris underneath them, and stimulate the formation of exuberant granulation tissue. In view of these problems cyanoacrylates are an ideal dressing after gingivectomy. As soon as the material is applied as a spray or on a piece of gauze, the bleeding stops immediately (Fig. 12-4). On the attached gingiva (which is firm and nonmobile) the dressing lasts from 4 to 7 days. In 7 days healing is far advanced and usually no additional dressing is necessary. Follow-up studies on these patients for up to 4 years have failed to reveal any undesirable effects. As a matter of fact it is the clinical impression of more than one dentist that the healing under the cyanoacrylate is faster than under conventional dressings.

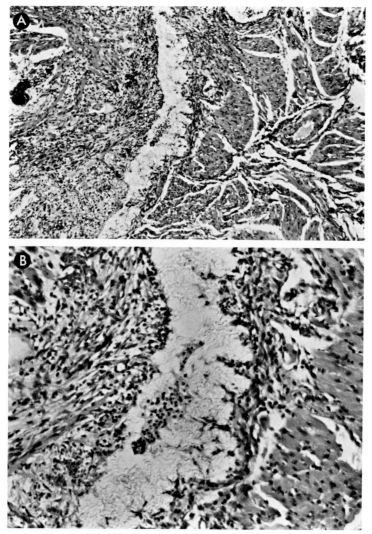

Fig. 12–2.—Low **(A)** and high **(B)** power photomicrographs of a bisected rat tongue held together with butyl cyanoacrylate. Note the minimal inflammatory response.

Gingivoplasty. Application of adhesives in gingivoplasty procedure and the findings are identical to those described for gingivectomy.

Mucogingival Surgery. In mucogingival surgery a full thickness mucoperiosteal flap is usually raised from the bone and after removing the periodontal defects the flap is repositioned at a predetermined position. Usually this procedure not only requires a number of peripheral and interproximal sutures but in addition it is necessary to "dress" these areas with one of a variety of so called "perio-

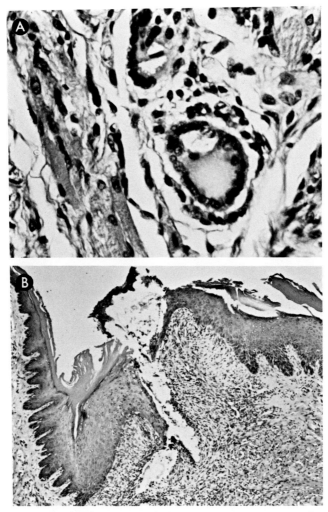

Fig. 12–3.—**A**, giant cell in an area of isobutyl cyanoacrylate implant showing phagocytosed material. **B**, sequestration of cyanoacrylate at the suture line.

dontal packs". In a series of studies involving this surgical procedure, the mucogingival flaps were repositioned with one or two retaining sutures, the flap held in place as desired, and the area was sprayed or covered with isobutyl cyanoacrylate. Clinical observations have shown that the use of this material enhances the reparative processes and is certainly far more convenient for the patient and the operator.

In mucogingival surgery there are occasions when a portion of the alveolar bone has to be left uncovered. In these cases the isobutyl cyanoacrylate was applied as usual and it did not cause any undesirable reaction. Healing progressed as expected. This however is not surprising because in a series of studies

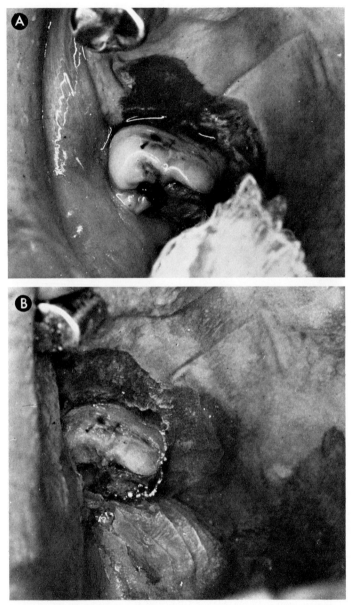

Fig. 12–4.—A, photograph of a surgical site around an upper molar tooth. B, surgical site shown in A after the application of the adhesive.

on the monkey and the rat the acceptability of these materials has been demonstrated.

Pedicle Grafts. One of the surgical procedures performed in the oral cavity consists of removing a full thickness pedicle gingival graft from one part of the mouth and stabilizing it over a denuded tooth surface. This graft requires a number of interproximal sutures as well as a periodontal surgical dressing. Isobutyl cyanoacrylate has been employed in these cases with remarkable success. In this procedure, after the pedicle graft has been moved to the recipient site a single suspensory suture is put around the area and the graft is pressed in place for two minutes. Upon removal of the compression the area is immediately sprayed with the adhesive. Following this, a small piece of gauze inpregnated with isobutyl cyanoacrylate is placed over the wound. The procedure has been consistently successful.

Free Grafts. Free mucosal grafts in the oral cavity are used for a variety of reasons. Essentially the procedure consists of removing tissue from one part of the mouth and placing it at a recipient site. As a rule, the graft requires numerous sutures for adequate stabilization. Since the grafts are of very small size it takes a great deal of time and dexterity. Under the currently employed procedures, suturing the area is followed by the use of a surgical dressing which in turn is protected by tinfoil or rubber dam. The technique is therefore cumbersome and time consuming.

Using isobutyl cyanoacrylate a series of free grafts has been successfully established in human patients. After the graft is placed in the recipient site the area is merely sprayed with adhesive without any sutures. In this particular procedure the operator can cut down the surgical time from 45 to less than 20 minutes.

Surgery on the Palate. On surgical and biopsy sites of the palate it is difficult or impossible to place an adequate surgical dressing. The use of the cyanoacrylates however makes it easy to cover these areas.

Extraction Wounds. One of the complications in dental extractions is the loss of the blood clot and subsequent development of alveolar osteitis. This condition is referred to as the "dry socket". Isobutyl cyanoacrylate has been employed as a dressing following surgical removal of teeth. After a tooth has been extracted the surrounding tissue is sutured, if necessary, and the socket is allowed to fill with blood. At this time, a piece of gauze inpregnated with isobutyl cyanoacrylate is placed upon the wound. *Extraction wounds however should not be sprayed* in order to prevent the incorporation of the adhesive in the socket.

SUMMARY

This report deals with a summation of a series of studies with chemical adhesives of the cyanoacrylate group. Studies done on a number of species of animals and on man show that the butyl and isobutyl cyanoacrylates are excellent surface dressings for orofacial wounds.

REFERENCES

1. Coover, H. W., Jr., *et al.*: Chemistry and Performance of cyanoacrylate adhesives, Soc. Plastic Eng. J. 15:413, 1959.

2. Bhaskar, S. N., Jacoway, J. R., Margetis, P. M., Leonard, F., and Pani, K. C.: Oral tissue response to chemical adhesive (cyanoacrylates), Oral Surg. 22:394, 1966.
3. Bhaskar, S. N., Frisch, J., Margetis, P. M., and Leonard, F.: Application of a new chemical adhesive in periodontics and oral surgery, Oral Surg. 22:526, 1966.
4. Bhaskar, S. N., Frisch, J., Margetis, P. M., and Leonard, F.: Response of rat tongue to hextyl, heptyl and octyl cyanoacrylates, Oral Surg. 24:137, 1967.
5. Bhaskar, S. N., and Frisch, J.: Free mucosal graft with tissue adhesive; Report of 17 cases, J. Perio. 39:190, 1967.
6. Bhaskar, S. N., Frisch, J., and Cutright, D. E.: Effect of butyl cyanoacrylate on the healing of extraction wounds, Oral Surg. 24:604, 1967.
7. Bhaskar, S. N.: Butyl Cyanoacrylate as a Surface in Human Oral Wounds, Amer. Assoc. Advanc. Sci., Symposium, 1967.
8. Bhaskar, S. N.: Use of normal butyl cyanoacrylate in the oral cavity; Experimental and clinical studies, *Annual Report to the R&D Command,* Army Medical Service, Dept. of the Army, 1968.
9. Bhaskar, S. N., and Frisch, J.: Use of cyanoacrylate adhesives in dentistry, J.A.D.A. 77:831, 1968.
10. Bhaskar, S. N.: Tissue response of rat tongue to normal and isobutyl cyanoacrylate, Oral Surg. 26:573, 1968.
11. Bhaskar, S. N., Frisch, J., and Margetis, P. M.: Tissue response to a butyl cyanoacrylate containing dental cement, J. Dent. Res. 48:57, 1969.
12. Bhaskar, S. N., and Cutright, D. E.: Healing of skin wounds under a butyl cyanoacrylate dressing, J. Dent. Res. 48:294, 1969.
13. Bhaskar, S. N., Cutright, D. E., and Beasley, J. D.: Oral spray of isobutyl cyanoacrylate and its systemic effect, Oral Surg. 29:313, 1969.
14. Beasley, J. D., Bhaskar, S. N., Gross, A., and Cutright, D. E.: Effect of antibiotics and chemical adhesives on infected wounds, (In press).
15. Bhaskar, S. N.: Unpublished Data.
16. Hunsuck, E. E., Cutright, D. E., and Bhaskar, S. N.: Modified delayed closure of facial wounds with isobutyl cyanoacrylate, Oral Surg. 29:305, 1969.
17. Bhaskar, S. N., Cutright, D. E., Boyers, R. C., and Margetis, P.M. Pulp capping with isobutyl cyanoacrylate, J.A.D.A. 79:639, 1969.
18. Bhaskar, S. N., Cutright, D. E., Beasley, J. D., and Boyers, R. C.: Pulpal response to four restorative materials, Oral Surg. 28:126, 1969.
19. Levin, M. P., and Cucolo, F. I.: Pulpal response of isobutyl cyanoacrylate in human deciduous teeth, Int. Assn. Dent. Res., Supplement 48:180.
20. Bhaskar, S. N., and Ward, J. P.: Pulp capping with isobutyl cyanoacrylate, Int. Assn. Dent. Res., Supplement 48:180.

13

Bacterial Infection of Superficial Wounds:
A Human Model for *Staphylococcus Aureus*

Richard R. Marples, B.M., M.Sc.* and
Albert M. Kligman, M.D., Ph.D.*

Skin which is covered with an intact epidermis probably very rarely becomes infected since no crevices exist which would enable microbes to enter deeper tissues. Moreover virulent organisms do not ordinarily find conditions on the intact surface suitable for multiplication and no matter how many cells arrive they cannot become established and soon disappear. The establishment of an infection requires a physical breach of the integument. Experience with *S. aureus,* the commonest cause of wound infections, great and small, has indicated that breaking through the epidermal barrier is by itself rarely sufficient. In fact, experimenters have had extraordinary difficulties in producing cutaneous infections. Many investigators [1, 2] tried to transmit impetigo but success was not frequent. Elek and Conen [3] found it necessary to inject more than a million organisms intradermally to create even a transient pustule. Maibach applied large numbers of cells to skin traumatized in a variety of ways but infections rarely followed [4]. Duncan's success rate of about 30% does not seem impressive in the light of the exceptional circumstances required [5]. Undiluted broth cultures were applied to stab wounds of the lower legs and covered with an impermeable dressing for several days. Elsewhere on the body the infection rates were even lower.

In our laboratories Singh and co-workers finally did develop a technique for creating *S. aureus* infections consistently, without traumatizing the skin [6]. The cells were applied to degermed normal skin kept moist under an occlusive dressing for at least 3 days. The importance of eliminating bacterial competitors was a key finding in that study. Nonetheless, takes were uncommon when less than 10^5 organisms per square centimeter were applied. In the developing infection, the organisms reached levels of $10^7/cm.^2$ in about 5 days. They did not invade the tissue but elaborated diffusible toxic products which provoked a papulo-pustular irritant dermatitis.

---

*Department of Dermatology, University of Pennsylvania School of Medicine, Philadelphia, Pennsylvania.

The circumstances necessary to induce such infections are entirely artificial and do not obtain in real life. One cannot imagine a situation where hundreds of thousands of organisms would congregate in a small area. Yet everyone knows that many kinds of minor skin trauma may be followed by infection: abrasions, cuts, burns, insect bites, scratches, etc. Somehow these trivial insults to the integument create an opportunity for few organisms to undergo unrestrained multiplication.

Our objective was to develop a realistic human model for studying infections of superficially wounded skin. We elected to use the technique of stripping away the horny layer barrier with cellophane tape—a simple procedure which has been of inestimable value in dermatologic investigations of many kinds [7]. It is important to realize that stripping does more than remove the stratum corneum; it damages the viable epidermis much more than originally believed. The retraction of desmosomes into the cytoplasm enables the intercellular spaces to become distended with fluid from leaky dermal vessels [8]. A burst of mitotic activity occurs which reaches a peak at about 48 hours. Diffusional water loss is very high but the formation of a parakeratotic layer provides a temporary barrier which even 24 hours later is much less permeable [9]. The anatomic regeneration of a new horny layer takes about 10 days.

METHODS

Subjects. The subjects were healthy adult male prisoner volunteers, accepted only after the following laboratory tests were found to be normal: CBC, urinalysis, SGOT and fasting blood sugar.

Stripping. Up to four sites were marked out on the forearm and the stratum corneum removed with cellophane tape until the glistening layer was reached. Two assistants alternately applied 1 inch wide strips of cellophane tape at right angles preparing thereby a square area with a moist surface. The strips were firmly applied and briskly ripped off since we wished to promote transudation of serum. A period of twenty-four hours was usually permitted to elapse before inoculation.

Inoculation. A non-typable skin strain of *S. aureus* susceptible to all common antibiotics was used throughout. Cells from an overnight surface growth on Trypticase Soy Agar were suspended in saline to form a turbid suspension. This was diluted till just hazy. Volumetric dilutions were prepared from the latter. The number of viable cells per ml. was established by counting in culture [6].

A volume of 0.01 ml. was applied by micropipette to the stripped skin which was then covered with a 2 cm. square of poly(vinylidine chloride) film (Saran Wrap®). This was sealed to the skin under regular cloth adhesive tape (Zonas Brand®). The latter does not allow the growth of organisms beneath it [10].

Assessment of Bacterial Growth. The quantitative detergent scrub technique was used in the initial phase of this study [11]. The method for estimating the number of aerobic organisms per cm.² has been described previously. Later, the procedure was simplified by using touch plates containing selective and nonselective media. The density of growth in the center of 4 sq. cm. was estimated on a 6-point scale [12]:

0	10 colonies
+	10–100 colonies
++	more than 100 colonies
+++	some colonies touching
++++	growth not quite confluent
+++++	confluent growth

Cytological Study. After 24 hours of occlusion clean slides were applied to the stripped surface or to the contact side of the Saran film. The limits of the area under plastic film were marked on the back of each slide which was stained with May Grunwald-Giemsa for study of leukocytes and bacteria.

Clinical Evaluation. The sites were scored on a 5-point scale based upon the intensity of erythema and suppuration twenty-four hours after inoculation. The estimates were in relation to the appearance of uninoculated stripped sites which were somewhat reddened and moist but usually not suppurative. All but the mildest infection evoked a thin serosanguineous exudate over a strongly erythematous base. Grade 5 infections showed ulceration and extension beyond the inoculation site.

RESULTS

Bacteriological and Clinical Effects in Stripped Sites

The procedure finally adopted was to delay inoculation for one day after stripping and then to apply an occlusive dressing for 24 hours only. One must also have an appreciation of what happens in uninoculated stripped sites.

Uninoculated Sites. When left unoccluded resident organisms, chiefly coagulase negative staphylococci, were present on the stripped site but in lower numbers than the surrounding normal skin only in the first 24 hours. Microbial numbers then rose above control levels by the second or third day and thereafter slowly declined. Rarely, perhaps once in fifty subjects a spontaneous *S. aureus* infection occurred during the unoccluded 24 hour waiting period, this being clinically evident by tenderness, greater redness and a moist exudate. *S. aureus* is obviously plentiful in the particular environment where the experiments were carried out. In the absence of infection the sites rapidly lost redness, developed a brownish leathery crust and healed without scarring.

When a site stripped one day earlier was occluded without inoculation its appearance 24 hours later showed a mild reddish-brown color and a moist shiny surface. Again, and somewhat more frequently, spontaneous infection could occur during this 24 hour period. *S. aureus* was the usual invader but various gram-negative organisms usually enterobacteria sometimes became established. Spontaneous infections were much more frequent when uninoculated stripped sites were occluded immediately after stripping. Twenty-six sites were studied in this way. *S. aureus* became dominant in 5 and was recovered in moderate numbers in another five sites. Enterobacteria dominated the flora in one site and were present in 4 others. *Pseudomonas* was recovered in moderate numbers from one site. Coagulase negative staphylococci were overwhelmingly the dominant organism in 20 cases. Diphtheroids, common members of the normal flora were rare on stripped sites. In this series clinically apparent infection (grade +++) occurred

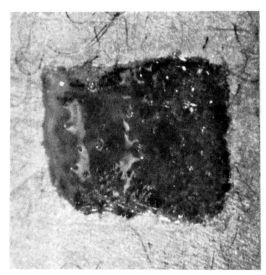

Fig. 13–1.—Infected lesion. *S. aureus* inoculated 24 hours after stripping. Note the seropurulent exudate and ulcerated base.

but once in a site which yielded 8×10^6 *S. aureus* per sq. cm. and no other organisms. An exudate was seen in touch smears only three times, from the site containing *Pseudomonas,* the *S. aureus* infection and, inexplicably, from a site which yielded only a modest number of resident coagulase negative cocci on culture.

Occlusion immediately after stripping thus sometimes led to abnormal bacterial populations and to actual clinical infections. By delaying the occlusion for one day, there was uneventful recolonization on the site by resident skin organisms. As a consequence, uninoculated stripped sites occluded 24 hours later could serve as negative controls.

Inoculated Sites. *S. aureus* produced characteristic clinical changes within 24 hours when sites were inoculated and occluded one day after stripping.

Most sites were distinctly moist. A visible exudate, usually serosanguineous, but occasionally purulent was also present (Fig. 13-1). In mild infections, touch smears were more informative of the presence of numerous leukocytes than naked eye evaluation. In more severe infections the exudate was often purulent and copious enough to seep out around the occlusive dressing. Sometimes a red and tender lesion developed with multiple small erosions, occasionally culminating in ulceration. Edema, as a rule, was not prominent. Ordinarily tenderness was too great to permit standard scrubbing for quantifying bacteria. Light scrubbing often accentuated epidermal denudation and a serous exudate rapidly reappeared. After removal of the occlusive patch most sites rapidly dried up and healing followed promptly. Because a few lesions did not respond in this way it became our practice to treat each site with a neomycin cream (Neosporin®) twice daily for 2 days.

When occlusion was maintained for 2 days instead of one the lesion usually did

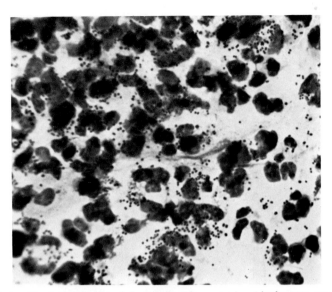

Fig. 13–2.—Contact slide of an infected site. Many cocci and leukocytes are present.

not become much more inflamed. Nonetheless, severe ulcerative infections occurred in 2 subjects requiring oral antibiotics.

Bacteriology of Inoculated Sites. After 24 hours of occlusion, the density of *S. aureus* was quite high, more than 10^6 per sq. cm. In the presence of copious exudate the bacterial population was sometimes substantially less. Coagulase negative cocci and enterobacteria were occasionally present. The former often reached very high densities early in the occlusion period (see below). Sites sampled at different times on the same individual yielded consistent results.

Cytological findings. Three patterns could be recognized in touch slides:

1. The usual picture was a microscopic exudate of polymorphonuclear leukocytes and many cocci whether or not frank pus was evident clinically. Phagocytosis was very evident and the leukocytes were rather well preserved (Fig. 13-2). Some proteinaceous amorphous material was present. This picture was interpreted as a balance between host and pathogen though one or the other might be dominant in some instances.

2. Less commonly, the smear showed innumerable bacteria with a few degenerated granulocytes and considerable amorphous material (Fig. 13-3). An occasional macrophage could be recognized. This was the typical picture with a 48-hour delay before inoculation. It may be interpreted as an overgrowth of bacteria in a privileged situation more or less inaccessible to phagocytes. The host remains indifferent.

3. In the sites showing the greatest signs of inflammation with a copious exudate, the cytologic scene consisted of many leukocytes and few organisms (Fig. 13-4). The leukocytes were excellently preserved and a few red cells could sometimes be identified. This is the picture of a successful response on the part of the host which has vanquished the bacterial invader.

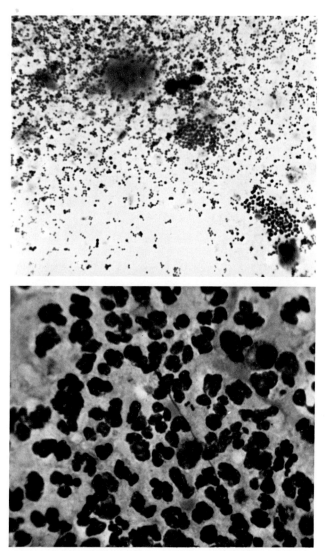

Fig. 13-3 (top).—Contact slide of uninoculated site immediately occluded for 24 hours. There are huge numbers of resident cocci and a few degenerate leukocytes.

Fig. 13-4 (bottom).—Contact slide of purulent exudate. Many leukocytes and few surviving bacteria are evident.

There was usually close correlation between the clinical and cytologic appearances. The cytological response was more sensitive. On the other hand the number of organisms could not be consistently correlated with either clinical or cytologic findings. This is not surprising in view of the 3 different patterns described above.

Experiments

Experiment 1—Inoculation Immediately after Stripping. In 5 subjects 10^5 cells were applied under occlusion to freshly stripped sites. Within 6 hours two of these subjects complained of pain and swelling associated with slight fever. Palpable nodes were present in the axilla. The skin around the inoculum site was hot, reddened and sore. Clinical signs of a spreading cellulitis were apparent in all five. Systemic penicillin was immediately administered and the occlusive dressings removed. This brought about immediate regression of the signs and symptoms.

On a later occasion, a similar situation arose by accident. Again all five subjects showed clinical signs of spreading infection within hours, requiring intercession as above.

Subsequently we cautiously applied 10^3 cells to freshly stripped skin. While this lower dose did not provoke a spreading cellulitis local ulceration occurred. Further study with very low inoculum size is in progress. Some bacterial species can be safely inoculated onto freshly stripped skin; these studies are in progress.

Experiment 2—Inoculation at Various Times after Stripping. Four sites were marked out on the upper back of two subjects. On four successive days one site was stripped. On the fifth day, each site was inoculated with 50,000 *S. aureus* cells and occluded for 48 hours.

Both the day-old and 2-day-old stripped sites were more inflamed than the others. The organism had multiplied at all sites but to progressively lesser extents with lengthening of the interval (Table 13-1). Normal skin residents were insignificant with the 24 hour wait. Thereafter, they were always present but never attained a majority. Even after a 4-day interval, *S. aureus* made up 92% of the microflora in one subject and 59% in the other. When uninoculated but similarly occluded sites were studied it was found that recolonization by normal skin residents did occur within this time.

Thus, with a one-day delay, *S. aureus* attained high densities of 10^7 per cm.^{2}

Table 13-1
Influence of Interval Between Stripping and Inoculation
Inoculum 50,000 Cells—48 Hours Occlusion*

Time Since Stripping	Subject 1			Subject 2		
	Total	S. aureus	% S. aureus	Total	S. aureus	% S. aureus
1 day	409	407	99.5	198.8	198.8	100
2 days	93.4	88.4	94.6	131.3	131.3	100
3 days	112.2	97.1	86.6	507	44.9	88.5
4 days	3.45	2.05	59.4	70.2	64.6	92.0

*Density in millions/cm.^{2}

Table 13-2
Effect of Inoculum Size 48 Hours after Stripping

Inoculum	Subjects	Dense Growth	Poor Growth
4×10^5	20	16	4
6×10^4	10	10	0
10^3	10	10	0
4×10^2	12	10	2
10^1	12	4	8

during a 48-hour occlusion. A considerable increase of the original inoculum occurred even when there is a two-day interval between stripping and inoculation.

Experiment 3—Dose Effects. This early experiment was conducted before the advantages of a 24-hour delay after stripping were realized. Sites were inoculated after a 48-hour delay with various numbers of *S. aureus* cells and occluded for 24 hours. Sampling was performed with Rodac plates containing media selective for *S. aureus*.

With this interval between stripping and inoculation, clinical lesions were few. The data gathered related to bacterial multiplication only. Above 10^3 there was a dense growth of *S. aureus* irrespective of inoculum size (Table 13-2). Only when the inoculum was approximately 10 cells was poor growth a majority finding. Even in the latter group dense growth, indistinguishable from that following higher inocula, occurred at 4 sites.

These findings indicate an essentially "all or none" type of phenomenon. If the inoculum survives the shock of transplantation it will multiply to a dense population of more than a million cells per sq. cm. within 24 hours.

A dose response relationship is therefore difficult to demonstrate. Had we used our more usual 24-hour delay the increased frequency of clinical infections might have shown such a relationship. If bacterial growth is the parameter to be measured it would be necessary to sample the sites within a few hours of inoculation.

Experiment 4—Cytologic Observations. Sites were inoculated with 10^5 *S. aureus* cells 24 and 48 hours after stripping and occluded for 24 hours.

Of the 21 sites inoculated 24 hours after stripping, 15 showed a leukocytic exudate. However only 3 of 22 sites in one study and only 2 of 20 in a repeat experiment showed a polymorph exudate with the 48-hour delay. Bacteria were very common as judged from cultures or from stained slides. Where granulocytes were numerous the sites were clinically infected and of a severity similar to infections produced 24 hours after stripping.

Experiment 5—Dynamics of Early Colonization. In five subjects four stripped sites were prepared and inoculated with 4,000 *S. aureus* cells per sq. cm. after a 24-hour delay. One site each was sampled at 20 minutes and at 2, 6 and 24 hours. The density of all organisms, *S. aureus* and residents, at these various times is shown in Figure 13-5. After 20 minutes, only low numbers were recovered. The total was 4700/cm.² of which 360/cm.² were *S. aureus*. By 2 hours, the total population was 57,300 and *S. aureus* had reached 1150 organisms per sq. cm. At 6 hours, the density reached 10^8/cm.² in 3 subjects, 2 of whom carried 10^7 *S. aureus*. The geometric mean, however, was 3.53×10^6 organisms of which

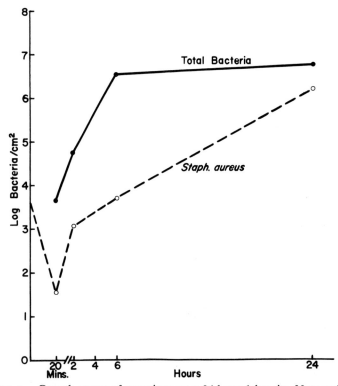

Fig. 13–5.—Growth curves of organisms on a 24-hour delay site. Note early diminution of inoculum and the steady increase in their number to more than 10^6 twenty-four hours later.

S. aureus made up only 5700. At 24 hours, all 5 sites yielded more than 10^6 cells with a geometric mean density of 5.84×10^6. More than 10^6 *S. aureus* were present in 4 of the 5 sites with a mean density of 1.64×10^6 cells per sq. cm. The exudate corresponded closely to the microbial density. Foci of polymorphonuclear leukocytes were detected microscopically in 3 subjects—in one of whom pus was present clinically at 6 hours and in 3 at 24. Two of these bore more than 10^7 *S. aureus*. In one subject a copious exudate was associated with only 10^5 *S. aureus*.

Table 13-3
Prophylaxis of S. aureus Infections by Antibiotic Cream

	Neomycin-gramicidin	Cream Base	Untreated
Number of sites	13	13	13
S. aureus positive	5	13	13
Mean density (positive sites)	1.09×10^4	7.41×10^6	4.36×10^6
Cytological exudate	1	8	10
Clinical severity	1.2	2.3	3.0

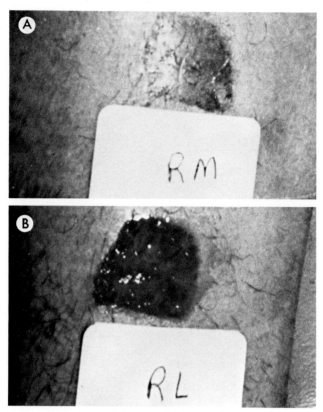

Fig. 13–6.—A, suppression of infection with neomycin-gramicidin cream. B, intense inflammatory reaction in untreated infected site.

Experiment 6—Prophylaxis by Topical Antibiotic. An antibiotic active in the presence of skin secretions should prevent multiplication of *S. aureus* and forestall infection.

Three 24-hour-old stripped sites on the forearms of 13 volunteers were inoculated as above with 4×10^5 *S. aureus* cells. Six hours later one site was treated with a neomycin-gramicidin cream (Spectrocin Cream®), the second with the cream base and the third was an untreated control. The sites were occluded for a further 18 hours before sampling with the detergent scrub technique.

S. aureus was recovered in huge numbers from all 13 sites which were not treated or those which received the cream base. The geometric mean density was of the order of millions per sq. cm. The antibiotic treated site, however, yielded *S. aureus* only five times in quite low numbers (Table 13-3). Microscopically a leukocytic exudate was present in 10 of the 13 untreated sites, 8 of the cream base sites but in only 1 site treated with the antibiotic. A typical clinical appearance is shown in Figure 13-6.

DISCUSSION

The results of this study indicate that a crisp, swiftly developing infection with *Staphylococcus aureus* can be induced by inoculating tape stripped skin with relatively few organisms. Thus, the gap between clinical and experimental experience has been closed. Though the most trivial of superficial injuries may be complicated by infection, a generation of experimenters has been frustrated in vigorous attempts to induce infections at will [4]. Success was achieved by extreme tactics such as injecting millions of organisms [3], applying dense suspensions to puncture stabs [5] or contaminating a silk thread before suturing it into the skin [3]. Some forward movement was registered when it became possible to produce infections without damaging the skin [6]. That model still did not clarify how pyogenic infections followed superficial insults. The requisite conditions, days of occlusion and many thousands of organisms, certainly did not resemble real life.

The crux of the problem was to create an infection with small numbers of organisms. *S. aureus* is omnipresent in man's environment, but ordinarily does not live on normal skin. By zealous sampling of many sites repeatedly, small numbers of *S. aureus* can be isolated from the integument of practically anyone [13]. Despite the most scrupulous aseptic technique, surgical wounds will almost always yield *S. aureus* during the course of operations [14]. In these instances, the number of cells is usually very small. Clearly, very special circumstances must obtain to enable a few organisms to multiply so rapidly as to reach an infective level.

The present observations afford some insight into the details of pathogenesis. However, it is only by hindsight that we perceive the peculiar advantages of strip wounding followed by a 24-hour delay before inoculation. Immediate inoculation after injury was found to be hazardous and difficult to control. When the delay was lengthened to 48 hours the healing process had restored an effective barrier to leukocytes and although the inoculum regularly colonized the site the host remained indifferent. By 24 hours after stripping, resident organisms have recolonized the site but are still present only in low numbers. We showed previously the ecologically important advantage conferred by reducing competitors by prior ethanol degerming [6]. Secondly, stripping calls forth a serous exudate. This event is of paramount importance for serum is a splendid nutrient for *S. aureus* whereas it is often bactericidal for nonpyogenic organisms. Serum also promotes growth by keeping the surface wet, thus approximating the effect of occlusion. Dryness is extremely antithetic to the multiplication of bacteria on skin. We of course guaranteed a wet environment by an impermeable covering but even without this measure spontaneous *S. aureus* infections sometimes occurred in stripped sites. Last, but not least, the viable epidermis remains after stripping. It serves as a partial barrier to the free emigration of leukocytes. In short, the pathogen is in an ideal situation for multiplying in pure culture out of reach of granulocytes, the chief instrument of the body for destroying pyogenic bacteria. By the time leukocytes arrive in numbers a vast bacterial population has come into being. Even though resident coagulase negative staphylococci usually dominate the flora, particularly in the early hours after occlusion, *S. aureus* surmounts this competition and multiplies steadily throughout the 24 hours.

That an intense inflammatory lesion develops so speedily even with twenty-four hours delay is noteworthy. The reason for this is the immense expansion in the numbers of *S. aureus* within a few hours. Within a day the numbers are of the order of 10^6 per sq. cm., a near maximum density. In the previous study on normal skin [6] saturation levels of about $2 \times 10^7/\text{cm.}^2$ were attained in about 4 days and did not materially increase thereafter even when occlusion was maintained for two weeks.

It is not hard to understand why the severity of the reaction at 24 hours whether estimated clinically, cytologically or bacteriologically was not particularly dose dependent. Even with very small inocula unrestrained growth will result in a huge population within a period of hours, obliterating the initial advantage of a much larger inoculum. Since the development of a clinically or cytologically apparent infection is the sum of two interacting populations, leukocytes and organisms, the killing of leukocytes by staphylococcal leukocidins and the simultaneous killing of cocci by leukocytes may produce a variety of results depending to a large degree on incidental random factors. Had we maintained the infection for 48 hours, there is little doubt that the severity of infection would be the same for any infective dose. We did not actually ascertain the number of organisms that would produce lesions 50% of the times. This is all but impossible with our techniques, for the counting error becomes very large in the case of small numbers. What we designate to be 100 organisms might very well be 10. It seems a likelihood that even less than 10 organisms would sometimes be infective, especially with longer occlusion. To test this assumption would require a prohibitive number of inoculated sites. The reasons for failure of colonization at higher inocula were usually technical. Occlusion is critical for success and loose dressings were noted in most failures.

We can conceive that conditions approximating those of stripping could occur naturally so that in a privileged site a handful of organisms might undergo such rapid growth as to cause an infection. Scrapings, scuffings, grazes, abrasions, burns, cuts and all manner of minor skin injuries sometimes obviously do create the right opportunities. The association of wound infections with razor preparation before surgery has pertinence here [15]. Moisture is probably the decisive factor after minor injury. In relation to the frequency of such trauma, infection is uncommon. It is the first few hours which all the necessary conditions have propitiously converged; moisture, nourishment, separation from phagocytes and relative absence of rivals.

It is instructive to compare our experiences with those of Foster and Hutt who applied many *S. aureus* cells to skin freshly denuded of epidermis [16]. To be sure, a suppurative reaction occurred. Still it seems that their infections were less severe than those we encountered when *S. aureus* was applied to freshly stripped skin. Indeed, toxemia and spreading cellulitis evolved so dramatically that we were forced to intervene after a few hours. Very likely bacterial multiplication was not nearly so great in denuded skin because of the immediate influx of granulocytes. Further studies of the effect of very small inocula of *S. aureus* and other organisms on freshly stripped sites may be very informative and useful in the study of the initiation of natural infections but should be undertaken with care and recognition of the risks. Very different circumstances prevail if one waits 24 hours before inoculating the pathogen. The parakeratotic layer which forms in that time provides a temporary barrier which limits the inward diffusion of toxins. This ad hoc barrier increases over the next few days so that inoculations 2, 3 and 4 days after stripping evoke progressively lesser reactions. Moreover, the resident flora have returned to the scene and often dominate.

The following guidelines are suggested for utilizing this model. Strip smartly to the glistening layer, wait 24 hours and apply 10^3–10^5 organisms. Occlude for 24 hours and terminate. Simple removal of occlusion will generally suffice. It is the better part of discretion, however, to apply an antibiotic cream twice daily for the next two days. We have routinely used a neomycin cream.

Though safety is the compelling factor in terminating the infection after 24 hours, one usually has all the desired data by that time. Several kinds of appraisal are possible, clinical, bacteriological and cytological. Clinical appearance only may be misleading since true infections may be overlooked if the exudate is not voluminous and all three methods are complementary. Touch plates are not troublesome and rather reliably indicate the amount of bacterial growth particularly when antibacterial agents are being studied.

The immediate uses for this model are to study the pathogenesis of pyogenic infections and to appraise the effectiveness of topical or systemic antibiotics in superficial *S. aureus* infections. Important measures of host resistance may be determinable with this technique including the effects of underlying disease (diabetes, lymphoma), sex, age, race, etc. on natural resistance.

SUMMARY

A human model has been developed for creating *S. aureus* infections after superficial wounding. The technique entails the application of a few thousand organisms to skin stripped of its horny layer twenty-four hours earlier. The site is then covered with an impermeable dressing for 24 hours. This results in a bright red, exudative lesion which generally shows great numbers of leukocytes and bacteria; the density of the latter commonly exceeds $1 \times 10^6/$cm.^{2}.

The high proportion of takes with small numbers of organisms, 100 or less, is attributable to four conditions which stripping peculiarly provides: moisture, serum nutrient, absence of phagocytes during rapid growth and few competing organisms.

REFERENCES

1. Bigger, J. W., and Hodgson, G. A.: Impetigo contagiosa its cause and treatment, Lancet 1:544, 1943.
2. Sheehan, H. L., and Fergusson, A. G.: Impetigo: aetiology and treatment, Lancet 1:547, 1943.
3. Elek, S. D., and Conen, P. E.: The virulence of *Staphylococcus pyogenes* for man, Brit. J. Exper. Path. 38:573, 1957.
4. Maibach, H. I.: Experimentally induced infections in the skin of man, in Maibach, H. I., and Hildick-Smith, G. (eds.): *Skin Bacteria and Their Role in Infection* (New York: McGraw-Hill Book Company, Inc., 1965).
5. Duncan, W. C., McBride, M. E., and Knox, J. M.: Experimental production of infections in humans, J. Invest. Dermat. 54:319, 1970.
6. Singh, G., Marples, R. R., and Kligman, A. M.: Experimental *Staphylococcus aureus* infections in humans, J. Invest. Dermat. (In press).

7. Pinkus, H.: Tape stripping in dermatological research. A review with emphasis on epidermal biology, Gior. ital. dermat. e sif. 107:1115, 1966.
8. Mishima, Y., and Pinkus, H.: Electron microscopy of keratin layer stripped human epidermis, J. Invest. Dermat. 50:89, 1968.
9. Matoltsy, A. G., Schragger, A., and Matoltsy, M. N.: Observations on regeneration of the skin barrier, J. Invest. Dermat. 38:251, 1962.
10. Marples, R. R., and Kligman, A. M.: Growth of bacteria under adhesive tapes, Arch. Dermat. 99:107, 1969.
11. Williamson, P., and Kligman, A. M.: A new method for the quantitative investigation of cutaneous bacteria, J. Invest. Permat. 45:498, 1965.
12. Marples, R. R., and Kligman, A. M.: In vivo methods for appraising antibacterial agents, T.G.A. Cosmetics J. 1:26, 1969.
13. Williams, R. E. O.: Skin and nose carriage of bacteriophage types of *Staphylococcus aureus,* J. Path. & Bact. 58:259, 1946.
14. Burke, J. F.: Identification of the sources of staphylocci contaminating the surgical wound during operation, Ann. Surg. 158:898, 1963.
15. Seropian, R., and Reynolds, B. M.: Wound infections after preoperative depilatory versus razor preparation, Am. J. Surg. 121:251, 1971.
16. Foster, W. D., and Hutt, M. S. R.: Experimental staphylococcal infections in man, Lancet 2:1373, 1960.

14

The Effect of Climate on the Repair
of Cutaneous Wounds in Humans

James W. Bothwell, Ph.D., David T. Rovee, Ph.D.*,
Anne Marie Downes, B.A.*, Patricia A. Flanagan, R.N., B.A.* and
Carole A. Kurowsky, R.N.**

The microclimate created by wound covers has been shown by a number of investigators to exert a marked effect upon epidermal repair both in experimental animals and in man [1–6]. Repair has been observed to be more rapid under occlusive or semi-occlusive covers than when the wound is exposed to its atmospheric environment. It is generally agreed that the difference in repair rate result from a difference in the maintenance of moisture at the wound site. A moist environment maintains viability of the exposed cells. When desiccation to varying degrees is encountered, inhibition of epidermal repair results. When the defect is protected from drying by a suitable wound cover, desiccation does not occur and epidermal repair can begin rapidly and proceed without interference. It follows that wound covers with varying capacity to prevent desiccation should offer different degrees of protection from drying and that exposure to different drying forces should result in varying degrees of inhibition of epidermal repair. However, little direct experimental information is available on the effect of such environments on epidermal repair. Rovee [7] reported that epidermal repair in the ear of germfree rats living in isolators at high relative humidity was the same as that of conventional rats in the same warm moist environment. At the same time the repair of similar wounds in conventional rats housed in normal but much dryer animal quarters was slower. Spruit [8] observed a seasonal effect on the repair of the exposed tape stripped wound. He found that in Nijmegen, Netherlands the fastest epidermal regeneration occurred in the spring and the slowest in autumn. The report of Baker and Kligman [9] indicates a slower healing of the tape stripped wound than does that of Matoltsy *et al*. [10]. Although these differences might be explained by differences in the TWL (transepidermal water loss) measuring equipment used, it has been our experience using these two kinds of equipment that this is unlikely. Absolute values of a given measure-

---

*Skin Biology Department, Johnson & Johnson Research, New Brunswick, New Jersey.

ment may vary but the relative changes during repair remain much the same. Another possible explanation for the difference would be that of climatic environment. The Matoltsy studies were done in Miami while those of Baker and Kligman were done in Philadelphia.

The following studies were undertaken in an effort to determine whether the macro environment as represented by different climates would result in significant repair differences as determined in two human epidermal wound models for which reasonable quantification of repair is available.

METEOROLOGICAL OBSERVATIONS

Studies were conducted in three climates: 1) hot, wet, subtropical—Miami, Florida—August, 1969; 2) dry, desert—Yuma, Arizona—June, 1971; 3) cold, winter—Fairbanks, Alaska—February, 1970, New Brunswick, New Jersey—January, 1970 and Roscoe, New York—February, 1971.

Two kinds of records were kept in order to establish the nature of the climatic environment to which the experimental wounds were exposed during these studies.

Hourly weather station readings were recorded for temperatures and dew point. From these, relative humidity was calculated and the Humidity Ratio was derived from a psychometric chart. Humidity Ratio (W) is defined as the mass

Table 14-1
Meteorological Measurements and Humidity Ratios at Each of the Study Sites
During the Experimental Period

Location	Day 1		Day 2		Day 3		Day 4	
	Temp. °F	$W \times 10^3$	Temp. °F	$W \times 10^3$	Temp. °F	$W \times 10^3$	Temp. °F	$W \times 10^3$
Miami, Fla.	85	19	86	18	86	18	83	16
Fairbanks, Alaska	6	0.9	15	1.1	26	1.4	27	1.8
New Brunswick, N.J.	20	1.3	19	1.4	14	1.1	13	0.9
Roscoe, N.Y.	11	.7	20	1.6	—	—	—	—
Yuma, Ariz.	78	9	82	8	86	7	90	7

Table 14-2
Daily Humidity Ratios Calculated from Detailed Records
of Life Environment in Fairbanks

Humidity Ratio W $\times 10^3$—lb. moisture/lb. dry air
Wound Age in Days

Subject	1	2	3	4
JB	3.2	2.2	3.0	3.1
RA	3.0	3.2	3.8	3.2
BK	3.0	3.2	3.8	3.2
WV	2.7	3.2	3.8	2.8
TB	2.7	3.2	3.8	2.8
RK	3.7	3.7	2.6	3.2
Average	3.0	3.1	3.5	3.0

Table 14-3

Relationship between Epithelial Repair of Incision Wound and Humidity Ratio

Location	Humidity Ratio		Percent Incisions Epithelialized at 2 Days	Mean Gape of Incision at Day 2
	Weather Station	Life Environment		
Miami	18	17*	100	0
Yuma	8	8.5†	50	108
Fairbanks	1	3.1†	0	400
New Jersey	1	2.5‡	0	300

†Calculated from records of temperature and humidity made during study.
‡Estimated assuming 8 hours in laboratory at 72°F and 10% R.H., 2 hours exposed to outside environment and 14 hours in hot air heated home at 72°F and 20% R.H.
*Estimated assuming 8 hours in non air conditioned hospital at 85°F and 80% R.H., 4 hours exposed to outside environment and 12 hours in air conditioned home at 78°F and 55% R.H.

of water associated with a unit mass of dry air and represents a measure of the absolute humidity. These data are summarized in Table 14-1.

A second and more realistic value of the environmental moisture is shown in Table 14-2 as the Humidity Ratio (W) for the life environment of the subjects. The Fairbanks data are considered the most reliable because portable psychrometers were carried by each of the subjects and temperature and humidity entered in a notebook at each change of location. Thus, a running account of environmental conditions was obtained. Table 14-2 shows the daily Humidity Ratios for each of the subjects. In the subsequent Yuma and Roscoe studies, four to six temperature and humidity readings per day were made, representative of the various changes of location, and the Humidity Ratio for the group was calculated.

Because of less subject control in the early Miami and New Jersey studies, estimates of the life environment were made as noted in Table 14-3.

Although there is a difference between life environment measurements and the weather station readings, a clearcut difference in climate is seen, using either criterion.

TAPE STRIPPED WOUND MODEL

The tape stripped epidermis first described by Wolf and studied carefully by Pincus [11] has been extensively used by dermatologists as an example of very superficial ($10–15\mu$ deep) epidermal trauma.

Early measurements of healing based on water barrier function of the stratum corneum were made by Fallon and Moyer [12] who trapped moisture from air blown over the wound. Matoltsy et al. [10] measured the change of moisture in a closed cylinder held over the healing stripped site and reported healing as a function of reduction in the insensible water loss. More recently advanced systems using flowing air and various water detection methods have been reported by Spruit [8, 13, 14], Baker and Kligman [9], Jelenko [15] and Johnson and Shuster [16]. The insensible water loss thus measured is generally referred to as transepidermal water loss (TWL).

Because there is a great difference in TWL values between the intact and the damaged skin (50–100 fold) the time of return to normal which takes about ten to fourteen days is reasonable to measure. However, the final point of return to normal approaches asymptotically and there is also some variation in the normal intact skin. This makes it difficult to determine a specific time of complete repair. Spruit [8] describes half regeneration times for the early parakeratotic barrier and reports $_pt^{1/2}$ values that vary from 0.7 to 2.3 days. The second or final barrier formation showed $t^{1/2}$ values closer to 5 days. Possible environmental effects that would delay repair would most likely be seen as influencing the early phase $(_pt^{1/2})$.

Thus, studies were undertaken in two distinct climates, one a cold weather study in Roscoe, New York and the second in the hot, dry season of Yuma, Arizona.

Because an occlusive and a semi-occlusive wound cover would be expected to exert different levels of control of moisture loss to a drying environment these two types were included in the study.

The occlusive dressing was constructed of a 1 inch square of Saran Wrap® film adhered to the center of a 2 × 2 inch section of a surgical tape. The semi-occlusive dressing was a commercially available 1 inch wide first aid bandage (Band Aid® Sheer Strip with Keypak® pad). It consisted of a perforated plasticized vinyl backed pressure sensitive tape to which an absorbent pad covered with a polyethylene coated nonwoven fabric is attached. The dressing is designed to adhere to two sides of a wound.

Methods

The tape stripped wound was produced using strips of an industrial pressure sensitive tape (Permacel P-69 Plastic Coated Cloth Tape). The tape was faced to silicone release paper and cut to 1 × 2 inch segments for repeated stripping of horny layers. A stripping tape was placed on the surface to be stripped and outlined at the corners with a ball point pen to define the area. The tapes were applied, pressed down firmly and removed sequentially until a smooth, even glistening surface was achieved. This usually required about 20–30 strips, but varied with the subjects used. Biopsy sections have demonstrated that at that point the stratum corneum has been completely removed, exposing moist underlying nucleated cells of the malpighian layer.

For these studies, three wounds were created on the outer aspect of the upper arm of four adult volunteer subjects. The initial TWL values for the stripped areas and an adjacent intact site were measured using an air flow hygrometer system (Model 154 Sweat Rate Apparatus, Sage Instruments) as originally described by Baker and Kligman [9] with modifications as recommended by Spruit to minimize air leak through the tubing noted during very low air flow rates.

Following initial TWL readings, two of the wounds on each arm were covered with test dressings while the third served as an untreated control. Subsequent readings were taken over the treated as well as adjacent skin sites at 6 hourly intervals in one study (Roscoe) and at 8 hourly intervals in the second (Yuma) for a total of 48 hours. During this period, the water barrier function usually returned to about 80% of normal.

A "percent damage" value was calculated for each of the TWL readings to relate each value to its own initial reading according to the formula:

"Percent Damage" = x/y × 100
  where x = TWL value at each of the 6 or 8 hourly time periods
    y = TWL value for time 0

"Percent damage" as a function of time was plotted for each wound, the best straight line determined by linear regression analysis and $t^{1/2}$ values calculated. These values are equivalent to the $_p t^{1/2}$ values reported by Spruit and represent the early or parakeratotic repair phase.

Results

Table 14-4 reports the $t^{1/2}$ values for the covered and uncovered stripped wounds in a winter and a hot desert climate. The uncovered wounds show a significantly slower repair ($p < .01$) in the cold climate as compared to the rate in the desert climate.

When the wound microclimate in each of the dissimilar macroclimates was controlled by means of an occlusive saran dressing, repair rates were similar and significantly more rapid than in the untreated control wounds. In the desert climate of Yuma, the partially occlusive commercial dressing was as effective as the occlusive when compared to the uncovered control, but in the colder region, the degree of protection afforded by the partially occlusive dressing was less than that of the occlusive dressing. Although the degree of protection was less than that of the occlusive cover, the repair rate was significantly better than in the exposed control wound.

Table 14-4
Effect of Climate on Repair of Tape Stripped Wounds

Time for Half Repair (t½) in Hours*

	Roscoe			Yuma		
Subject	Untreated	Occluded	Partially Occluded	Untreated	Occluded	Partially Occluded
JB	38	15	22	18	11	9
RA	25	10	21	25	11	13
AD	33	22	29	21	14	20
RK	43	30	30	23	17	16
Aver.	35	19	25	22	13	15

*Each figure represents mean value for left and right arm.

LINEAR INCISION WOUND MODEL

Earlier studies [6] have shown that a split thickness linear incision is sensitive to a drying environment even though it has a low exposed surface area compared to the tape stripped wound. The availability of a set of objective criteria utilizing biopsy procedures at daily intervals following wounding makes possible better assessment of environmental effects on various repair phases. The studies were repeated in Miami, Fairbanks, New Jersey and Yuma.

Method

Incisions 15 mm. long and approximately 300μ deep were made on the forearms of 4 to 15 adult volunteer subjects depending upon the particular study. Wounds were made with a sterile scalpel and bleeding other than slight oozing was controlled by firm pressure with a gauze sponge for three minutes. The wounds were left uncovered and observations of all wounds were made daily. Biopsies were taken at daily intervals and fixed in Bouin's solution. The samples were subsequently returned to the laboratory, prepared and routinely stained with hematoxylin and eosin. Assessment of epithelial repair, measurement of gape and estimation of degree of polymorphonuclear leukocyte response were made microscopically and complemented the gross observations made daily.

The intensity of inflammatory infiltrate composed mainly of polymorphonuclear leukocytes was estimated on a 0 to $+++$ scale, where 0 equals no observable infiltrate, $+$ equals slight infiltrate, $++$ equals moderate infiltrate, and $+++$ equals severe or intense infiltrate.

A retrospective survey for each subject was done at the completion of the biopsy schedule to determine living habits, general activity and special exertion during the experimental period. This was particularly important in the Miami and in the early New Jersey studies because the daily activities of the volunteer subjects were not as well controlled as in subsequent studies.

Results

Epithelialization. Table 14-5 reports the time required to establish complete epithelial continuity as determined microscopically from the biopsy sections. It is clear that the cold-dry environment of Fairbanks and New Jersey exerted a delaying effect on the capacity to reestablish epithelial cover. The Miami climate allowed the most rapid repair, while at the desert site, the rate was intermediate.

A similar relationship is seen in Figure 14-1 which shows the effect on the gape of the incisions. The wounds in Fairbanks and New Jersey developed a marked gape within the first 24 hours, while in Miami at the same time period those not already closed showed little gape between the epidermal edges. The desert wounds again showed an intermediate response.

The actual moisture content of the air as expressed by Humidity Ratio at each location is compared with these two repair parameters in Table 14-2. Whether the comparison is made against data derived from the meteorological measurements at the local weather station or against measured or estimated life environ-

Table 14-5
Effect of Climate on Time Required to Reestablish Epithelial Continuity

Epithelialization Complete / Total Sites

Wound Age in Days	Miami	Fairbanks	New Jersey	Yuma
1	3/9	0/7	0/10	0/8
2	5/5	0/4	0/6	3/6
3	3/4	5/5	5/6	5/6
4	4/4	1/3	2/2	4/4

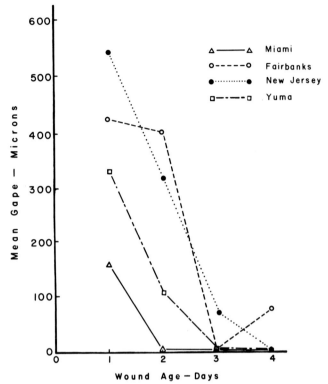

Fig. 14–1.—Mean wound gape of incisions as a function of wound age in three climates. Gape was measured in microns microscopically from biopsy section of uncovered wounds.

ments, the repair was much slower in the dry environments than in the moist.

Inflammatory Response. In Figure 14-2, the gross erythemal response decreased rapidly in the Miami wounds but was present for 3–4 days in both of the dry environments. This rapid reduction in gross inflammation in Miami was nearly but not quite as rapid as seen when the wounds are covered with an occlusive saran dressing [6]. In microscopic section the polymorphonuclear leukocyte response (Fig. 14-3), although about the same in all wounds at 24 hours, showed a rapid reduction in the Miami wounds and a far slower reduction in those in the dry climates.

DISCUSSION

The effort to establish valid relationships between climate and epithelial repair is fraught with a long list of problems when one attempts to do the studies on a group of human subjects over a period of several days. Even when valid quantitative and semi-quantitative wound repair models are available, the list of uncontrollable variables makes it nearly impossible to develop unassailable experimental procedures. Air velocity over the wound is certainly an important factor

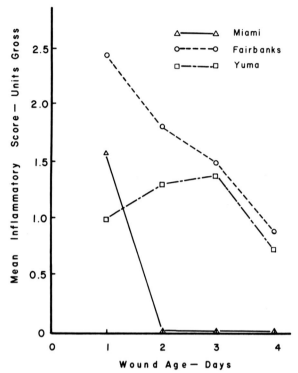

Fig. 14–2.—Gross inflammatory response of incisions in three climates as a function of wound age. The degree of visible erythema was recorded in arbitrary units of 0 to +3.

in desiccation but cannot be controlled in a real life situation, nor can measurements of the velocity be even reasonably estimated [17].

The fact that results were obtained that show a consistent macro environmental (moisture) impact on two exposed repairing epidermal wound models suggests that the effect of wound desiccation on epidermal repair is profound and perhaps so dominated by environmental moisture that it can be demonstrated in spite of an array of variables.

Even though people tend to compensate for climatic extremes with air conditioners in hot climates and indoor confinement in cold climates, the measurements of absolute humidity demonstrate that the life environment can be reasonably that as judged by the meteorological measurements. This was true at least for sedentary individuals used in these studies.

The results with the tape stripped wound model indicate that in addition to a microclimate impact, wound covers with varying degrees of occlusiveness show varying capacity to protect against wound desiccation when the drying impact is large, as in the cold winter climate.

Unreported studies in our laboratory using the incision model as well as a cantharadin blister model have also demonstrated this differential effect. Dress-

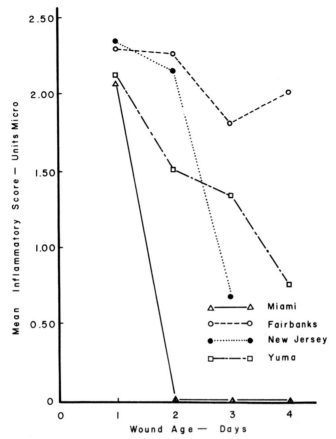

Fig. 14–3.—Inflammatory response of incisions in three climates as a function of wound age. The extent of polymorphonuclear infiltration was estimated microscopically from biopsy sections on an arbitrary scale of 0 to +3.

ings that allow varying air circulation around a wound show varying protection from desiccation, particularly in cold weather.

The moisture in the air of the homes of many people in winter in the northern tier of states in the United States is well within the range of Humidity Ratios reported for the cold climate studies. Thus, a hot-air-heated home without a humidifier maintained at 72°F will often have a relative humidity of 10%. The Humidity Ratio under these conditions is $W = 1.8$. This is similar to the reported data that demonstrate impaired epidermal repair.

Factors other than environmental moisture may well affect the repair process and have not been measured in these studies. The surface temperature and immediate subsurface temperature of a repairing epidermal wound may well exert an influence. Studies are currently underway to measure wound temperatures both for exposed and covered defects.

Temperature changes that could alter skin temperature and the microcirculation may contribute to the availability of moisture from beneath the wound and accentuate desiccation.

Physical activity is likely a factor in some of the parameters reported here. The wounds slowest to epithelialize in the Miami study were those of physical therapists who encountered considerable patient lifting during the study.

The microbiological content of the wounds was likely different in the various environments encountered during these studies. No sign of infection was seen in any of the experimental wounds.

In spite of the many uncontrolled variables in this type of study, we believe that the results give support to the concept that environmental moisture has major impact upon the repair of small epithelial wounds and that the effect is seen as wound desiccation. This desiccation can to a large extent be altered by wound covers.

SUMMARY

Studies were undertaken using two epidermal wound models in humans to assess the effect of three climatic environments on epidermal repair.

Results demonstrated a correlation of repair with absolute humidity of the environment measured as Humidity Ratio (W).

Control of the microclimate by means of wound covers reduced wound desiccation under drying conditions and allowed for improved repair.

In spite of the many uncontrollable variables in a human study of this type, the results support the concept that environmental moisture has impact upon the repair of small epithelial wounds, that this impact is seen as wound desiccation and that this desiccation can to a large extent be altered by wound covers.

ACKNOWLEDGMENTS

The authors wish to recognize and show appreciation to others whose help made these studies possible: to Mr. E. Artz and Mr. R. Kennedy for their technical assistance in transporting bulky equipment to remote locations and in taking TWL readings at abnormal hours; to the volunteer subjects without whose contribution these studies could not have been done; to Miss J. Labun for preparation of tables and graphs; and to Miss E. Hahn for her help and forbearance in typing this manuscript.

REFERENCES

1. Winter, G. D.: Formation of the scab and the rate of epithelization of superficial wounds in the skin of the young domestic pig, Nature 193:293, 1962.
2. Winter, G. D., and Scales, J. T.: Effect of air drying and dressings on the surface of a wound, Nature 197:91, 1963.
3. Hinman, C. D., and Maibach, H. I.: Effect of air exposure and occlusion on experimental human skin wounds, Nature 200:377, 1963.
4. Harris, D. R., and Keefe, R. L.: A histologic study of gold leaf treated experimental wounds, J. Invest. Dermat. 52:487, 1969.
5. Krawczyk, W. S.: A pattern of epidermal cell migration during wound healing, J. Cell Biol. 49:247, 1971.

6. Bothwell, J. W., and Rovee, D. T.: The effect of dressings on the repair of cutaneous wounds in humans, in Harkiss, K. J. (ed.): *Surgical Dressings and Wound Healing* (London, Bradford University Press, 1971).
7. Rovee, D. T., Kurowsky, C. A., and Flanagan, P. A.: Bacterial Burden and Wound Repair in Conventional and Germfree Rats, in Miranda, G. (ed.): *Germ Free Biology* (New York: Plenum Press, 1969).
8. Spruit, D., and Malten, K. E.: Epidermal water barrier formation after stripping of normal skin, J. Invest. Dermat. 45:6, 1965.
9. Baker, H., and Kligman, A. M.: Measurement of transepidermal water loss by electrical hygrometry, Arch. Dermat. 96:441, 1967.
10. Matoltsy, A. G., Schragger, A., and Matoltsy, M. N.: Observations on regeneration of the skin barrier, J. Invest. Dermat. 38:251, 1962.
11. Pinkus, H.: Examination of the epidermis by the strip method of removing horny layers. I. Observations on thickness of the horny layer and on mitotic activity after stripping, J. Invest. Dermat. 16:383, 1951.
12. Fallon, R. H., and Moyer, C. A.: Rates of insensible perspiration through normal, burned, tape stripped and epidermally denuded living human skin, Ann. Surg. 158:915, 1963.
13. Spruit, D., and Malten, K. E.: The regeneration rate of the water vapor barrier of heavily damaged skin, Dermatologica 132:115, 1966.
14. Spruit, D.: Measurement of the water vapor loss from human skin by a thermal conductivity cell, J. Appl. Physiol. 23:994, 1967.
15. Jelenko, C., III: Studies in burns. I. Water loss from the body surface, Ann. Surg. 165:83, 1967.
16. Johnson, C., and Shuster, S.: The measurement of transepidermal water loss, Brit. J. Dermat. 81:40, 1969.
17. Tromp, S. W., and Weihe, W. H. (eds.): Proceedings of Fourth International Biometeorological Congress, Internat. J. Biometeorology 11 (Suppl.), 1967.

15

Local Antibiotic Treatment of Wounds

Norton G. Waterman, M.D., F.A.C.S. and
Nina Tyler Pollard, Ph.D.†*

Wound infections have continued to be a significant problem to physicians despite the development of antibiotics and improved surgical and aseptic techniques. The persistence of this problem has resulted in continued experimental and clinical efforts in the treatment of both contaminated and uncontaminated wounds to reduce or eliminate infection which adversely affects wound healing.

Semmelweis introduced disinfection of surgeons' hands with chlorinated lime in order to prevent the occurrence of puerperal fever in 1847. For many years antisepsis was not generally recognized until Lister, with great persistence, was able to overcome the opposition to this concept. This new idea gave the first hope that infections in wounds could be eliminated. This did not and has not occurred.

Chemotherapy of infections began after the introduction of salvarsan for the treatment of syphilis in 1909. When the search for chemical agents acting on pathogenic bacteria began, it was found that compounds which were highly active in vitro were completely inactive in humans and animals. Subsequently, a large variety of chemicals and agents too numerous to mention, were employed. Faulty laboratory work and incredible clinical observations resulted in the perpetration of a great number of therapeutic frauds. Very little good was accomplished by the application of these agents. The period was more of a tribute to the capacity of the body to withstand insult than it was to antimicrobial chemotherapeutics.

The presently employed techniques for the treatment and care of wounds, both surgical and traumatic, were developed principally in the period between the two World Wars during the first half of the twentieth century. These consisted essentially of thorough debridement and gentle care of the tissues. The modern age of chemotherapy began with the introduction of the sulfonamides in 1935 and penicillin in 1940.·

---

*Associate Clinical Professor of Surgery, University of Louisville School of Medicine, Louisville, Kentucky.

†Clinical Associate in Surgery, University of Louisville School of Medicine, Louisville, Kentucky.

It was natural that topical antibiotics would be employed during World War II. The sulfonamides were used indiscriminately by both physicians and nonmedical personnel. Due to the enthusiasm of investigators, poor impressions derived from limited periods of observation and studies lacking untreated controls and follow-up, resulted in the wide employment of the sulfonamides and of sulfonamides in combination with penicillin. The study reported by Meleney [1] done after World War II by nine different hospital groups in various parts of the United States showed that sulfonamides used locally and/or systemically did not reduce the incidence of local infections in civilian wounds. The results were no better than when wounds were treated with the accepted principles of wound care. The utilization of wound irrigation with antibiotics or other methods of local application fell into disrepute.

The recent success of topical antibiotics in the prevention of infection by the gram negative enteric bacteria in burn patients has produced a resurgence of interest in the use of antibiotics to prevent wound infections—a factor in delaying normal wound healing. The literature is extensive and a complete review is not possible in the allotted space. Consequently, this chapter is concerned with antimicrobial agents and wounds produced by controlled and uncontrolled trauma and does not include burns.

GENERAL CONSIDERATIONS

Infection rates continue to be between 5 and 10% as reported by most reliable institutions. Studies of the bacteriology of fresh surgical wounds done prior to World War II are similar to the one reported by Ives and Hirshfeld [2]. They found that cultures containing potential pathogens are present on the skin in 86% of the patients at the start of an operation and 100% at the close of the operation. These figures indicate that the skin is not sterile at the beginning of the operation and is very heavily contaminated at the termination of the operative procedure. Positive cultures were obtained from the fascia in 44% of the cases early in the operations after the incisions had been made, and in 83% at the close of the operations. This, of course, indicates that the number of bacteria in the wounds increases with the length of the operation and that the fascia layer is also heavily contaminated.

The ad hoc Committee of Trauma, National Academy of Science-National Research Council in a national study in 1964 [3], reports that the frequency of recovery of bacteria from postoperatively infected and uninfected wounds shows that staphylococci remain the most important organisms found in postoperative wound infections—coagulase-positive staphylococci were isolated from 31% of the infected wounds and from 14% of the clinically uninfected wounds. The coliform bacilli, proteus and pseudomonas had incidences of 22, 13 and 13% respectively.

Studies done prior to this decade showed that a large percentage of the microorganisms isolated were gram-positive cocci. To determine if the gram-negative enteric organisms are now present more frequently than staphylococci in the operative incision it would be necessary to repeat operating room studies of the wounds.

The physician has known that the employment of techniques to handle the tissue gently, to remove foreign materials and blood clots and to obliterate dead space would reduce the incidence of infection. Condie and Ferguson [4] have shown in experimental studies on dogs of the closure of incisions heavily contaminated with staphylococcus, that the quantity of suture material and trauma was of less consequence than obliterating potential dead space in the genesis of wound infections. This concept has generally been accepted by the more knowledgeable and experienced surgeons as being correct. Certainly, contaminated incisions occurring in the great majority of all wounds do not become infected. The reported infection rate is usually less than 10%.

The early sequence of events and the period of development of occurring inflammations secondary to bacterial infection have been studied extensively by Miles and associates [5–7] and Burke [8]. These studies have been the basis for the rational explanation of the inability to prevent the occurrences of wound infections and indicate that bacterial infection can be stopped or modified during the early period after wounding occurs. If interference with the wound tissue defenses against bacterial invasion and multiplication occurs during the first few hours, there is an enhancement of the bacterial lesion. Enhancement of the defense mechanisms after this period produces no discernible effect. Both the vascular and biochemical events which inhibit the infection occur during the first few hours and apparently become inoperative after this time. From these studies most investigators state that they believe that the time of maximum antibiotic effect in preventing infections must exist soon after the bacteria contaminate the tissues. The earliest opportunity to prevent infection is during this time. It is from these studies that the failure of prophylactic antibiotics have been explained. The problem of the prevention of infections by antibiotics, of course, is complex. Other factors such as host resistance, tissue trauma, the existence of foreign material and hematoma and the degree of contamination associated with the specific pathogenicity of the invading bacteria, are all definite factors.

These general considerations show in part the multiplicity of existent factors, each having its own variables. Because clinical and experimental studies are so complex, it is doubtful that most studies can be absolutely valid. These investigations generally only indicate that which may be of value.

EXPERIMENTAL LOCAL ANTIBIOTIC STUDIES

A moderate number of studies have been done utilizing local antibiotic treatment of contaminated wounds in experimental animals to prevent infection. The numerous methods of study used resulted in a wide and varied experience by the different investigators. The methods most commonly employed are irrigation with antibiotics, aerosol antibiotic sprays, powdered antibiotics, tissue infiltration (injection) with antibiotics and irrigation with antibiotic and detergent combinations.

A report on the results of the irrigation of contaminated experimental wound incisions with saline, soap solutions and chemical germicides is not the purpose of this paper. However, contaminated wounds irrigated with salt-containing solutions and soaps have been used as controls along with untreated wound incisions for comparison with wounds treated with antibiotics. Therefore, a comment on

representative studies would be of value. Peterson [9], in 1945, studied the efficacy of preventing wound infection in Staphylococcus aureus contaminated
wounds in dogs. He found that wounds irrigated with saline were less infected
than wounds washed with soaps and that those washed with soaps had a greater
incidence of infection than did the untreated controls. In a similar study, Falconer, Liljedahl and Olovson [10] found that there was no significant difference
between saline irrigations and soap irrigations. Taylor [11] thought that wound
irrigation with isotonic saline was an inefficient means of removing bacteria and
would actually force bacteria into deeper crevices not previously infected. She
believed the most important benefit derived from irrigation was the removal of
blood clots and necrotic tissues which acted as foreign bodies and as a media for
the growth of bacteria. It is evident that earlier studies express widely conflicting
opinions. Subsequent studies by Singleton, Davis and Julian [12] comparing untreated controls and saline irrigation with antibiotic irrigation of wounds indicated that the saline irrigation of the wounds was certainly beneficial. Gingrass,
Close and Ellison [13, 14], however, showed that saline irrigation of wounds to
remove the contaminating bacteria was not beneficial. The last two cited studies
were better controlled because they standardized the species and quantity of the
bacterial inoculum, time intervals between inoculation and treatment, treatment
technique and the location, size and method of closure of the incisions.

Singleton and Julian [15] found that washing wounds contaminated with
feces with gauze and soap was significantly more effective than soap instilled
into wounds alone. The newer soaps containing detergents reduced the incidence
of infection better than green soap. They found that irrigation with a 20% mefenide (sulfamylon) solution had a significant benefit. The best results were
obtained by irrigating the wounds contaminated with feces by utilizing a 1%
neomycin or kanamycin solution. Though differences were noted between the
different solutions, no attempt was made to determine the species of bacteria
causing the infections. Aseptic techniques were not employed and the quantity
of bacteria was probably variable in each study group.

Casten, Nach and Spinzia [16] found that the addition of penicillin to irrigating fluid notably reduced the incidence of wound infections. The reduction was
correlated with the concentration of penicillin. When penicillin resistant organisms were used, wound irrigation with or without antibiotics was ineffectual in
their opinion. Gingrass, Close and Ellison [14] inoculated standardized wound
incisions in guinea pigs with specified concentrations of bacteria and permitted
an eight-day period for observations of wounds which were treated with antibiotic irrigated solutions containing neomycin. They compared this antibiotic solution with saline irrigation, saline irrigation with scrubs and with hexachloraphene
as a detergent and soap. They found that the neomycin solutions were significantly more effective in preventing the development of infection than irrigation
with hexachloraphene. They also stated that when parenteral neomycin was employed in combination with the antibiotic irrigation, there was a significant
reduction in the percentage of wound infections. Hopson et al. [17] employed
kanamycin and cephalothin for the irrigation of wounds contaminated with
Staphylococcus aureus and E. coli. The incidence of infection was markedly reduced by elimination of such factors as necrotic tissue, foreign body, host re-

sistance, skin contamination and variation in the number and types of bacteria. The controlled untreated contaminated incisions were made on the same animals so each animal would serve as its own control. They believed that it was important that each animal serve as its own control because a small but significant number of animals did not develop wound infections in the untreated controls. This, in their opinion, was necessary to eliminate absorption of the antibiotic as a factor in preventing infection in the untreated control. This study and the study of Gingrass *et al.* [14] permitted the bacterial inoculum to remain in place for one hour prior to the irrigation. This was done in order to allow the bacteria to invade and become imbedded in the incised tissues. Wound infections which were present but not seen on the third day became evident by the eighth day. The last two studies cited showed the necessity for longer periods of observation of contaminated wounds, a factor not observed by many earlier investigators.

The recent experimental investigation by Glotzer, Goodman and Geronimus [18] employed both irrigation and scrubbing of the contaminated experimental wounds with antibiotics in guinea pigs. The wound infections were produced using an inoculum of penicillin resistant staphylococci or a mixture of six strains of intestinal bacteria collectively resistant to ten commonly used antibiotics. They found that infections were prevented by scrubbing the wounds with a bacitracin-neomycin polymyxin B solution one hour after contamination. Even with the presence of a silk suture acting as a foreign body and with strangulated fat in the wound, this regime maintained its effectiveness. They also found that antibiotics did not prevent infections remote from the treated wounds and believed this indicated that systemic absorption did not play a part in the prevention of the wound infection. They did not determine the serum antibiotic concentrations.

Other means of applying antibiotics directly to contaminated wounds or incisions have been employed. The utilization of topical sprays has been studied extensively by military medical groups. These studies were the result of interest in war injuries that occurred in Korea and Vietnam. Mendelson [19] studied the effect of massive wounds in goats produced by explosives to determine the prolongation of survival time in lethal open wounds. He compared irrigations of normal saline, azochloramidex in combination with hexachloramine and bacitracin-neomycin solutions with a penicillin and a bacitracin-neomycin spray. Only the bacitracin-neomycin and penicillin sprays significantly prolonged the immediate survival time. The penicillin spray produced the most significant benefits and was consistently more beneficial than the bacitracin-neomycin spray. It should be noted that prolongation of survival time correlated with the decrease in the growth of *Clostridium welchii*, an insignificant cause of infections in humans and other experimental animals. They also found that there was no evidence that local antibiotic application by itself would produce as good a result as adequate removal of the debris and devitalized tissue. In a related study Brinkley, Bailey and Mendelson [20] found there was extensive contamination of high explosive-induced wounds by both clostridia and staphylococci. Both topical penicillin and mefenide sprays were effective in inhibiting the growth of clostridia. Neither agent effectively inhibited the multiplication of staphylococci. More recently, studies by Matsumoto *et al.* [21] at the Walter Reed Army Institute of Research found that the topical application of a neosporin spray containing neomycin, polymyxin B and bacitracin, to large contaminated crushing wounds on the thighs of rabbits reduced the mortality from 64% to 4% if the wounds were sprayed shortly after injury.

The value of the direct deposition of a known quantity of powdered antibiotic into contaminated wounds prior to closure has recently been studied by two groups. Both groups believed that the use of the powdered form would be more advantageous than irrigation with an antibiotic solution, because the concentration in the wound would be greater at the termination of the closure. Gray and Kidd [22] found that combinations of neomycin, polymyxin and bacitracin had a wide range of antibacterial activity with little adverse local tissue and systemic toxic effect, allergenicity, or the development of bacterial resistance or superinfection. This combination prevented wound infections by staphylococci and a number of gram-negative enteric bacteria. Studies by Waterman, Howell and Babich [23] found that cephalothin reduced the incidence of infection by staphylococci, streptococci and coliform bacilli in experimental wound incisions in guinea pigs. An assay of the microbiologic tissue cephalothin activity present 24 hours after the introduction of the powder in the wounds showed it was still at a level considered adequate to prevent wound infections. The antibiotic remained in concentration for a sufficient length of time to kill the pathogenic bacteria present and had no adverse effect on wound healing.

Grunberg and Schnitzer [24] attempted to establish a standard method for the screening of compounds for local antibacterial activity. This study was carried out by injecting a bacterial culture containing *Staphylococcus hemolyticus* and *Staphylococcus aureus* into the subcutaneous tissue of the abdominal wall of mice. The bacterial injection was followed immediately by an infiltration of the same tissue with 1 ml. of graded concentrations of the antibiotic tested. This study allowed no time for the bacterial infection to be seeded prior to the treatment with the antibiotic. The antibiotics used were nitrofurazone, polymyxin B, neomycin, bacitracin and penicillin. They were able to show a reduction of the incidence of infections at the treated sites when compared to the untreated controls. The best results were obtained with neomycin and polymyxin B. A similar study as early as 1946 was carried out by Howes [25] employing mefenide. Rabbits were wounded by excising a 3 cm.^{2} of skin from their backs and crushing the underlying muscle. The wounds were contaminated with staphylococci or laboratory floor dirt. The latter method has been little employed. The wounds were then infiltrated with combinations of mefenide and streptomycin. This antibiotic combination prevented infection in the crushed wounds of the treated group when compared to the controlled untreated group. Although this study contained too few animals and little knowledge of the types or quantity of bacteria present in the inoculum, they noted that there was a failure to prevent infection in wounds treated three hours after their infliction and contamination. This observation was made prior to the aforementioned studies showing that after a certain time period infections will occur whether the wound is treated or not.

The utilization of antibiotic detergent solutions for irrigation has been used by orthopedic surgeons at various institutions in the United States. Brunner and associates [26] determined that aqueous tridecyl-2-sulfate solutions inhibited or prevented the formation of penicillinase when detergents were added to solutions containing penicillin. This solution would be just as effective against highly resistant strains of staphylococci in vitro as against sensitive strains. Similarly,

Compere *et al.* [27] suggested that other antibiotics would become more effective when used in solutions containing a surface active detergent. They believe that the detergent acted as both a mucolytic and wetting agent permitting the antibiotic to reach bacteria in more inaccessible areas.

In general, it is likely that saline irrigation of contaminated wounds in experimental animals is beneficial in reducing the incidence of infection as compared to controlled untreated infections in a variety of experimental animals. Antibiotics, employed in irrigation solutions, topical sprays and in powder forms, appear to be beneficial in the prevention of infection in experimental animals. Although actual blood levels of antibiotics have been studied extensively, it would appear that the quantity of absorption of the antimicrobial agent in treated wounds is not sufficient to prevent infections in untreated contaminated incisions located in a different site in the same animal.

It can be seen that varied and sometimes confusing experiences are represented in this summary of representative studies using local antibiotics in the treatment of induced experimental wound infections. This is also reflected in clinical studies carried out on humans.

CLINICAL LOCAL ANTIBIOTIC STUDIES

In general, most studies have shown some value from the use of topical antibiotics in the prevention of wound infections. Only a few studies have found little or no value in the use of local antibiotics. Caro and Reynolds [28] found no significant difference in the sepsis rate in a study of superficial wounds in which deep hemostatic sutures were excluded. They utilized an aerosol spray containing neomycin, polymyxin B and bacitracin. The infection rate was the same in both the treated and untreated wounds. The incidence of infection was similar to that reported by the ad hoc Committee on Trauma [3] in a national study which found that nonspecific prophylactic antibiotic therapy did not reduce wound sepsis rates. Many other studies, however, have found that the utilization of topical antibiotics by either irrigation, spray or tissue injection is of value.

Mountain and Seal [29] studied a group of patients having appendectomies. These patients had bacterial contamination of their wounds by potential pathogens due to spread from the acutely inflamed appendix. They found that instillation of ampicillin in 500 mg. quantities significantly reduced the incidence of wound sepsis. A double blind study by Brockenbrough and Moylan [30] included 240 patients with contaminated surgical incisions. Seventy-seven percent of the wounds had growth in bacterial cultures obtained prior to the wound closures. Wound infections occurred in 20% of the patients who had been treated with a saline irrigant and in 10% of those treated with a kanamycin irrigation. Seidenstein *et al.* [31] also reported a study using the double blind approach on 311 patients. One-hundred-and-fifty-five patients had a kanamycin irrigation of the incisions and 156 patients' wounds were irrigated with a placebo containing no antibiotics. There were six wound infections in the kanamycin group and 11 in the group irrigated with saline. This was a 50% reduction in the infection rate in the antibiotic treated group. The total number of patients treated in these studies was quite small. Analysis has shown that the data were not statistically conclusive. Though the latter two studies cited indicate that antibiotic irrigation was of value, the authors acknowledge that no significant difference existed. There are many studies with fewer cases recommending antibiotic irrigation as being of great value.

Aerosol antibiotic combinations of polymyxin B, bacitracin and neomycin were used during the 1950 decade. This combination, known as polybactrin, was used in treating wounds in a large number of studies. The report of Forbes [32] is representative of these studies. He found that three-quarters of the infections were caused by *Staphylococcus aureus* either alone or in combination with other bacteria. There was no case of allergy or other side effect from the antibiotics in the investigation. From the period 1957–1960, the infection rate fell progressively from 6.7%, which is consistent with both the British and North American national averages, to 1.8%. Similar studies by Fielding, Rao and Davis [33] had an infection rate of 0.9% when topical antibiotics were used compared with 3.8% in control untreated wounds in clean operations where contamination was not likely to occur, and a rate of 12.8% compared with 16.1% in potentially infected wounds. Most of the wound infections were caused by staphylococci. Gibson [34] had a similar experience. Stoller [35] did a double blind study on patients with acute appendicitis. The wound incisions were treated with an aerosol polybactrin spray or etherialized starch. The results showed that there was no significant difference between the two groups, although there were fewer infections in the antibiotic treated groups of patients. This investigation did not include a bacteriologic study of the causative microorganisms. It has been shown in other studies, however, that wound infection following appendectomy is not usually staphylococcal. None of the studies determined if polybactrin was more effective against gram-positive cocci than the gram-negative bacilli. These factors may account for the difference in this report when compared to others.

A recent study by Mack and Cantrell [36] showed that an aerosol containing neomycin, polymyxin B and bacitracin was effective in eliminating bacterial infections of granulating wounds populated by a variety of gram-positive and -negative microorganisms. There were two significant observations in this study. The first was that an overgrowth of resistant bacteria did not occur during a ten-day period in the antibiotic treated wounds. The second observation was that a remarkable variation in the species and the number of bacteria occurred spontaneously in the untreated control group.

The experimental studies on war type injuries in animals resulted in clinical studies on patients in Vietnam. Heisterkamp *et al.* [37] studied the effect of a topical oxytetracycline aerosol and the combination of neomycin, bacitracin and polymyxin aerosol on war wounds in soldiers where debridement was delayed. They found that infection occurred in 16% of the oxytetracycline treated group, 16% of the combination antibiotic treated group, and in 39% of the untreated group.

Local antibiotics have been employed in forms other than as irrigants and topical sprays. Ryan [38] infiltrated the soft tissues about the incisions in hernia operations with penicillin G in order to increase the concentration of antibiotic in the soft tissues of the wounds. There was a statistically significant decrease in the infection rate when comparisons were made with the untreated controls. In a different approach, Nash and Hugh [39] placed 1 Gm. of ampicillin in wound incisions in patients having colon operations. These investigators believed that a greater concentration of antibiotic would remain in the sutured incisions than would be present when antibiotic aerosols and irrigations were employed. The results of their study showed a significant reduction in wound sepsis. Of those patients not treated with the antibiotic powder, 40% developed infections, while only 3% developed infections in the treated group. Clinical studies reporting antibiotic-detergent combinations contain too few patients to be of significance.

Most clinical reports state that there have been no adverse effects from local antibiotic treatment of wounds. There have been no reports of allergic reaction or retardation of wound healing. One frequently cited report [40] described a loss of hearing in one patient from a neomycin irrigation of a granulating wound. Complications are rare, not recognized or have not been reported.

Multiple variables are involved in these clinical studies. The processes are complex and are not susceptible to adequate controls. Since many factors such as the species of bacteria, the degree of wound contamination, and the bacterial antibiotic sensitivity are not known statistical correlation would seem unlikely.

PARENTERAL ANTIBIOTICS

The studies on the utilization of parenteral antibiotics to prevent wound infections are closely related to local antibiotic treatment. Comment is necessary on this controversial subject. Until recently, most clinical studies have concluded that prophylactic antibiotics have not decreased the incidence of postoperative wound infection. This conclusion is the result of a number of clinical reports [41–44] from reliable institutions. However, in these studies antibiotic therapy was begun at the time of contamination or after the wounding occurred. They are also open to criticism because they are retrospective and poorly controlled.

Recently, the studies of Bernard and Cole [45], Bernard *et al.* [46], Polk and Lopez-Mayor [47], and others [48, 49] have shown that a decrease in the incidence of wound infections occurs in patients if they were given prophylactic antibiotics prior to operation. The apparent success of this approach has been explained by findings from previously cited studies [5–8]. These studies show that suppression of infection occurred immediately after wounding because tissue defenses against bacteria are established during this period. Factors influencing resistance to bacteria were inoperative after this time. The experiments showed that antibiotics are effective in supplementing the host defenses during this initial period, but apparently become ineffective later. When antibiotics were utilized after the bacteria had become established, the host defenses had become inadequate. Utilization of antibiotics did not prevent the development of wound infections in this circumstance. The experimental study of Gingrass, Close and Ellison [14] appears to substantiate this concept. They found that a significant decrease in infections occurred in wounds in experimental animals when combinations of parenteral antibiotics were given prior to the injury. A significant decrease was observed when parenteral antibiotics were given prior to wounding and were followed by antibiotic irrigation.

These recent reports indicate that the proper timing of the antibiotic administration is an essential factor for effective prophylaxis. If this concept is valid, antimicrobial agents should apparently be given before the bacterial contamination occurs. This is a very recently developed approach and it certainly merits further study.

EFFECT OF ANTIBIOTICS ON WOUND HEALING

There have been a number of reports on the inhibition of protein synthesis in rats by penicillamine, an in vivo product of the hydrolysis of penicillin. Penicillamine delays the intermolecular covalent bonding in collagen. It has been estimated that approximately 40% of the injected penicillin is hydrolyzed into penicillamine. Pohl and Hunt [50] found that there was little evidence of interference and decreased wound strength if doses corresponding to 80 million units per day in a man weighing 70 kilograms were given. In another study, Seifter *et al.* [51], reported that penicillin would reduce the tensile strength of healing wounds if doses approximating 600 million units per day were given to man. The authors in both studies agree that neither study indicated that penicillin used in maximum therapeutic dosage in man would affect or interfere with collagen metabolism.

Chloramphenicol and tetracycline have shown inhibition of protein synthesis. Chloramphenicol has been shown to inhibit protein synthesis in a mammalian cell free system as well as in bacterial systems. This antibiotic also inhibits antibody synthesis as well. Tetracycline, which influences both nitrogen and electrolyte balances in man, inhibits growth of bone in embryonic rats and in cell tissue cultures. Bloom and Grillo [52] used the tensile strength of wounds in guinea pigs to measure the effect of both of these antibiotics on collagen synthesis. There was no significant difference in the wound tensile strength of animals treated with these antibiotics when compared to the untreated controls. They believed that the fibroblastic system is considerably less sensitive to the effect of these drugs than in other tissue systems which have been studied.

Histologic examination [15] of wounds treated with high concentrations of cephalothin have been done at the end of the first, second, third and seventh days and compared to untreated controls. One hundred milligrams of powder was placed in each treated incision and the skin closed with nylon sutures. Little difference was noted between the treated and untreated groups. On the seventh day marked reparative fibrosis was present in both groups.

Various antibiotics have been shown to affect nutrition in animals and man. All antibiotics can produce adverse effects such as allergy, renal tubular necrosis, etc. There is not sufficient evidence at present to show that any antibiotic presently employed for the treatment of infection affects wound healing when used in therapeutic quantities.

COMMENTS

It is doubtful that any clinical or experimental comparison can be made from the studies that have been done to date. Many factors play a role in the development of infections which affect wound healing in both patients and experimental animals. The different results obtained by various experimental studies are good examples. The conflict of opinions is probably the result of data obtained from experiments in which a great number of experimental and bacteriologic variables exist. A variety of experimental animals have been employed, including mice, guinea pigs, rabbits, goats and dogs. Many of the studies neglected to show how bacteria present on the skin were reduced or altered prior to incision. Some studies required an enormous number of human pathogens, between 5 million and 500 million, to induce infections in experimental animals. The human pathogens employed were often not normal pathogens for the experimental animals. The size of the inoculum varied and it was not determined whether the number of organisms used was viable or not. Other investigators smeared feces in the wound. One ingenious investigator used the dirt from the laboratory floor as the inoculum.

Some investigators determined whether the microorganisms used were sensitive or resistant to the antibiotic employed; others did not. Frequently, the time factor between inoculation and treatment was not recorded, though the more recent studies have tried to permit sufficient time for the initiation of infection to occur prior to treatment. Many types of local, intravenous and general anesthesia were used. It was not determined whether the animals were in shock—a factor proven to inhibit the normal host tissue resistance to infection.

Some investigators placed suture material in the depths of the wound; others ligated portions of the subcutaneous tissue in order to produce tissue necrosis. Many authors sutured the skin without obliteration of the dead space or evacuation of hematomas which may have occurred beneath the sutures. The location of the incision as well as the size and depth were not described or were different. Systemic absorption of local antibiotics is generally accepted as having no discernible effect on the infection occurring in the untreated wounds when the treated contaminated incisions were used in the same animals. However, there is some conflict of opinion in this matter, as others were able to determine that there was some systemic effect from the local treatment.

Analysis of the clinical studies showed that many of the group studies were not comparable. Sepsis is not a uniform and distinct entity. Underlying diseases and the state of the health of the patients were not noted. The operative material was frequently not defined and was heterogenous. The factors within the fluctuation of the monthly and yearly sepsis rates make it difficult to accept retrospective and uncontrolled studies of antibiotics as being other than misleading.

It is needless to further belabor the fact that many variables exist. The literature, however, does leave an impression. The mass of literature indicates that:

1. Antibiotic irrigations, sprays or aerosols and powders do reduce the incidence of wound infections in experimental animals.

2. Local antibiotics reduce the incidence of wound infections in humans.

3. Parenteral antibiotics given after injury and contamination occur do not reduce infections in experimental animals or humans.

4. Parenteral antibiotics given prior to injury and contamination do reduce the incidence of wound infection.

Some of the impressions are correct and others will no doubt be proven false. A critical review can also lead to a statement that neither the experimental nor the clinical literature convincingly demonstrates that antibiotics given either parenterally or employed topically can or cannot prevent infection.

It would be improper to become disheartened. The problems of coping with infections occurring in skin burns had at one time appeared to be insurmountable. The success of topical antibiotic agents in the treatment of burns in recent years should give us hope that local treatment of wounds to prevent infections can be solved. More clinical and experimental studies are necessary. It is our opinion that the efficacy of local treatment of wounds with antibiotics should be investigated with a national study involving a number of reliable institutions.

REFERENCES

1. Meleney, F. L.: A statistical analysis of a study of the prevention of infection in soft part wounds, compound fractures and burns with special reference to the sulfonamides, Surg. Gynec. & Obst. 80:263, 1945.
2. Ives, H. R., and Hirshfield, J. W.: The bacterial flora of clean surgical wounds, Ann. Surg. 107:607, 1938.
3. Report of the Ad Hoc Committee of the Committee on Trauma, Division of Medical Sciences, National Academy of Sciences-National Research Council: Postoperative wound infections, Ann. Surg. 160 (Supp. 2): 1, 1964.
4. Condie, J. D., and Ferguson, D. J.: Experimental wound infections: Contamination versus surgical technique, Surgery 50:367, 1961.
5. Miles, A. A., Miles, E. M., and Burke, J.: The value and duration of defence reactions of th e skin to primary lodgement of bacteria, Brit. J. Exper. Path. 38:79, 1957.
6. Miles, A. A.: Non-specific defense reactions in bacterial infections, Ann. New York Acad. Sc. 66:356, 1956.
7. Miles, A. A., and Niven, J. F.: The enhancement of infection during shock produced by bacterial toxins and other agents, Brit. J. Exper. Path. 31:73, 1950.
8. Burk, J. F.: The effective period of preventive antibiotic action in experimental incisions and dermal lesions, Surgery 50:161, 1961.
9. Peterson, L. W.: Prophylaxis of wound infection, Arch. Surg. 50:177, 1945.
10. Falconer, B., Liljedahl, S., and Olovson, T.: On the effect of treatment of traumatic wounds with soap solution, Acta. chir. scandinav. 103:222, 1952.
11. Taylor, F. W.: An experimental evaluation of operative wound irrigations, Surg. Gynec. & Obst. 113:465, 1961.
12. Singleton, A. O., Jr., Davis, D., and Julian, J.: Prevention of wound infection following contamination with colon organisms, Surg. Gynec. & Obst. 180:389, 1959.
13. Gingrass, R. P., Close, A. S., and Ellison, E. H.: Experimental wound infection and its prevention by topical and parenteral techniques, Wisconsin M. J. 62:501, 1963.
14. Gingrass, R. P., Close, A. S., and Ellison, E.: The effect of various topical and parenteral agents on the prevention of infection in experimental contaminated wounds, J. Trauma 4:763, 1964.
15. Singleton, A. O., Jr., and Julian, J.: Experimental evaluation of methods used to prevent infection in wounds which have been contaminated with feces, Ann. Surg. 151:912, 1960.
16. Casten, D. F., Nach, R. J., and Spinza, J.: On experimental and clinical study of the effectiveness of antibiotic wound irrigation in preventing infection, Surg. Gynec. & Obst. 118:783, 1964.
17. Hopson, W. B., Britt, L. G., Sherman, R. T., and Ledes, C. P.: The use of topical antibiotics in the prevention of experimental wound infection, J. S. Res. 8:261, 1968.
18. Glotzer, D. J., Goodman, W. S., and Geronimus, L. H.: Topical antibiotic prophylaxis in contaminated wounds. Experimental evaluation, Arch. Surg. 100:589, 1970.
19. Mendelson, J. A.: Topical therapy as an expedient treatment of massive open wounds, Surgery 48:1035, 1960.
20. Brinkley, F. B., Bailey, J. A., and Mendelson, J. A.: Comparative duration of the antibacterial effect of topical penicillin and mafenide on experimental animals, J. Lab. & Clin. Med. 62:286, 1963.
21. Matsumoto, T., et al.: Topical antibiotic spray in contaminated crush wounds in animals, Military Med. 133:869, 1968.
22. Gray, F. J., and Kidd, E. E.: Topical chemotherapy in prevention of wound infection, Surgery 54:891, 1963.

23. Waterman, N. G., Howell, R. S., and Babich, M.: The effect of a prophylactic topical antibiotic on the incidence of wound infection, Arch. Surg. 97:365, 1968.
24. Grunberg, E., and Schnitzer, R. J.: Experimental approach to topical antibacterial therapy, Ann. New York Acad. Sc. 82:114, 1959.
25. Howes, E. L.: Prevention of wound infections by injection of non-toxic antibacterial agents, Ann. Surg. 124:268, 1946.
26. Brunner, R., Kraushaar, A., and Prohaska, E.: Inhibition of penicillinase and reduction of resistance in surface-active substances, Antibiotic Ann. 1:169, 1959-60.
27. Compere, E. L., Metzger, W., and Miltra, R.: The treatment of pyogenic bone and joint infections by closed irrigation with a non-toxic detergent and one or more antibiotics, J. Bone & Joint Surg. 49A:614, 1967.
28. Caro, D., and Reynolds, E. W.: Prevention of wound sepsis in a casualty department, Brit. J. Clin. Prac. 21:605, 1967.
29. Mountain, J. C., and Seal, P. V.: Topical ampicillin in grid-iron appendectomy wounds, Brit. J. Clin. Prac. 24:111, 1970.
30. Brockenbrough, E. C., and Moylan, J. A.: Treatment of contaminated surgical wounds with a topical antibiotic—a double-blind study of 240 patients, Am. J. Surg. 35:789, 1969.
31. Seidenstein, M., Salomons, M. M., Herbsman, H., et al.: Evaluation of local antibiotic instillation in extremity wounds, Surgery 68:809, 1970.
32. Forbes, G. B.: Staphylococcal infection of operation wounds with special reference to topical prophylaxis, Lancet 2:505, 1961.
33. Fielding, G., Rao, A., Davis, N. C., and Werner, N.: Prophylactic topical use of antibiotics in surgical wounds: A controlled clinical trial using polybactrin, M. J. Australia 2:159, 1965.
34. Gibson, R. M.: Application of antibiotics (polybactrin) in surgical practice, using the aerosol technique, Brit. M. J. 1:326, 1958.
35. Stoller, J. L.: Topical antibiotic therapy in acute appendicitis, Brit. J. Clin. Prac. 19:687, 1965.
36. Mack, R. M., and Cantrell, J. R.: Quantitative studies of the bacterial flora of open skin wounds: The effect of topical antibiotics, Ann. Surg. 166:886, 1967.
37. Heisterkamp, C., Vernick, J., Simmons, R. L., et al.: Topical antibiotics in war wounds—a re-evaluation, Military Med. 134:13,1969.
38. Ryan, E. A.: Wound infection prevention by topical antibiotics, Brit. J. Surg. 54:324, 1967.
39. Nash, A. G., and Hugh, T. B.: Topical ampicillin and wound infection in colon surgery, Brit. M. J. 1:471, 1967.
40. Kelly, D. R., Nilo, E. R., and Berggren, R. B.: Brief recording-deafness after topical neomycin wound irrigation, New England J. Med. 280:1338, 1969.
41. McKittrick, L. S., and Wheelock, F. C.: The routine use of antibiotics in elective abdominal surgery, Surg. Gynec. & Obst. 99:376, 1954.
42. Altemeier, W. A., Culbertson, W. R., and Vetto, M.: Prophylactic antibiotic therapy, Arch. Surg. 71:2, 1955.
43. Taylor, G. W.: Preventive use of antibiotics in surgery, Brit. M. Bull. 16:51, 1960.
44. Johnstone, F. R. C.: An assessment of prophylactic antibiotics in general surgery, Surg. Gynec. & Obst. 116:1, 1963.
45. Bernard, H. R., and Cole, W. R.: The prophylaxis of surgical infection: the effect of prophylactic antimicrobial drugs on the incidence of infection following potentially contaminated operations, Surgery 56:151, 1964.
46. Bernard, H. R., Clark, W. R., Jr., Leather, R. P., and Gray, V. C.: Chemoprophylaxis of postoperative infection—Cephalothin versus penicillin G, Arch. Surg. 99:388, 1969.
47. Polk, H. C., Jr., and Louez-Mayor, J. F.: Postoperative wound infection—A prospective study of determinant factors and prevention, Surgery 66:97, 1969.
48. Ketcham, G. F., Bloch, J. H., and Crawford, D. T.: The role of prophylactic antibiotic therapy in control of staphylococcal infections following cancer surgery, Surg. Gynec. & Obst. 174:345, 1962.

49. Todd, J. C.: Wound infection: Etiology, prevention, and management, Surg. Clin. N. Am. 48:787, 1968.
50. Pohl, R., and Hunt, T. K.: Penicillin G and wound healing, Arch. Surg. 101:610, 1970.
51. Seifter, E., Morris, J. J., and Levenson, S. M.: Effects of very large doses of penicillin G given orally to rats, Nature 217:1055, 1968.
52. Bloom, G. P., and Grillo, H. C.: The influence of tetracycline and chloramphenicol on the healing of cutaneous wounds, J. S. Res. 10:1, 1970.

16

Keloids and Hypertrophic Scars

Jose Garcia-Velasco, M.D., F.A.C.S. *

Hypertrophic scars and keloids are an abnormal proliferation of dense fibrous tissue which develops in the dermis, usually covered with a thin layer of epidermis. They are characterized by an elevation, extension into surrounding normal tissue and a tendency to recur after excision [1].

Histologically the young keloid is a connective tissue proliferation with many fibroblasts, edema, new blood vessels and a characteristic lack of elastic tissue. As it gets older the vascularization is less apparent, the fibroblasts decrease in number and the collagen is totally or partially hyalinized [2].

The first clear description of a keloid was given by Alibert in 1806. He termed the lesions "les cancroides", but it wasn't until 1817 that he used the term "cheloide" [3]. The word keloid is derived from the Greek *chele,* meaning crab's claw, and *oid* meaning like [1].

There are many theories regarding the etiology and pathology of hypertrophic scars and keloids. In patients with keloid and hypertrophic scars there appears to be some abnormality in the second and third phases of wound healing (fibroblast proliferation with collagen formation, and maturation of the scar), with the process of fibroplasia continuing beyond the usual final point to produce a benign fibrous tumor [1]. Among the factors associated with hypertrophic scars or keloid type of healing, we find: skin color, race and heredity, hormonal factor, tension on the wound, the wound's orientation in relation to skin lines, local infection, absence of primary healing, foreign body reaction, hair and keratinized material of endogenous origin [3–10]. Though keloid and hypertrophic scars can be found in the skin of almost any part of the human body, the most frequent areas are the face, the neck, the anterior chest and the shoulder (from vaccination). They often appear after ear piercing (Fig. 16-1A). These scars are less frequently seen in other places (Fig. 16-1B) and very seldom on mucosal surfaces.

Sometimes it is difficult to make a definite clinical differentiation between keloids and hypertrophic scars. In hypertrophic scars, the second phase of healing appears to be an overreactive type of response which is self limiting, and the

---
*Department of Plastic and Reconstructive Surgery, Hospital General, Centro Medico Nacional, Instituto Mexicano Del Seguro Social.

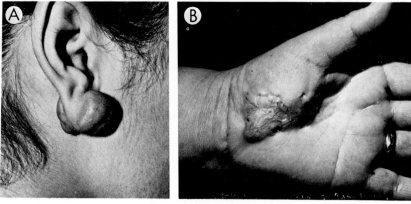

Fig. 16–1.—A, typical keloid following ear piercing. **B**, unusual keloid scar on the palm of the hand.

scar eventually undergoes some degree of maturation. Hypertrophic scars never invade the surrounding tissue as a true keloid does [1]. In keloids, the process of fibroplasia continues on and on enlarging the scar and even involving areas of skin that were not damaged by the original trauma. Conway *et al.* [11] tried to establish the difference by tissue culture techniques, but the difficulties of technique made their results of little value from the clinical point of view.

TREATMENT

The treatment of keloids and hypertrophic scars has been a challenge to the specialist dealing with wound healing and skin problems. If the problem is mainly functional as in the case of scar contractures caused by trauma, burns or badly placed incisions, a treatment consisting of contracture relief by Z-plasty, skin flap or skin graft is in most cases very successful (Fig. 16-2). The problem arises when the patient seeks more than a good functional result and desires a better cosmetic result. The most advisable types of treatment for keloids are surgery combined with radiotherapy, surgery combined with corticosteroids, or corticosteroids alone. Even though many workers report good results with radiotherapy [12], the hazards of its use are well known and recently fewer specialists use this kind of treatment [13]. Surgery alone generally has very little chance of success, but the method recommended by Conway *et al.* [11] to excise the lesion within its area margin to get a smaller scar may be used in extremely large keloids.

Even though surgery combined with steroid compounds is probably the most recommended treatment at present, the result is not perfect. Steroid compounds have been used alone with similar results [1, 5, 11, 14–28]. Conway and Stark [29] observed that ACTH improved the symptoms of itching and pain when injected into keloids, but no change in the lesion was observed. Their results encouraged others to try various other anti-inflammatory agents including hydro-

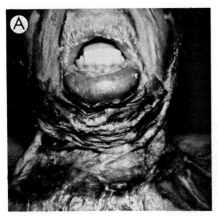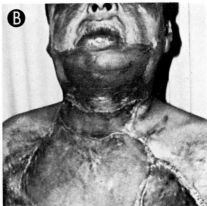

Fig. 16–2.—A, post burn scar contracture of the neck. **B**, after treatment with excision and split thickness skin grafts.

cortisone acetate, dexamethasone and triamcinolone acetonide. These have been used for the treatment of keloids by direct injection into the scar using a regular syringe or the Dermojet syringe [30], or by injection into the wound margins prior to suture. Similar results have been reported with both techniques giving satisfactory responses—the only interesting side effect was local skin and subcutaneous tissue atrophy.

Among several experiments carried out to study the mechanism of the action of topical corticosteroids on inflammation and wound healing, Berliner reported [14, 17–19, 26, 27, 31] the effect of these compounds in the wound healing process and concluded that an appropriate and well controlled therapeutic treatment of keloids and hypertrophic scars with corticosteroids can be achieved. Various studies have been carried out with different products to illustrate the wound healing process under topical corticosteroid therapy. Studies on the skin of female CBA mice were conducted to evaluate the effect of topically applied anti-inflammatory corticosteroids on healing wounds. The animals were treated with various anti-inflammatory corticosteroids in propylene glycol buffered with 0.01% citrate once daily for the duration of the experiment, after a wound had been made on the dorsal midline. The wound area was removed after killing the animals at 4, 8, 12, 16 and 20 days after treatment. A control group of animals was treated in the same fashion. Tensile strength was determined. In the control wounds tensile strength reached its maximum at 16 days with a slight decrease at 20 days. The treated wound tensile strength remained relatively low for 16 days. At 20 days there was no significant difference between the tensile strength of control and treated wounds. Gross examination of the wounds at 20 days showed less scar in the treated wounds.

Histological studies of healing wounds were carried out in dogs [27]. Two incisions were made on the back of the animals; one was swabbed with fluocinolone acetonide 0.025% in propylene glycol buffered with 0.01% citrate and the other with a placebo solution three times a day for 20 days. Fluocinolone acetonide was chosen in this experiment as it was shown to be 40 times more potent than cortisol in inhibiting fibroblast growth in vitro [15]. Biopsy specimens were taken at 8, 13 and 20 days and histological specimens were prepared and stained with hematoxylin and eosin or Mowry's mucopolysaccharide stain, and examined in normal and polarized light. All histological specimens consistently showed a marked decrease in the width of the forming scar in the steroid treated wounds. Additionally, examination of the hematoxylin and eosin stained sections showed a drastic diminution in the number of fibroblasts in the steroid treated scar with respect to the control. In the placebo treated wounds, the newly formed collagen at the site of the wound was fibrillar and oriented in the same plane as the epidermis. However, with fluocinolone acetonide the collagen was much less dense and the fine fibrils were oriented more in the same direction as the incision. Examination of the scar with polarized light again showed that the extent of the wound, as indicated by old collagen at the edges of the wound, was smaller in steroid treated wounds. Sections from wound tissues treated with fluocinolone acetonide showed very little mucopolysaccharide staining material while those with no steroid treatment had an abundance of this material [32]. In summary, the width of the scar, the amount of collagen present, the amount of mucopolysaccharide staining material and the number of fibroblasts at the site of the wound were markedly decreased in wounds treated with the steroid from 13 days of treatment on.

Based on these studies, a clinical study was conducted in patients with keloids using the synthetic corticosteroid compound in different routes and dosage forms

Fig. 16–3.—**A**, keloid on the forearm. **B**, treatment by excision and injection of the wound's margins with a suspension of F.A. 40 mg./ml. Note the remission on one portion and the recurrence of the rest.

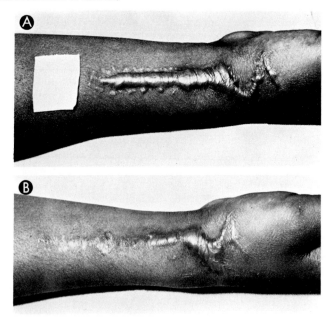

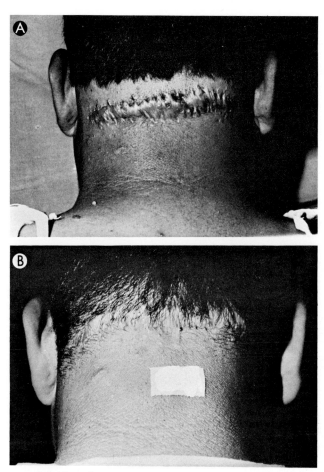

Fig. 16–4.—A, keloid on the nape of the neck. B, after treatment with excision and injection of the wound's margin with a suspension of F.A. 40 mg./ml.

[33, 34]. The solution of fluocinolone acetonide (F.A.) at 0.025% in propylene glycol was tested clinically. Surgery was performed to remove the lesion, direct careful closure without tension was made when possible, or a split thickness skin graft was placed over the defect if the area was too extensive to suture. The wound was swabbed with the solution once a day for one month. In all cases the lesion reappeared and in some instances it was larger. Therefore, this solution was considered to be clinically ineffective.

A more concentrated medication was tested in a group of 15 patients where the scars were excised and the wounds carefully closed using subdermal sutures to minimize the tension and a continuous intradermal suture with 4-0 nylon to permit it to be left a longer time. The suture line was left intact for 12 hours, 0.2% F.A. cream was applied to the wound and then an occlusive dressing (Saran Wrap® sealed with adhesive tape) was applied for 72 hours. The dressing

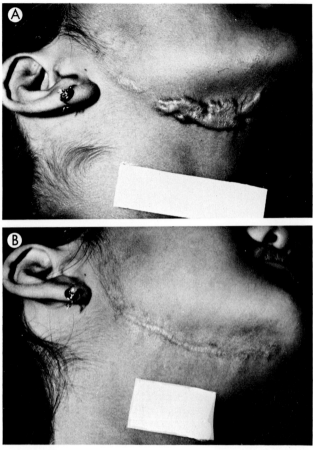

Fig. 16–5.—**A**, post burn keloid of the neck. **B**, after treatment with excision and injection of the wound's margin with suspension of F.A. 40 mg./ml.

was removed, the wound was left exposed for 8 hours to avoid maceration and then the same occlusive dressing applied. This procedure was repeated for 6 weeks. All the wounds healed uneventfully, the follow-up showed that the keloids appeared again but less extensively and after a longer period of remission. An overall study of the patients showed that the remission of the lesion was present during the time the cream was used. In some cases, the longer remission demonstrated the effect of the compound, but showed that by this procedure selection of dosage form and time of use are difficult to determine.

A different group of 15 patients was treated the same way as far as the removal of the scar and suturing of the wound was concerned, but in these cases the steroid compound was a suspension of F.A. 40 mg./ml. injected into the wound margins prior to the suture. Here again the results were very similar to the previous group, the healing was normal and the scars remained flat for a

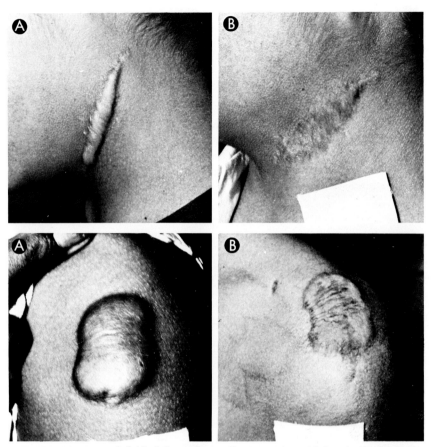

Fig. 16–6 (top).—**A**, keloid of the neck. **B**, after treatment with intralesional injection of 3 doses of a suspension of 40 mg./ml. of F.A.

Fig. 16–7 (bottom).—**A**, post vaccination keloid of the shoulder. **B**, after treatment with intralesional injection of one dose of a suspension of F.A. 40 mg./ml. Note the skin atrophy around the treated lesion.

longer period of time, but the final result was a hypertrophic lesion of some degree. Some slight improvement was found nevertheless (Figs. 16-3 to 16-5).

The same 40 mg./ml. suspension was used in the classical intralesional injection when the lesion was very extensive and the surgical removal impractical. A total of 30 patients was treated by impregnating the lesion with the compound. Results similar to those found by other authors who have worked on this problem were seen in this group of patients where there was an improvement of the symptoms and a softening of the lesion after the first dose making the subsequent injections easier (Figs. 16-6 and 16-7). The maximum dose was 2 ml. repeated as necessary every month—in some cases as many as 5 times.

Generally, we can say that when hypertrophic scars were treated, the results were better than those of a true keloid. At the end of our study, the observations were quite satisfactory, with results in 50% of the cases showing flattening of the scars and disappearance of itching and pain. In 30% of the patients studied, the scars were softer with some improvement of symptoms and 20% evidenced no improvement. Long term follow-up has shown recurrence in a few cases (Fig. 16-6). The complications were a slight degree of skin and subcutaneous tissue atrophy which could be controlled. No systemic effects were seen (Fig. 16-7).

Our general feeling is that the steroid compounds are presently the best treatment for keloids and hypertrophic scars, although they are not the last word. The general problems in all the cases were the difficulties in selecting the correct dose and the right duration of treatment to prevent the appearance of new keloids or hypertrophic scars. In conclusion, a new progressive and systematic form of administration must be developed to distribute the drug "in situ" in the exact dose and during the correct period of time.

REFERENCES

1. Smith, J. W., and Conway, H.: In Grabb, W. C., and Smith, J. W. (eds.): *Plastic Surgery* (Boston: Little, Brown and Company, 1968).
2. Gonzalez, A.: Personal communication.
3. Cosman, B., Crikelair, G. F., Ju, D. M. C., Gaulin, J. C., and Lattes, R.: The surgical treatment of keloids, Plast. & Reconstruct. Surg. 27:335, 1961.
4. Crikelair, G. F., Ju, D. M. C., and Cosman, B.: Scars and Keloids, in Converse, J. M. (ed.): *Reconstructive Plastic Surgery* (Philadelphia: W. B. Saunders Co., 1964).
5. Garb, J., and Stone, M. J.: Keloids: Review of literature and report of eighty cases, Am. J. Surg. 58:315, 1942.
6. Trusler, H. M., and Bauer, T. K.: Keloids and hypertrophic scars, Arch. Surg. 57: 539, 1948.
7. Asboe-Hansen, G.: Hypertrophic scar and keloids, Dermatología 120:178, 1960.
8. Glucksman, A.: Local factors in the histogenesis of hypertrophic scars, Brit. J. Plast. Surg. 4:88, 1951.
9. Fajer, C. M., and Zederfeldt, B.: Studies on wound healing and trauma, Acta path. et microbiol. scandinav. 47:225, 1959.
10. Patterson, W. B. (ed.): *Wound Healing and Tissue Repair* (Chicago: University of Chicago Press, 1956).
11. Conway, H., Gillette, R., Smith, J. W., and Findley, A.: Differential diagnosis of keloids and hypertrophic scars by tissue culture technique with notes on therapy of keloids by surgical excision and Decadron, Plast. & Reconstruct. Surg. 25:117, 1960.
12. Fischer, E., and Strock, H.: Roentgen therapy of keloid, Schweiz. med. Wchnschr. 87:1281, 1957.
13. Conway, Herbert, and Hugo, Norman E.: Radiation dermatitis and malignancy, Plast. & Reconstruct. Surg. 38:3, 1966.
14. Ruhmann, A. G., and Berliner, D. L.: Effects of steroids on growth of mouse fibroblasts in vitro, Endocrinology 76:916, 1965.
15. Schlagel, C. A.: Comparative efficacy of topical anti-inflammatory corticosteroids, J. Pharm. Sci. 54:335, 1965.
16. Tonelli, G., Thibault, L., and Ringler, I.: Bioassay for the concomitant assessment of the antiphlogistic and thymolytic activities of topically applied corticoids, Endocrinology 77:625, 1965.
17. Baker, B. L., and Whitaker, W. L.: Interference with wound healing by local action of adrenocortical steroids, Endocrinology 46:544, 1950.
18. Ruhmann, A. G., and Berliner, D. L.: Influence of steroids on fibroblasts. II. The fibroblast as an assay system for topical anti-inflammatory potency of corticosteroids, J. Invest. Dermat. 49:123, 1967.

19. Castor, C. W., and Muriden, K. D.: Collagen formation in monolayer cultures of human fibroblasts. The effects of hydrocortisone, Lab. Invest. 13:560, 1964.
20. Castor, C. W.: Adrenocorticoid suppression of mucopolysaccharide formation in human connective tissue cell cultures, J. Lab. & Clin. Med. 60:788, 1962.
21. Griffith, B. H.: The treatment of keloids with triamcinolone acetonide, Plast. & Reconstruct. Surg. 38:202, 1966.
22. Ketchum, L., Smith, J., Robinson, D. W., and Masters, F. W.: The treatment of hypertrophic scar, keloid and scar contracture by triamcinolone acetonide, Plast. & Reconstruct. Surg. 38:209, 1966.
23. Maguire, H. C., Jr.: Treatment of keloids with triamcinolone acetonide injected intralesionally, J.A.M.A. 192:325, 1965.
24. Murray, R. D.: Kenalog and the treatment of hypertrophied scars and keloids in Negroes and whites, Plast. & Reconstruct. Surg. 31:275, 1963.
25. Pariser, H., and Murray, P. F.: Intralesional injections of triamcinolone, Arch. Derm. 87:183, 1963.
26. Campos, J. S., and Berliner, D. L.: Acción de la aplicación tópica de fluocinolona en el proceso de cicatrización en humanos. Reporte preliminar, VI Reunión Anual Soc. Mex. Nut. y Endoc. 59, 1966.
27. Berliner, D. L., Williams, R. J., Taylor, G. N., and Nabors, C. J., Jr.: Decreased scar formation with topical corticosteroid treatment, Surgery 61:619, 1967.
28. Griffith, B. H., Monroe, C. W., and McKinney, P.: A follow up study on the treatment of keloids with triamcinolone acetonide, Plast. & Reconstruct. Surg. 46:145, 1970.
29. Conway, H., and Stark, R. B.: ACTH in plastic surgery, Plast. & Reconstruct. Surg. 8:354, 1951.
30. Vallis, Charles P.: Intralesional injection of keloids and hypertrophic scars with the Dermojet, Plast. & Reconstruct. Surg. 40:255, 1967.
31. Berliner, D. L., and Ruhmann, A. G.: Influence of steroids on fibroblasts. I. An in vitro fibroblast assay for corticosteroids, J. Invest. Dermat. 49:117, 1967.
32. Berliner, D. L., Williams, R. J., Taylor, G. N., and Nabors, C. J., Jr.: A histological and histochemical investigation concerning the effects of topically applied fluocinolone acetonide on scar formation, VI Reunión Anual Soc. Mex. Nut. y Endoc. 41, 1966.
33. García-Velasco, J.: Tratamiento de cicatrices queloides con el uso del acetonido de fluocinolona, Revista Médica I.M.S.S. (In press).
34. García-Velasco, J.: Cirugía Reconstructiva en Dermatología Fasciculo de Actualización de Dermatología, I.M.S.S. 1971.

17

Oxygen Tension and Epithelialization

I. A. Silver, M.D. *

There are many widely scattered references to the effects of oxygen on healing phenomena in different tissues [1–5] but relatively few which refer specifically to the epidermis [6, 7]. Many of these latter are empirical observations on the clinical response of nonhealing, open or infected wounds to treatment by various forms of hyperbaric oxygen application [8–10]. There are also many reports on the effects of oxygen on the healing of burns [11–13] and others particularly on the beneficial results that may attend hyperbaric oxygen therapy in cases of skin grafting [14–16].

With regard to the general oxygen environment of the various layers of the skin little has been published beyond measurements of diffusion of oxygen through intact skin during a search for suitable methods of measuring arterial Po_2 without surgical interference to patients [17–19]. This type of work has been extended by Fatt [20] who has also examined oxygen diffusion through the conjunctival epithelium, and by others who have examined oxygen diffusion and uptake in various layers of the cornea [21, 22].

The original work on the diffusion of oxygen into the deeper layers of the skin was performed by Montgomery and Horwitz [23–25] and continued by Penneys [26, 27].

No measurements of the relative oxygen permeability of the different layers of intact human skin have been reported except by Evans and Naylor [18] in relation to tape stripped skin and by Penneys [28] on isolated human stratum corneum.

The relationship of local wound environment to speed of epithelialization has been considered by Winter [29–31] in the pig and by Hinman and Maibach [32] in man through observations on epidermal regeneration under inert films. Although a relationship between oxygen permeability of the films studied and the rate of repair was noted, no measurements of the actual oxygen environment of the cells were made.

A major effort to measure oxygen tension during subepidermal wound healing has been carried out by Hunt, Zederfeldt *et al.* [33, 34] and contributions in this

---

*Department of Pathology, University of Bristol, England.

field have also been made by Niinikoski [35, 36], Remensnyder and Majno [37] and Silver [38–40]. This work has established the value of the oxygen electrode for investigations on healing tissue, and it seemed appropriate to utilize similar well tested methods, where appropriate, to establish (a) what is the normal range of oxygen environment of intact skin, (b) what changes in the environment can be expected in normal epidermal healing, (c) if imposed changes in this environment can affect healing rates, (d) what conditions exist in naturally slow healing skin defects such as burns and chronic ulcers, (e) the source of the normal epidermal O_2 supply—whether it is mostly from the blood or from the air, (f) if the supply differs in damaged epidermis, (g) what is the effect of traditional and more recently developed surgical dressings and (h) what happens during the development of superficial infections.

MATERIALS AND METHODS

Two types of oxygen electrodes were constructed and used for this investigation. The first was an ultramicro needle electrode based on the design of Silver [41] and the second was a multi-cathode Clark-type electrode [42] based on the designs of Lübbers *et al.* [43] and Evans and Naylor [44]. The needle electrodes were inserted into the skin to investigate the oxygen microenvironment at different depths below the surface, whereas the multiwire cathode was applied to the surface of intact, stripped or wounded skin to measure an "averaged" oxygen availability on a relatively gross area (about 5 mm.²).

Attempts were made to measure Pco_2 by means of macro and semimicro CO_2 electrodes [45] but these proved to be rather unreliable in the situations studied.

Oxygen Probes

Microelectrodes. These were prepared from 300μ or 12.5μ 30% iridium-platinum wire (Johnson Matthey Ltd., London, England). Both sizes of wire were electropolished to pencil point tips of between 0.5 and 2.0 μ. They were then coated with glass so that only the extreme tip of the electrode was uninsulated. The glass near the tip was very thin, and the diameter of glass and metal together did not exceed 3μ; in most cases it was about 1.5μ. The needle was coated with a thin hydrophylic film and was then inserted into a glass capillary so that its point projected from the glass for a few microns. After filling the outer capillary with electrolyte, a second oxygen permeable, but water repellent, film was deposited over the end of the outer capillary and the protruding tip of the microelectrode. A silver wire was inserted into the electrolyte from the back of the capillary to form the indifferent electrode. This system is essentially an ultramicro Clark electrode.

A second, simpler microelectrode was also used. Insulated needles were made as described above, silver was then deposited on the glass starting 50μ from the tip, and this was connected via a conducting epoxy resin (Ciba-ARL, Duxford, England) to a silver contact wire attached to the back of the electrode. The tip was dipped in the resin Rhoplex AC35 (Rohm and Haas Co., Philadelphia, Pa.) to produce a diffusion membrane.

Microelectrodes of $0.5–1.5\mu$ tip diameter collect their oxygen from a very small volume of tissue, of the order of $3–10\mu$ diameter. Thus, they can easily resolve differences of oxygen availability in various layers of the epidermis. However, because of their good resolution, if they are measuring in a nonhomogeneous environment, they may give accurate information about conditions in their immediate vicinity, but be misleading about the general condition of the epidermis over a slightly wider area. They are therefore best used in groups rather than singly so that a histogram of Po_2 values can be obtained [46].

Macroelectrodes. Multi-cathode electrodes were made by inserting a number of 5 or 10μ platinum wires into individual glass capillary tubes which were subsequently fused together. The end of the platinum-in-glass assembly was ground flat and the free wires at the back of the capillaries were twisted carefully together. The electrode assembly was placed inside a Perspex housing 5 mm. in diameter and fixed with adhesive so that the electrode tips protruded slightly below the casing. A silver wire was included in the adhesive and extended into the space between the electrodes and the casing. Contact with the backs of the electrode wires was made with a mercury seal. Electrolyte was introduced between electrodes and the casing, and the open end of the case was sealed with a 12 or 25μ Teflon membrane secured by an O ring.

Both macro and microelectrodes were polarized with a D.C. potential of between 600 and 800 mV., which was determined by the individual electrode characteristics. The current output from the electrodes, which was directly proportional to the oxygen concentration in the electrolyte between the electrode tip and the membrane, was fed to a high input impedance DC amplifier. Microelectrodes gave a current of about 10^{-13} A/mm. Hg Po_2 whereas multiwire electrodes gave relatively large currents of the order of 10^{-5} A/mm. Hg Po_2, although this varied according to the size and number of the wires used to make the cathodes.

Carbon Dioxide Probes

Pco_2 electrodes were based on a flat ended glass pH electrode placed in a housing behind a CO_2 permeable membrane. The housing contained a very weak solution of $NaHCO_3$, and pH changes reflected the amount of CO_2 dissolved in the electrolyte in front of the electrode. Until the present time it has been impossible to make such electrodes smaller than about $50–80\mu$ diameter, but recent developments in the field of ion specific microelectrodes suggest the possible availability of probes in the 1μ range [47].

Pco_2 electrodes have a very poor resolution and since CO_2 is so highly diffusible in tissue, it is very difficult and probably not very profitable to measure CO_2 gradients.

Electrodes were applied to the skin with a micromanipulator. Macroelectrodes were placed with great care to insure that they did not cause local pressure and thus affect the microcirculation of the region being measured. The method described by Huch [19] was found to be satisfactory. This involved a thick silicone rubber pad around the electrode which distributed its weight over a large area and minimized oxygen diffusion from the air under the electrode.

Skin Coverings

Skin dressings tested were standard hospital gauze swabs, Nonad-tulle (Allen and Hanbury), 12 and 6μ Teflon Film, Polythene film and Melinex polyester film (I.C.I.).

Short term alterations in wound oxygen tension were achieved by altering the respiratory gas composition, by enclosing the wounded area in a plastic bag whose gas content could be varied and by altering both respiratory gas tension and the atmosphere over the wound. With small animals the last alteration was achieved by enclosing the animal in a case inside a gas filled bag.

The investigation of oxygen permeability of skin and healing processes was carried out on small laboratory animals (rats, mice and rabbits) and on human volunteers. A few measurements were also made on pigs.

Skin stripping was carried out with standard commercial cellophane tape.

OBSERVATIONS

Oxygen Diffusion through Intact Skin

Measurements were made at the surface of skin with multi-cathode electrodes under different conditions of oxygen breathing, skin temperature and physiological states. Further observations were carried out with microelectrodes inserted into the upper layers of the dermis and deep layers of epidermis when respiratory gas tensions were kept constant and changes in Po_2 were made in the gas over the skin at the electrode site. The most striking feature of these measurements was the rather low oxygen permeability of normal human skin under resting conditions, a feature shared with the pig, as compared to the more oxygen permeable characteristics of the skin of the small laboratory animals.

A further point of some interest was that oxygen breathing in man did not necessarily elevate the Po_2 in the epidermis although it almost invariably did so in small animals.

In contrast to oxygen breathing, vasodilatation induced by warming the body or limb some distance from the measuring site always raised the Po_2 in normal human skin, but warming the skin locally near the electrode site did not have a constant effect. There was an apparent difference in permeability between subjects of about 20 years old and those of 40 years; the younger skin appeared to be more permeable. However, with the small number of subjects examined the difference was not statistically significant. Different skin areas also showed considerable variation in oxygen transmission and this seemed to be correlated with the thickness of the cornified layer.

Figures for surface Po_2 of different species breathing air and 100% O_2 for 15 minutes are given in Table 17-1. Each figure is the mean of 30 readings. The ambient air temperature was 20°C but the skin temperature was not measured.

Table 17-1
Po_2 (mm. Hg) at the Skin Surface

Species	Site	Air	O_2 for 15 Min.
Man	Medial forearm	7 ± 4.3	21 ± 10.8
	Palm	5.2 ± 3.8	12.0 ± 8.2
	Earlobe	18.1 ± 7.1	32.4 ± 14.4
Mouse	Back	28 ± 7.7	$123 \pm 21.2*$
Rabbit	Ear	25.3 ± 8.4	$125 \pm 24.1*$

*Depilated

Table 17-2
Effect of Ambient Temperature on Po_2 (mm. Hg)
at the Skin Surface of Man

Ambient Temperature	Air	O_2 for 15 Min.
4°C	2.1 ± 1.3	2.2 ± 1.5
20°C	7.0 ± 4.3	21.0 ± 10.8
37°C	40.3 ± 14.8	97 ± 30.7

The human subjects exhibited a mild degree of vasodilatation as judged by skin color before oxygen breathing. This indicates the variability of Po_2 of the human skin but does not give a guide to the Po_2 in the basal layers, nor does it show the considerable effects of temperature.

A series of experiments to show the effect of temperature on medial forearm skin Po_2 in man is summarized in Table 17-2. The subjects were in a sitting position and had been exposed to the ambient temperature for 15 minutes before measurements were started. These figures indicate the quantity of oxygen reaching the outer layers of the skin from the dermal capillary bed in varying conditions.

Diffusion of oxygen in the opposite direction was measured with microelectrodes in the basal layer of the epidermis of the forearm after occlusion of the circulation by tourniquet. Before application of the tourniquet the skin around the electrode was covered with a thick melinex film and as soon as the Po_2 in the basal layer of the skin had fallen to zero after the cessation of circulation (about 2 min.) the melinex was removed to allow access of air to the skin surface near the electrode. In 8 out of 20 observations the basal layer Po_2 remained at zero, and in 2 cases it rose to 8 mm. Hg. In the remaining 10 cases the values were between 3 and 5 mm. Hg. It seemed likely, therefore, that although O_2 did penetrate the stratum corneum it was very rapidly used by the deeper living layers of epidermis which therefore kept the Po_2 low. The major source of error in these measurements was the exact placement of the electrode point in relation to the basal layers of the skin. The electrodes were inserted to a standard depth and then withdrawn until there was no dimpling of the skin. Records from electrode tracks that showed bleeding were discarded.

In contrast to the observation above, it was noticed in rat, rabbit, and mouse, that microelectrodes in the upper dermis as well as in deep epidermis registered oxygen tensions of up to 25 mm. Hg even after the death of the animal, which indicated considerable inward diffusion of oxygen.

Microelectrode measurements in the basal layer of intact human forearm skin at an ambient temperature of 20°C showed variable oxygen tensions, with a mean value in the region of 20 mm. Hg.

An attempt to obtain a more reliable average Po_2 for the basal layers was made by examining fluid from suction blisters and also from spontaneous friction blisters. Unfortunately, even the most gently produced suction blister induced local dermal hyperemia and readings of Po_2 blister fluid were uniformly high— around 40–50 mm. Hg. Similar hyperemia was also seen after cellophane tape stripping of the epidermis.

Diffusion through Stripped Skin

After stripping with cellophane tape to the glistening moist layer, large multi-point electrodes were placed on the exposed surface of the skin and air diffusion was minimized by application of a heavy mineral oil with low oxygen solubility around the electrode, then covering this with a polyester film. The stripped skin had a high Po_2, of the order of 40 mm. Hg and showed brisk response to the breathing of oxygen, presumably because local vasodilatation had been induced by the stripping. The day after stripping, the Po_2 at the skin surface had fallen to around 25 mm, Hg, and a day later was only 10 mm. It remained at about this level thereafter.

Oxygen Environment in Superficial Wounds

Loss of continuity of epidermis inevitably caused some vascular response in the dermis as well as destroying the barrier properties of the epidermis, both with respect to water loss and oxygen trapping.

In small incised wounds reaching the dermis in human skin, and to a lesser extent in laboratory animals, the first environmental effect was the reversal of the oxygen gradient in the cut skin edge, and the exposure of dermis and basal layers of epidermis to atmospheric oxygen tension and also to drying by evaporation. This loss of the oxygen diffusion barrier was very short lived, even if there was no gross hemorrhage. Within a few minutes of incision the cut edges were accumulating debris, either from clothing, blood or plasma oozing into the wound cavity. As soon as a clot was established the oxygen tension at the bottom of the wound began to fall. Within a few hours of wounding the Po_2 at the dermo-epidermal junction was often less than 10 mm. Hg. This appeared to be due partly to the relatively low O_2 permeability of the scab that had formed over the incision and partly to the changes in the dermal blood flow that occurred during the inflammatory response. The small amounts of fluids that leak from inflamed capillaries are quite sufficient to increase diffusion distances significantly and to cause drastic alterations in dermal tissue Po_2 [39, 40]. Added to this is the accumulation of polymorphonuclear cells which have a high O_2 uptake. Polymorphs are subsequently replaced by macrophages which act as an oxygen sink [39] between the capillaries and the epidermal cells. Nevertheless, the basal cells of the epidermis started to move across the wound under the base of the scab, through the upper, desiccated layers of the dermis in what seems to be a relatively hostile environment. These migrating cells are presumably capable of using oxygen although little seemed to be available from the capillary bed. Oxygen breathing at this time, 12 to 24 hours after wounding, had little or no effect on the epidermal Po_2 at the wound edge. Diffusion of oxygen from the air was also severely limited by the scab, and again only a very slow effect could be observed from increasing the O_2 concentration in the air above the wound. Oxygen supply to the basal layers did not appear to increase until about 4 days after wounding, when fibroblast and endothelial proliferation in the dermis was well established. By this time the epidermis was several cells thick and was rapidly reestablishing its own normal structure.

In thin skinned animals the scab was less permeable to oxygen than the normal skin.

Table 17-3
Effects of Hemorrhage on Epidermal Wound Po$_2$ in Rabbits when O$_2$ Diffusion
from Air is Excluded, Measured with a Surface Electrode (mm. Hg)

State	Number of Animals	Air Breathing	Oxygen Breathing for 15 Min.
Normal anesthetized	20	20.0 ± 7.4	83.7 ± 24.6
15 min. at blood pressure 55 mm. Hg	10	0.0	1.3 ± 0.5
15 min. at blood pressure 55 mm. Hg + reinfusion to B.P. > 90 mm. Hg	10	5.6	23.2 ± 7.8
45 min. at blood pressure 55 mm. Hg	10	0.0	0.0
45 min. at blood pressure 55 mm. Hg + reinfusion to B.P. > 90 mm. Hg	10	0.0	0.0

Effect of Shock

A limited number (20) of measurements of wound Po$_2$ were performed on anesthetized rabbits during acute hemorrhage and early hemorrhagic shock to determine the effects of cardiovascular changes on the oxygen supply to superficial wounds. Atmospheric air was excluded by a melinex film. It appeared that one of the first responses to bleeding was a reduction in blood flow to, and Po$_2$ in, the wound area. During the acute phase of hemorrhage, a mean arterial pressure of 55 mm. Hg was observed and the Po$_2$ fell to zero in all wounds studied. Reinfusion of blood within 15–20 min. resulted in reestablishment of normal tension during a half-hour period. If blood was withheld for more than three-quarters of an hour, no short term recovery of wound Po$_2$ occurred during reinfusion, although normal blood pressure was reestablished. Previous observations of deeper wounds in rabbits indicated that these remained hypoxic for at least 48 hours after 45 min. of lowered blood pressure [40]. Rabbits are particularly susceptible to hemorrhage and form a good model system for studying the early effects of shock on wounds. They will not however tolerate arterial pressures below about 50 mm. Hg. The observations are summarized in Table 17-3.

Measurements under Occlusive Films and Wound Dressings

Some occlusive films have been reported as markedly affecting epithelial migration rates in the pig and man [29–32]. On superficial abrasions on human skin covered by Teflon, Polythene or polyester films and also on abrasions covered with gauze swabs, measurements were made by means of microelectrodes inserted through the covering into the surface across which epithelial migration was occurring. Similar observations were carried out on depilated rabbit skin bearing superficial incisions reaching the upper layer of the dermis. The measurements obtained are summarized in Table 17-4.

It was possible in human skin to manipulate a microelectrode under direct vision and to measure first the Po$_2$ above epithelium and below the dressing,

Table 17-4
Oxygen Tension under Wound Dressings (mm. Hg)

Wound Covering

Species	Site	Teflon	Poly-ethylene	Polyester	Gauze Swab (Under Scab) Dry	Wet	Nonad. Tulle
Man	Above epithelium	135	123	21	5	2	0
	Below epithelium	108	89	4	—	—	—
Rabbit	Wound cavity	128	113	18	20	7	8

then to advance the electrode tip through the newly migrated epithelium near the wound edge. This was feasible in the case of the transparent plastic coverings but was impracticable for the swabs or paraffin tulle. It can be seen from Table 17-4 that oxygen permeable films allowed the development of a completely different type of epithelial environment than is present in naturally healing wounds under a scab, whereas films of low oxygen permeability such as polyester allow the development of an oxygen environment very similar to that under a scab. The situation under a gauze dressing may be of some significance. Under a dry swab there is normal scab formation and the oxygen environment is similar to that in an uncovered wound with a scab. In wounds where there has been fluid loss into a swab, whether or not a scab was present, the Po$_2$ in the wound surface was so low as to be difficult to measure with the techniques that were used. Exudate soaked swabs can therefore form a considerable barrier to oxygen diffusion from the air.

If the Po$_2$ of the gas above a wound covered with a dressing was changed, the expected alterations were found below the dressing according to its properties. Thus, pure oxygen directed onto Teflon covered wounds raised the epidermal Po$_2$ to nearly 700 mm. Hg while similar treatment of polyester or wet swab-covered wounds resulted in very much smaller changes (Table 17-5).

When epidermal continuity was reestablished the oxygen gradient within the

Table 17-5
Effect of 5 min. exposure of Wound Area to Pure O$_2$ Atmosphere, on Po$_2$ of Wound Surface Below Various Dressings

Dressing	Po$_2$ (mm. Hg)
Teflon	685
Polythene	628
Polyester	173
Nonad. tulle	151
Dry swab (measured under scab)	48
Wet swab	35

epithelium began to change so that by 4 days after incision or abrasion a contribution to the basal epidermal layers of oxygen from the vasculature of the dermis could be detected by covering the wound surface with an oxygen barrier and then having the subject breathe pure O_2 for 5 minutes. By 8 days the wound Po_2 gradients had been reversed due to the relatively impermeable nature of the newly established cornified layer, and achieved gradients similar to those found in normal skin.

Effects of Minor Stress on Skin Wound Po_2

Skin circulation in man is notoriously responsive to emotional stress, and it can also be shown that regenerating connective tissue vessels in experimental animals are particularly sensitive to environmental stress. Vasoconstriction of healing dermal wounds in rabbits is a feature commonly associated with the retardation of wound healing which may occur if an animal is placed in unfamiliar surroundings or is exposed to noise or physical disturbance. Using a surface electrode, a few measurements were therefore made on Po_2 of stripped epidermis, in man and in rabbits, to test the effect of very minor stress on oxygen supply from the dermis. Measurements were obtained from 6 people, three of whom were familiar with the investigation and quite relaxed, and three who were new to the situation and mildly apprehensive. In the case of the rabbits, measurements were made in an unfamiliar room with a high intermittent noise level which had previously been shown to be associated with contraction of blood vessels in healing connective tissue. The results, which form only a very small group, are shown in Table 17-6.

Each figure represents a mean of 6 readings on each subject, thus the figures for the rabbits are a mean of 18 readings.

Effects of Infection

Occlusive plastic skin dressings in man are frequently associated with superficial wound infections and destruction of epidermis. Similar infections may develop on depilated rabbit skin where a superficial abrasion is covered by plastic film. Measurements of Po_2 under occlusive dressings on rabbit skin wounds indicated that even when oxygen permeable films were used, developing bacteria were able to lower skin surface oxygen concentrations very considerably. An

Table 17-6
Po_2 (mm. Hg) in Stripped Skin during Mild Stress

	Subjects	Po_2 Breathing Air	Po_2 Breathing O_2 for 5 min.
Experienced Group	A	28	98
	B	42	163
	C	36	148
Naive Group	D	15	43
	E	7	16
	F	11	14
Familiar room	Rabbits (3)	45 ± 4.0	189 ± 17.3
Noisy room	Rabbits (3)	12.6 ± 4.7	40 ± 6.7

interesting feature of such measurements was that the fall in Po_2 considerably preceded any visual indication of infection. The bacteria encountered under the films were *Proteus, Pseudomonas,* and *Staphylococci* spp. Epidermal cell detachment from the underlying tissue was a feature of infection under inert films and occurred soon after the rapid fall of Po_2 due to the bacteria. When infiltration of polymorphonuclear cells in the wound appeared, the Po_2 was further reduced and approached zero even under Teflon films. Spontaneous infections were most commonly seen under polyester film.

Measurements in Superficial Burns

Blisters were raised on human skin by mild thermal burns. Examination of the fluid in such blisters showed an oxygen environment quite different from that in suction or friction blisters. Po_2 in blister fluid was low initially although it rose after a few hours, apparently due to slow diffusion of O_2 into the fluid from the air. The damaged tissue under the blister exhibited a Po_2 of zero and no change could be elicited when oxygen was breathed for 15 minutes. Microelectrodes were also inserted into the reddened skin at the edge of the blister and again very low oxygen tensions were recorded which showed little or no alteration during oxygen breathing. The major difference in oxygen environment between incised or abraded wounds and minor burns was that very low tensions in burns persisted for five or six days after injury, whereas the other injuries reestablished normal Po_2 gradients after about 3 days, provided no infection developed.

DISCUSSION

Intact Skin

The findings reported here on the oxygen gradients of intact skin are in accord with the results of previous work [17–19] but they also emphasize the great variability of the normal epidermal environment as well as highlighting species differences in skin permeability. It has been shown by Huch [19] that the Po_2 at the skin surface of babies in the region of the medial malleolus of the ankle may be as high as 60 mm. Hg, whereas in adults considerable vasodilatation is necessary to raise the Po_2, even of thin skin of the ear lobe, to 40 mm. Hg. The breathing of pure O_2 does not necessarily raise the Po_2 at the skin surface in man, partly at least because of the marked vasoconstrictor action of oxygen on the peripheral capillary bed [48, 49]. However, when vasodilatation is present and a good dermal blood flow is maintained, large increases in epidermal Po_2 result. Much greater increases occur below the stratum corneum as was first shown by Montgomery, Howitz and Penneys [23–27].

Another feature of normal skin Po_2 is the great lability in its response to temperature change or pressure. In cold conditions accompanied by obvious vasoconstriction in the extremities, some parts of the epidermis must survive relatively long periods of almost complete anoxia. It should be remembered in this respect, however, that the reduced metabolic needs of skin during cooling may allow the relatively small amounts of oxygen that can diffuse through human skin from the air to assume a significant role which is not apparent during more favorable circulatory states or during higher metabolic rates. Starr [10] demonstrated the clinical use of surface application of oxygen in some cases of gangrene as long ago as 1932.

When Po_2 measurements at the surface of human skin are carried out over a period of about an hour in a constant temperature environment, a regular pattern of cyclical changes can be seen. These have also been reported by Evans and Naylor [18] and Huch [19] and apparently reflect cardiovascular regulatory rhythms. Similar rhythms are seen in animal skin but these disappear during hemorrhagic shock. They have also been described in other organs such as brain [41, 50].

The nature of the barrier to oxygen diffusion through intact human skin may be of some significance. The cornified layer appears to act as a mechanical barrier whereas the deeper layers act as an oxygen sink due to cellular oxygen uptake. The differing permeability to oxygen of different species seems to parallel the varying thickness of the stratum corneum, and similar variations can be found in human skin between one location and another on the same individual. Penneys *et al.* [28] have measured diffusion through isolated human stratum corneum in vitro and skin stripping has helped to demonstrate the degree of diffusion through the intact basal layers from the dermal blood vessels. The O_2 diffusion barrier in the upper epidermis may well be the same anatomically as the water barrier and its efficiency depends to some extent on the hydration of the stratum corneum. A similar oxygen barrier has recently been described around the carotid body [51] and in the middle meningeal artery [52].

The resting basal layers of the epidermis have a considerable oxygen uptake as judged by experiments in which skin circulation was occluded either by tourniquet to the limb or by local pressure. Within 1–1.5 min. of vascular occlusion in warm vasodilated skin, the basal layer Po_2 fell to zero, but the O_2 in the cornified layers was lost only slowly, even if diffusion in from the air was prevented. Thus, the nature of the cornified layer diffusion barrier seems to be almost entirely mechanical.

Damaged Skin

Minor superficial damage such as cellophane tape stripping of normal human skin produces marked changes in the oxygen permeability. The findings confirm those of Evans and Naylor [18]. Not only is the skin permeability increased, but the normal oxygen gradients may be reversed, especially where the dermal capillaries are not dilated. It might be reasonable to postulate that the control of epidermal growth and replacement could depend to some extent on the direction and steepness of oxygen gradients within the epidermis.

When more severe damage is considered and the movement of epidermal cells across a wound surface is examined, it appears that under a scab the conditions of oxygen supply are far from good. Epidermal cells before starting migration accumulate glycogen and it would seem that much of their energy requirement during migration under a scab must be derived from glycolytic activity. Nevertheless, epidermal cells in the migratory phase do have a considerable capacity for oxygen uptake as can be seen from Table 17-4 where a single layer of migratory cells is shown to modify considerably the amount of oxygen reaching the deeper tissue from the air.

Winter's observation on the healing rates of epidermal wounds in pig under different types of occlusive films and the effects of different oxygen atmospheres on such healing [53] strongly suggest that oxygen supply can be a major factor in determining the rates both of mitotic activity and of epithelial movement. The more limited data on movement of regenerating epidermis under inert films reported here support Winter's studies and also indicate that occlusive plastic skin dressings should probably be evaluated in terms of their oxygen permeability as well as water vapor and CO_2 permeability. Other factors which must also be considered are those of the heat retaining character of the film [54, 55].

The few measurements that have been made on superficial burns suggest that at least one aspect of the delayed healing characteristic of this type of injury, may be the inavailability of oxygen to the damaged tissue. Clearly, however, a great many more measurements of burn environment must be carried out before any firm conclusions can be reached, but the diffuse nature of burn injuries presents tissue with a special problem in that there is no clear, undamaged region from which regeneration can start. This unsatisfactory state is further complicated by the lack of early development of new blood vessels and a persistently low tissue Po_2. The divergent results from the use of oxygen in burn therapy show that more carefully controlled observations are necessary before the role of oxygen in burn healing can be properly evaluated.

Reports on the use of oxygen therapy for prolonging the survival of skin grafts have been generally encouraging. At first sight it may seem surprising that intermittent exposure of epidermis to hyperbaric oxygen for short periods at long intervals could have any lasting beneficial effect on cell renewal. However, if one considers the very fluctuating behavior of the natural environment of the deeper layers of the epidermis in terms of oxygen supply and the drastic reversals of O_2 gradients that occur during epithelial damage and repair, it may well be that external, artificially applied changes in gradient could provide a necessary stimulus to proliferation, as well as supplying some extra oxygen temporarily for metabolic usage.

The observations reported here on the relative ineffectiveness of short term oxygen breathing in changing wound Po_2 have also been noted in regard to dermal wounds [38, 58]. It seems that direct application of external oxygen to the wound surface by enclosing the treatment area in a plastic bag full of O_2 is a more certain, if rather slow, way of altering the wound environment than is oxygen breathing. Such locally applied oxygen will not have a great effect unless the wound is free of either natural or surgically applied oxygen diffusion barriers. Eschars and exudate-clogged gauze dressing are particularly good barriers whereas plastic films which allow water vapor and oxygen diffusion, and yet keep the wound surface moist and suitable for epidermal migration seem to provide almost ideal conditions. The problem of infection under such films still remains.

The information presented in this paper partially answers the questions posed in the introductory section but considerable scope is left for speculation on the question of whether or not the level of oxygen supply is a vital or merely secondary factor in epidermal regeneration.

SUMMARY

Oxygen tension measurements at the surface of, and at varying depths within the epidermis, indicated that there is a barrier to oxygen diffusion located in the stratum corneum.

Oxygen supply to the basal layers of human skin is almost entirely derived from the dermal capillary bed, but in small laboratory animals there is a considerable (50%) contribution from the air.

Oxygen tension in epidermal wounds varies according to the nature of the injury. Any wound that reaches the dermis usually results in a fall in Po_2 of the basal layers of the skin.

Epidermis migrating under a normal scab is moving in a low oxygen environment.

The migration rate of epidermis under occlusive plastic films is correlated with the oxygen permeability of the film. The more oxygen that is present, the faster is the reestablishment of epithelial continuity.

ACKNOWLEDGMENT

The work reported in this paper was made possible by support from the U.S. Army Research and Development Command under Contract DAJA 37-70-C-2328.

REFERENCES

1. Gage, A. A., Ishikawa, H., and Winter, P. M.: Experimental frostbite: The effect of hyperbaric oxygenation on tissue survival, Cryobiology 7:1, 1970.
2. Hunt, T. K., and Hutchison, J. G. P.: Studies on Oxygen Tension in Healing Wounds, in Illingworth, C. F. (ed.): *Wound Healing* (London: J. & A. Churchill, Ltd., 1966).
3. Hunt, T. K., and Niinikoski, J. H. A.: The role of oxygen in repair processes, Acta chir. scandinav. (In press).
4. Lundgren, C., and Sandberg, N.: Influence of Hyperbaric Oxygen on the Tensile Strength of Healing Wounds in Rats, in Ledingham, I. (ed.): *Hyperbaric Oxygenation* (Edinburgh: E. & S. Livingstone, Ltd., 1965).
5. Coulson, D. B., Ferguson, A. B., and Diehl, R. C.: Effect of hyperbaric oxygen on the healing femur of the rat, Surg. Forum 17:449, 1966.
6. Bullough, W. S., and Johnson, M.: Epidermal mitotic activity and oxygen tension, Nature 167:488, 1951.
7. Utkina, O. T.: Regeneration of the skin epithelium in healing wounds under normal conditions and at reduced barometric pressures, Biol. Abst. 45:78585, 1964.
8. Hall, A. D., Blaisdell, F. W., Thomas, A. N., Brandfield, R., McGinn, P., and Hare, R.: Response of Ischaemic Leg Ulcers to Hyperbaric Oxygen, in Brown, I. W., and Cox, B. G. (eds.): *Hyperbaric Medicine* (Washington, D.C.: N.A.S.-N.R.C., 1966).
9. Niinikoski, J.: Viability of ischaemic skin in hyperbaric oxygen, Acta. chir. scandinav. 136:567, 1970.
10. Starr, I.: On the conservative treatment of gangrene of the feet by selected temperature, oxygen and desiccation, Tr. A. Am. Physicians 47:339, 1932.
11. Gruber, R. P., Brinkley, F. B., Amato, J. J., and Mendelson, J. A.: Hyperbaric oxygen and pedicle flaps, skin grafts and burns, Plast. & Reconstruct. Surg. 45:24, 1970.
12. Ketcham, S. A., Zubrin, J. R., Thomas, A. N., and Hall, A. D.: Effect of hyperbaric oxygen on small, first, second and third degree burns, Surg. Forum 18:65, 1967.

13. Smith, G., Irvin, T. T., and Norman, J. N.: The Use of Hyperbaric Oxygen in Burns, in *Research in Burns* (Edinburgh: E. & S. Livingstone, Ltd., 1966).

14. Champion, W. M., McSherry, C. K., and Goulian, D'.: Effect of hyperbaric oxygen on survival of pedicled skin flaps, J. S. Res. 7:583, 1967.

15. McFarlane, R. M., and Wermuth, R. E.: The use of hyperbaric oxygen to prevent necrosis in experimental pedicle flaps and composite skin grafts, Plast. & Reconstruct. Surg. 37:422, 1966.

16. Perrins, D. J. D.: Hyperbaric Oxygenation of Ischaemic Skin Flaps and Pedicles, in Brown, I. W. Jr., and Cox, B. G. (eds.): Proceedings of the Third International Conference on Hyperbaric Medicine (Washington: N.A.S.-N.R.C., 1966).

17. Evans, N. T. S., and Naylor, P. F. D.: The systemic oxygen supply to the surface of the human skin, Resp. Physiol. 3:21, 1967.

18. Evans, N. T. S., and Naylor, P. F. D.: Skin Surface Po_2, in Bruley, D. F., Kessler, M., Silver, I. A., and Strauss, J. (eds.): *Oxygen Transport in Tissue* (In press).

19. Huch, R.: Po_2 Measurements on the Skin, in Bruley, D. F., Kessler, M., Silver, I. A., and Strauss, J. (eds.): *Oxygen Transport in Tissue* (In press).

20. Fatt, I., and St. Helen, R.: A multicathode polarographic oxygen sensor and its performance, J. Appl. Physiol. 27:435, 1969.

21. Barr, R. A., and Silver, I. A.: Oxygen diffusion through the cornea of the rat (In preparation).

22. Kwan, M., and Niinikoski, J. H. A.: Personal communication.

23. Montgomery, H., and Horwitz, O.: Oxygen tension in the skin of the extremities, J. Clin. Invest. 27:550, 1948.

24. Montgomery, H., and Horwitz, O.: Oxygen tension of tissues by the polarographic method, J. Clin. Invest. 29:1120, 1950.

25. Montgomery, H., Horwitz, O., and Penneys, R.: Polarographic measurement of oxygen in the skin of man and its circulatory implications, Tr. A. Am. Physicians 68:185, 1955.

26. Penneys, R., and Montgomery, H.: Oxygen tension of tissues by the polarographic method V. The rate of movement of oxygen from the peripheral artery to the skin, J. Clin. Invest. 31:1042, 1952.

27. Penneys, R. A.: Some Experiments on the Use of the Miniaturised Clark Electrode, and the Open-tip Electrode, for the Measurement of Tissue Oxygen Tension, in Hills, G. J. (ed.): *Polarography*, Vol. 2 (London: The Macmillan Company, 1964).

28. Penneys, R. A., Felder, W., and Christophers, E.: The passage of oxygen through isolated sheets of human stratum corneum, Proc. Soc. Exper. Biol. & Med. 127: 1020, 1968.

29. Winter, G. D.: Formation of the scab and the rate of epithelialisation of superficial wounds in the skin of the young Domestic Pig, Nature 193:293, 1962.

30. Winter, G. D.: *Communication* on wound healing, Nature 200:378, 1963.

31. Winter, G. D., and Scales, J. T.: Effect of air drying and dressings on the surfaces of a wound, Nature 197:91, 1963.

32. Hinman, C. D., and Maibach, H.: Effect of air exposure and occlusion on experimental human skin wounds, Nature 200:377, 1963.

33. Hunt, T. K., Twomey, P., Zederfeldt, B., and Conolly, W. B.: Respiratory gas tensions and pH in healing wounds, Am. J. Surg. 114:302, 1967.

34. Hunt, T. K., and Zederfeldt, B.: Nutritional and Environmental Aspects of Wound Healing, in Dunphy, J. E., and Van Winkle, W. (eds.): *Repair and Regeneration* (New York: The McGraw-Hill Book Company, Inc., 1969).

35. Niinikoski, J. H. A.: Effect of oxygen supply on wound healing and formation of experimental granulation tissue, Acta physiol. scandinav. 1-72, 1969.

36. Niinikoski, J. H. A., and Kulonen, E.: Reparation at increased oxygen supply, Experientia 26:247, 1970.

37. Remensnyder, J. P., and Majno, G.: Oxygen gradients in healing wounds, Am. J. Path. 52:301, 1968.

38. Silver, I. A.: The Measurement of Oxygen Tension in Healing Tissue, in Herzog, H. (ed.): *Progress in Respiration Research,* Vol. 3 (Basel: S. Karger, 1969).

39. Silver, I. A.: Wound Healing and Cellular Microenvironment 1. Final Technical Report, U.S. Army R. and D. Command, Contract DAJA 37-69-C-1169, 1970.
40. Silver, I. A.: Wound Healing and Cellular Microenvironment 2. Final Technical Report, U.S. Army R. and D. Command Contract DAJA 37-70-C-2328, 1971.
41. Silver, I. A.: Some observations on the cerebral cortex with an ultramicro, membrane-covered, oxygen electrode, Med. Electron. & Biol. Engineering 3:377, 1965.
42. Clark, L. C.: Monitor and control of blood and tissue oxygen tension, Tr. Am. Soc. Artif. Internal Organs 2:41, 1956.
43. Lübbers, D. W., Baumgärtl, H., Fabel, H., Huch, A., Kessler, M., Kunze, K., Riemann, H., Seiler, D., and Schuchhardt, S.: Principle of construction and application of various platinum electrodes, Prog. Resp. Res. 3:136, 1969.
44. Evans, N. T. S., and Naylor, P. F. D.: The use of multicathode surface oxygen electrodes for studying the microcirculation of human skin, Prog. Resp. Res. 3:161, 1969.
45. Silver, I. A.: Recent Developments in Po_2 and Pco_2 Electrodes, in Kaufman, R. L. (ed.): *Modern Technology in Physiological Sciences* (In press).
46. Lübbers, D. W.: The meaning of the tissue oxygen distribution curve and its measurement by means of Pt electrodes, Prog. Resp. Res. 3:112, 1969.
47. Eisenman, G.: Bioelectrodes, in Kaufmann, R. L. (ed.): *Modern Technology in Physiological Sciences* (In press).
48. Anderson, A., and Hillestad, L.: Hemodynamic responses to oxygen breathing and the effect of pharmacological blockade, Acta med. scandinav. 188:419, 1970.
49. Bird, A. D., and Telfer, A. B. M.: Effect of hyperbaric oxygen on limb circulation, Lancet 1:355, 1965.
50. Silver, I. A.: The Measurement of Oxygen Tension in Tissues, in Payne, J. P., and Hill, D. W. (eds.): *Oxygen Measurements in Blood and Tissues* (London: J. & A. Churchill, Ltd., 1966).
51. Acker, H., Lübbers, D. W., and Purves, M. J.: The distribution of oxygen tension in the carotid body of the cat, J. Physiol. (London) 216:78P, 1971.
52. Lübbers, D. W.: Unpublished observations.
53. Winter, G. D.: In Hunt, T. K., and Niinikoski, J. H. A. (eds.): The role of oxygen in repair processes, Acta. chir. scandinav. (In press).
54. Baron, H.: Die Bedeutung des Temperaturfaktors für Wunde und Haut bei Bedeckung mit "non-woven" und Folien-Schichten, unter besonderer Berücksichtigung von Kühlfarben, Arzneimittel Forsch. 17:1402, 1967.
55. Harris, D. R., and Keefe, R. L.: A histologic study of gold leaf treated experimental wounds, J. Invest. Dermat. 52:487, 1969.
56. Hunt, T. K., Zederfeldt, B., and Dunphy, J. E.: The role of oxygen tension in healing, Quart. J. Surg. (Banaras Hindu Univ.) 4:279, 1968.

Part VI

Supplementary Reports

Introduction

*David T. Rovee, Ph.D.**

Included in the text are four supplementary reports representing important contributions to the understanding of dermal-epidermal interactions, epithelial migration, the effects of clinically used hemostatic agents on epidermal healing, and observations on wounds in diseased skin (Darier's disease).

The importance of dermal-epidermal interactions in the conservation of epidermal specificities and epidermal organ formation unequivocally is well accepted. Students of wound healing only recently have applied some of the techniques of experimental embryology (e.g., recombinant grafting) to problems of repair. Although the interactions seen in adult skin may differ from those in embryonic tissues, they likely play an equally important role in the differentiation of wounded epidermis, and possibly in migratory patterns (through the collagenolytic activities†) or mitotic activity. The paper by Slavkin in this section suggests possible mechanisms for epidermal-dermal communications, some of which might act during wound healing.

In the following paper by Martinez, the mode of epithelial cell movement during the repair of gingival incisions gives insight not only into the healing of that tissue, but raises pertinent questions as to the impact of the intraoral environment on the patterns of response.

Harris examines the effects of commonly used and newer hemostatic agents on ensuing repair of cutaneous wounds, giving the biologist an appreciation of the clinician's need for a material that is not only a hemostat, but affords patient comfort and doesn't interfere with healing as well.

Peck has reported that epithelial migration, and perhaps mitotic and differentiative responses to wounding are enhanced in Darier's disease. The curious finding of remission of disease in the healed site and surrounding skin is also discussed.

---

*Department of Skin Biology, Johnson & Johnson Research, New Brunswick, New Jersey.
†See Grillo, H. C., and Gross, J.: Collagenolytic activity during mammalian wound repair, Developmental Biol. 15:300, 1967.

18

Intercellular Communication During
Epidermal Organ Formation

Harold C. Slavkin, D.D.S. *

THE PROBLEM

During development in metazoan organisms, a special class of interactions has been recognized (see Spemann [1] for comprehensive review) and labeled embryonic inductions. Recognition occurred largely because such phenomena appeared causally related to organ formation and to the differentiation of cells into various cell types. A major problem in developmental biology is to provide comprehensive descriptions and explanations of how changes at one moment affect subsequent events, and how might the interactions between dissimilar tissues (e.g., epithelium and mesenchyme, epidermis and dermis) be related to the differentiation of individual cells. How might extrachromosomal, extranuclear factors differentially effect specific gene activity—the so-called epigenetic influences upon cell differentiation? Although much has been learned about the molecular biology of the gene in prokaryotic cells [2] which often has created a misleading "sense of security" in what is known and actually understood, very little is yet known about cell differentiation in eukaryotic cells let alone within mammalian biological systems. The obvious clinical requirements to effectively treat patients on a basis supported by biological rationale has served as an immeasurable influence to rapidly synthesize and interpret information all too often obtained from quite simple systems (bacteria, yeast, slime molds, hydra, sponges) in an effort to enhance therapy. The following discussion attempts to relate recent advances in our understanding of intercellular communication among dissimilar cells within a mammalian epidermal organ system.

The mammalian integument demonstrates a remarkable degree of morphological and functional diversification, including mitotic activity, thickness, pattern of the dermal-epidermal interface, physical and chemical properties of the cuticle or stratum corneum, etc. In addition to these discrete variances in the superficial

---

*Chairman and Associate Professor of the Department of Biochemistry, School of Dentistry and Associate Professor, Graduate Program in Cellular and Molecular Biology, University of Southern California, Los Angeles, California.

epidermis, numerous regional variations in tissue thickness and dermal-epidermal interfaces can be observed. Another general feature of the unique qualities of epidermis is the distribution of specialized appendages in association with the integument (e.g., hair, nails, sebaceous, sweat, mammary and salivary glands, teeth, etc.). Exactly how this multiplicity of epidermal differentiation originates from an embryonic tissue of binary origin poses a significant problem to developmental biology.

Most of the experimental findings have been interpreted to suggest that there is no predetermined regional specificity in embryonic epithelia, both its differentiation into epidermis and its qualitative regional differentiation (such as hair or tooth formation) being initiated by morphogenetic directive stimuli from the adjacent mesenchyme [3].

Since the elegant experiments of Professor Hans Spemann [1] innumerable experimental embryologists and transplantation biologists have questioned the possible mechanisms of communication between epithelia (ectodermally derived) and the adjacent mesenchyme or dermis (mesodermally derived). The consequences of this heterotypic intercellular communication, if indeed an actual biological process, has been referred to as embryonic induction. Presumably developmental information of an epigenetic nature (outside the genome) is paramount to differential gene activity in eukaryotic cells within all types of metazoan development. A myriad of factors, substances and molecules have been implicated as the specific material or inducers prerequisite for cell differentiation and subsequent histogenesis, morphogenesis, organogenesis and ultimate functional activity with other organ systems within the organism [4–7].

Several questions appear quite appropriate: (1) is chemical information transferred between epithelia and mesenchyme during mammalian embryogenesis in any example of epidermal organ formation? (2) Is there a morphological criteria for the existence of chemical "information"? (3) What is the nature of the chemical information? (4) Of most importance, what is the biological consequence of transferred information and how specific is the information?

The answers to these questions, and many other obviously related questions remain, as yet, quite evasive in that selection of biological systems to obtain such information are derived from quite dissimilar species of animals, different organ systems and at different stages of development or maturation. The underlying assumption that there is a "universal" mechanism underlying all epithelial-mesenchymal interacting systems may, indeed, be fallacious. However, although incomplete, I wish to describe the recent progress made in our laboratory dealing with the possible transfer of information between epithelia and mesenchyme during embryonic mammalian tooth formation. In concert with many developmental biologists our primary objective has been to resolve embryonic morphological phenomena toward a molecular explanation of the events that underlly histological or ultrastructural images.

After a brief survey of the morphological parameters employed in studies of tooth development, I shall devote the remaining discussion toward relating recent observations which indicate that during epithelial-mesenchymal interactions chemical information may be transmitted between heterotypic cells within membrane limited vesicles. Intercellular communication within odontogenic epithelial-mesenchymal interactions may be comparable to interneuronal or neuromuscular transfer of chemical information packaged within synaptic vesicles—synaptic transmission [8].

EPITHELIAL-MESENCHYMAL INTERACTIONS DURING TOOTH FORMATION

In mammals, the formation of tooth development begins approximately mid-way through gestation. Early morphogenesis is comparable to all other epidermal organ systems. For the experimental embryologist tooth primordium offers unique biological opportunities generally not found in other epidermal organ systems: (1) two embryologically dissimilar tissues each form tissue-specific extracellular organic matrices in juxtaposition to one another without an intervening membrane (the dentine and enamel organic matrices); (2) a basement membrane (metachromatic) separates the epithelia from the adjacent mesenchyme throughout development and progressively becomes thicker and more complex with adjacent concomitant cell differentiation; (3) a gradient of increasing cell differentiation, rapidly dividing cells as well as terminally differentiated, nondividing, merocrine-type secretory cells (ameloblasts or odontoblasts); and (4) this epidermal organ system offers opportunities to study early cell differentiation, extracellular organic matrix formation and general morphogenesis, as well as the various stages of mineralization and calcification within the same biological specimen.

For much of our research we selected the cervical or germinative portion of the embryonic incisor tooth primordia (Hertwig's Epithelial Root Sheath region). This portion of a continuously developing rodent or rabbit incisor provides the entire gradient of cytodifferentiation within both inner enamel epithelia and adjacent odontoblasts (Fig. 18-1). Moreover, by excising this region from the whole organ rudiment, we selectively exclude the overt aspects of extracellular organic matrix formation, mineralization and calcification, phenomena which are fascinating in themselves yet provide additional complexity to the basic question being asked.

Many aspects of this work have been reported [9–11] and reviewed [12]. In this discussion I wish to briefly sketch several salient findings. Succinctly, the cervical or germinative portion of embryonic New Zealand white rabbit incisor tooth primordia can be cultured on the chick chorioallantoic membrane (CAM) for extended periods of time in organ culture and actually regenerate an entire tooth primordia. All of the developmental information for tooth development is inherent in those tissues which comprise this region. A mammalian rudiment without the in situ adjacent tissues or neuronal and humoral factors, can easily be cultured in an avian environment (CAM), and retain all of the essential regulatory mechanisms to ultimately express histogenesis, morphogenesis, organogenesis and mineralization and calcification of both enamel and dentine in vitro.

As in all other epidermal organ systems [13] embryonic tooth rudiments demonstrate epithelial-mesenchymal interactions which are reciprocal and interdependent; both tissues are critical for the differentiation within either tissue type (Fig. 18-2). Such interactions have been examined within recombinants of tissue and cell suspensions in vitro. Further, it has been elegantly demonstrated [14, 15] that mesenchyme instructs the adjacent epithelia as to what organ to form—

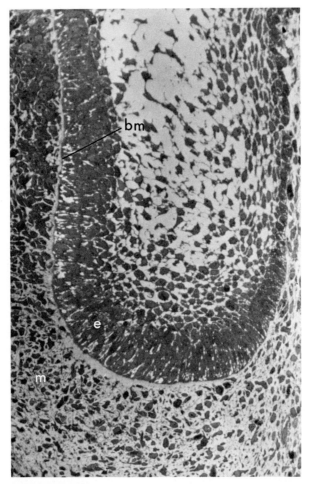

Fig. 18–1.—The germinative region (Hertwig's Epithelial Root Sheath) of rabbit incisor tooth primordia employed in many of our experiments. An exquisite gradient of cell differentiation is evident within each tissue, epithelia (*e*) and adjacent mesenchyme (*m*), separated by a metachromatic basement membrane (*bm*). Note that only those cells immediately in juxtaposition to the basement membrane or interface indicate overt cytodifferentiation and ultimately become the merocrine-type cells (ameloblasts and odontoblasts) synthesizing and exporting enamel protein and dentine tropocollagen, respectively. × 450.

mesenchymal specificity. The reader is encouraged to examine the exciting presentation dealing with mesenchymal specificity by Beer and Billingham (Chap. 9) and to evaluate an earlier discussion by Billingham and Silvers [3].

The technical requirements for isolating embryonic homotypic tissues or cells entails the employment of cation chelating agents or proteolytic enzymes (e.g., trypsinization). Obviously, such treatment "wounds" these embryonic tissues. The time required for these tissues to resume their interactions in vitro and sub-

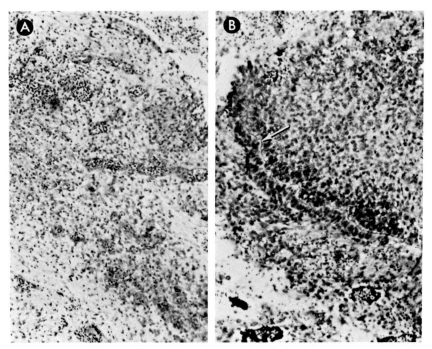

Fig. 18–2.—Epidermal organogenesis requires epithelial-mesenchymal interactions. **A**, if homotypic cell suspensions of either inner enamel epithelia or preodontoblasts are grafted to the chick chorioallantoic membrane (CAM) for periods up to 10 days, homotypic cells *do not indicate* cell differentiation. × 350. **B**, recombinant heterotypic cell cultures indicate the formation of a newly synthesized basement membrane (*arrow*) and the initiation of cytodifferentiation within 48 hours in vitro. Subsequent organ culture on the CAM shows the overt formation of a tooth rudiment. × 350.

sequently form an interface or basement membrane after recombination may actually be a measure of "wound healing" at the level of outer cell surfaces. Repeatedly, the formation of a metachromatic interface indicates the continuance of epithelial-mesenchymal interactions.

Three options seem quite evident: (1) examine the mesenchymal cells for a "mesenchymal factor" responsible for specificity; (2) examine the epithelial cells for "factors" involved in epithelial-mesenchymal interactions; or (3) examine the interface, basement membrane, or progenitor extracellular organic matrix for material(s) which may be transferred between heterotypic cells during development. We elected to pursue an examination of the interface for possible morphogenetic properties, chemical characteristics and the inclusion of "developmental information."

THE INTERCELLULAR MATRIX

It has been shown repeatedly in a variety of different epidermal organ systems that epithelial and mesenchymal tissues can be enzymatically separated, isolated and subsequently recombined in juxtaposition across a Millipore filter [13, 16]. Rodent embryonic incisor tooth rudiments have been dissociated into epithelia and mesenchyme and successfully cultured in juxtaposition to a Millipore filter using the transfilter induction approach [17]. In these experiments the inner enamel epithelia and adjacent mesenchymal cells (preodontoblasts) differentiated and synthesized their respective tissue-specific protein to form the dentine and enamel organic matrices; moreover, evidence for early mineralization was reported.

Reconsideration of transfilter induction experiments suggests that they could be explained through mesenchymal cell processes growing into the pores of the filters rather than diffusible "informational molecules" traversing distances of 25–70 microns (the thickness of the filters often used in these studies). However, electron microscopic observations of epithelial-mesenchymal interactions in situ or during transfilter induction experiments *do not indicate* heterotypic cell contacts [13]. The cell processes from the mesenchymal cells do not make contact with the basal lamina associated with the undersurfaces of epithelia! During transfilter experiments the inductive influence (presumably) had to traverse Millipore filter pores $25 \times 0.5 \mu$, yet it was significantly retarded by pores $70 \times 0.5 \mu$ or $25 \times 0.1 \mu$ [16]. In such experiments one would have to assume that diffusible agents would require the implausible diameter of nearly 0.1μ to explain all this data. Indeed, 0.1μ is an enormous dimension when considering even the size of macromolecules (proteins, nucleic acids, carbohydrates, lipids) with or without prosthetic groups. However, suppose the diffusible information was packaged within a membrane and then transferred between cells through the intercellular matrix as a vesicle.

In designing a series of experiments to examine this assumption several key points were considered: (1) a significant literature dealing with uni-direction, intercellular communication vis-a-vis synaptic transmission of chemical information enclosed within synaptic vesicles (500 Å to 4000 Å in diameter); (2) an appreciable literature in virology describing the entry and release of RNA-viruses in mammalian tissues—"informational molecules" enclosed in a protein core; (3) the implication of ribonucleic acids, proteins, lipoproteins and ribonucleoproteins as inducers in embryonic development [4–7]; (4) the repeated finding that RNA is a constituent of the outer cell surfaces of many types of mammalian cells [7, 17; and (5) that intercellular matrices or "substratum" enhance, invoke, complement or induce cell differentiation—the external milieu through which, or upon which, cells appear to differentiate [7].

With these points in mind we implemented several experiments which indicated rather surprising information. The interface or intercellular organic matrix, interposed between inner enamel epithelia and adjacent preodontoblasts, can be isolated so that it is devoid of adherent cells. In this experiment it is possible to isolate the matrix which is 10–20 microns thick, extremely porous (Fig. 18-3), is 80% water, weighs 80 μg. (dry weight/matrix isolated), is rich in collagen and noncollagenous protein and does not contain significant amounts of calcium. Once isolated, could this matrix be cultured with either tissue type to test if the matrix might enhance cell differentiation? If information is transferred between heterotypic cells and if this information traverses through the extracellular organic matrix, would the isolated matrix contain this material? If it does contain

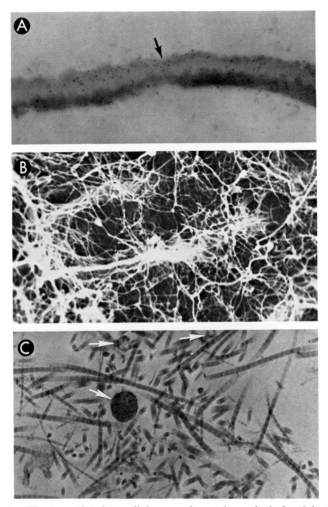

Fig. 18–3.—The progenitor intercellular organic matrix can be isolated devoid of cells and employed in studies designed to evaluate morphogenetic properties, chemical composition and the biochemical and radiochemical analyses of specific constituents. **A,** following an organ culture experiment which employed tritiated cytosine, the organic matrix was isolated and observed using autoradiographic criteria (the matrix shown here in longitudinal section is 15 μ thick). The *arrow* indicates surface shown in B and the area seen in cross section in C. × 1400. **B,** a topographical review of the mesenchymal surface utilizing the stereoscan electron microscope (courtesy of Dr. Alan Boyde, University College, London). Note the appreciable porosity of this biological matrix (80% water). × 5000. **C,** ultrastructural examination of the mesenchymal portion of the isolated matrices immediately following ultrasonication. Matrix vesicles (*arrows*) are retained within this material. × 39,000.

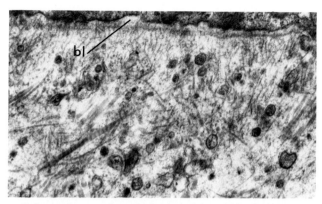

Fig. 18–4.—Prior to the cessation of mitotic activity within the inner enamel epithelia and adjacent preodontoblasts, numerous matrix vesicles are discernible within the intercellular organic matrix. Basal lamina (*bl*) adherent to the undersurface of the epithelia. × 37,000.

this material the matrix might support differentiation and histogenesis within either epithelia or mesenchyme. This was found to be the case.

When cell suspensions of either cell type were cultured within the boundaries of the isolated extracellular matrix, and this "assembly" cultured as a xenograft upon the CAM for periods up to 10 days, homotypic cells became tall columnar, merocrine-type cells analogous to those of normal tooth development [18]. Simple organ culture experiments employing radioactive precursors for RNAs (pulse/ chase experiments) indicated by autoradiography and direct biochemical and radiochemical analyses that RNAs were synthesized de novo within each cell type and transferred into the interface region [19]. The RNAs found within the intercellular matrix were low molecular weight, methylated RNAs and possessed electrophoretic mobilities of 2–7S [20]. These studies observed that RNAs found in the intercellular matrix were inhibited by Dactinomycin. Before the phenol extraction procedure electron microscopic examinations indicated the presence of membrane-limited, electron dense bodies (500 Å to 0.1 microns in diameter) which were discrete (step serial sections about 700 Å thick) and not part of cell processes. After phenol extraction these morphologically discernible images were not evident.

Recent ultrastructural studies indicate the matrix vesicles are seen in situ in the germinative region of embryonic incisor tooth primordia within both cell types (Fig. 18-4) and within the interface [21]. Moreover, Mr. Richard Croissant, a graduate student in our laboratory, recently was able to isolate matrix vesicles (Fig. 18-5) and found that some contain a liporibonucleoprotein complex [22]. Current efforts are directed toward isolation, characterization and, ultimately, what actually are the functions of matrix vesicles. The reader is encouraged to evaluate several recent papers describing matrix vesicles in other mammalian systems [23–25].

Are the matrix vesicles, isolated from odontogenic extracellular matrices analogous to synaptic vehicles? Is the RNA found within some of the vesicles "de-

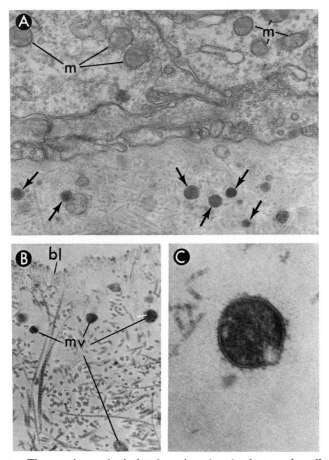

Fig. 18–5.—The matrix can be isolated, sonicated and subsequently collagenase digested in experiments designed to isolate the vesicles. **A**, the intercellular matrix in situ containing numerous matrix vesicles (*arrows*). Mitochondria (*m*) within secretory region of epithelial cells. × 20,250. **B**, the isolated intercellular matrix following ultrasonication. Note the numerous matrix vesicles (*mv*) included within this preparation. The basal lamina region (*bl*) is indicated. × 20,700. **C**, following digestion of the matrix, differential centrifugation affords an approach which enables the isolation of pellets of matrix vesicles. Note the integrity of the limiting trilaminar membrane. × 120,000.

velopmental information?" Are these vesicles actually transferred between heterotypic cells mediating a communication of developmental language or do they function in tissue-specific organic matrix formation? If vesicles which contain RNAs actually enter the adjacent cell type, do they function in protein synthesis through repression or derepression mechanisms? How significant are the qualitative aspects of the outer cell surfaces (histocompatibility antigens) and outer matrix vesicle surfaces? What might motivate vesicles to traverse through the extracellular milieu in discrete locations during embryogenesis? Are there comparable extracellular matrix vesicles in other epidermal organ systems? Could matrix vesicles play a role during epidermal wound healing? These are all questions that remain to be answered by future research.

ACKNOWLEDGMENTS

I wish to dedicate this contribution to Professor Lucien A. Bavetta, whose inspiration, friendship and many contributions to the original work reported here have been invaluable. My admiration and appreciation, also, to Messrs. Pablo Bringas, Richard Croissant, Philip Flores, John Lapyere, Ronald LeBaron, Richard Selmont and Steven Fowle, and to Mrs. Virginia Mansour for their competent technical assistance over the years. Thanks, too, to Miss Rita Bowman for typing this manuscript. The original work cited in this contribution has been supported by Research Grants DE-02848-03 and DE-0094-10 from the National Institute of Dental Research. The author is a recipient of a Research Career Development Award from the National Institutes of Health (DE-41739-04).

REFERENCES

1. Speman, H.: *Embryonic Development and Induction* (New Haven, Conn.: Yale University Press, 1938).
2. Watson, J. D.: *Molecular Biology of the Gene,* (2d ed.; New York: W. A. Benjamin, Inc., 1970).
3. Fleischmajer, R., and Billingham, R. E. (eds.): *Epithelial-Mesenchymal Interactions* (Baltimore: Williams and Wilkins Co., 1968).
4. Brachet, J.: *The Biochemistry of Development* (New York: Pergamon Press, 1960).
5. Tiedemann, H.: Inducers and Inhibitors of Embryonic Differentiation: Their Chemical Nature and Mechanism of Action, in Hagen, E., Wechsler, W., and Zilliken (eds.): *Morphological and Biochemical Aspects of Cytodifferentiation,* Vol. 1 (New York: S. Karger, 1967).
6. Yamada, T.: Differentiation of Lens Cells, in Hagen, E., Wechsler, W., and Zilliken, P. (eds.): *Morphological and Biochemical Aspects of Cytodifferentiation,* Vol. 1 (New York: S. Karger, 1967).
7. Slavkin, H. C.: The Dynamics of Extracellular and Cell Surface Protein Interactions, in Cameron, I. L., and Thrasher, J. D. (eds.): *Cellular and Molecular Renewal in the Mammalian Body* (New York: Academic Press, Inc., 1971).
8. Whittaker, V. P.: Synaptic Transmission, Proc. Nat. Acad. Sc. 60:1081, 1968.
9. Slavkin, H. C., and Bavetta, L. A.: Organogenesis: Prolonged differentiation and growth of tooth primordia on the chick-allantois, J. Anat. 86:12, 1952.
10. Slavkin, H. C., Beierle, J., and Bavetta, L. A.: Odontogenesis: Cell-cell interactions in vitro, Nature 217:269, 1968.
11. Slavkin, H. C., and Bavetta, L. A.: Odontogenic epithelial-mesenchymal interactions in vitro, J. Dent. Res. 47:779, 1968.
12. Slavkin, H. C., and Bavetta, L. A.: Morphogenic expressions during odontogenesis: A tool in developmental biology, Clin. Orthop. 59:97, 1968.
13. Grobstein, C.: Mechanisms of organogenetic tissue interaction, Natl. Cancer Inst. Monograph 26:279, 1967.
14. Kollar, E. J., and Baird, G. R.: The influence of the dental papilla on the development of tooth shape in embryonic mouse tooth germs, J. Embryol. & Exper. Morph. 21:131, 1969.
15. Kollar, E.: Histogenetic Aspects of Dermal-Epidermal Interactions, in Slavkin, H. C., and Bavetta, L. A. (eds.): *Developmental Aspects of Oral Biology* (New York: Academic Press, Inc., In press).

16. Saxen, L., Koskimies, O., Lahti, A., Miettinen, H., Rapola, J., and Wartiovaara, J.: Differentiation of Kidney Mesenchyme in an Experimental Model System, in Abercrombie, M., Brachet, J., and King, T. J. (eds.): *Advances in Morphogenesis,* Vol. 7 (New York: Academic Press, Inc., 1968).

17. Weiss, L.: Some Comments on RNA as a Component of the Cell Periphery, in Manson, L. A. (ed.): *Biological Properties of the Mammalian Surface Membrane* (Philadelphia: The Wistar Press, 1968).

18. Slavkin, H. C., LeBaron, R., Cameron, J., Bringas, P., and Bavetta, L. A.: Epithelial and mesenchymal cell interactions with extracellular matrices in vitro, J. Embryol. & Exper. Morph. 22:395, 1969.

19. Slavkin, H. C., Bringas, P., and Bavetta, L. A.: Ribonucleic acid within the extracellular matrix during embryonic tooth formation, J. Cell. Physiol. 73:179, 1969.

20. Slavkin, H. C., Flores, P., Bringas, P., and Bavetta, L. A.: Epithelial-mesenchymal interactions during odontogenesis. I. Isolation of several intercellular matrix low molecular weight methylated RNAs, Developmental Biol. 23(2):276, 1970.

21. Slavkin, H. C., Bringas, P., Croissant, R., and Bavetta, L. A.: Epithelial mesenchymal interactions during odontogenesis. II. Intercellular matrix vesicles, Developmental Biol. (In press).

22. Croissant, R.: Isolation of and intercellular matrix "RNA-protein complex" during odontogenesis, J. Dent. Res. (In press).

23. Bonucci, E.: Fine structure and histochemistry of calcifying globules in epiphyseal cartilage, Ztschr. Zellforsch. u. mikr. Anat. 103:192, 1970.

24. Anderson, H. C., Matsuzwa, T., Sajdera, S. W., and Ali, S. Y.: Membranous particles in calcifying matrix, Tr. N.Y. Acad. Sci. 32:619, 1970.

25. Ali, S. Y., Sajdera, S. W., and Anderson, H. C.: Isolation and characterization of calcifying matrix vesicles from epiphyseal cartilage, Proc. Nat. Acad. Sc. 67:1513, 1970.

19

Fine Structural Studies of Migrating Epithelial Cells Following Incision Wounds

I. Ricardo Martinez, Jr., M.D., Ph.D.

Stratified squamous keratinizing epithelium is a continuously renewing system in a steady state [1]. Under normal conditions mitotic reproduction, differentiation and desquamation are balanced in order to achieve the steady state. When the epithelium is wounded, the steady state is disrupted, and the cells acquire a new activity, that of migration [2–6]. Relative to this migratory activity, there is a diversity of opinion concerning: (1) the method by which epithelial cells migrate across the wound surface [3, 5, 7–13]; (2) the cell types which participate in the migratory process [10, 14–18]; (3) the plane of migration of the epithelial cells [6, 11–13, 19, 20]; (4) the mechanism by which the migrating epithelial cells invade through the fibrin, inflammatory exudate and cell debris of the wound [12, 13, 21, 22]; and (5) the mode of cessation of the migrating epithelium [23, 24].

This paper is concerned with the cellular activities and ultrastructure of migrating epithelial cells as they cover a wound defect and the cessation of migration when cells from opposing wound edges meet.

MATERIALS AND METHODS

Linear Incision Wounds in Albino Rat Incisor Gingiva

Male albino rats weighing approximately 150 Gm. were anesthetized with chloral hydrate. Linear incisions, 0.5 mm. deep, were made in the lingual incisor gingiva of the mandible. One linear incision per animal was made in the midline extending from the junction of the oral mucosa, lining the floor of the mandible, and the incisor gingiva to the base of the lower incisors. Reproducible wounds of 0.5 mm. depth were assured by the application of a blade guard to a curved #12 scalpel blade. The blade guard was constructed from the tip of a BEEM capsule.

---

*Department of Dermatology, Ochsner Clinic and Ochsner Foundation Hospital, New Orleans, Louisiana.

The smooth plastic guard apparently produced no additional trauma to the gingival epithelium. A curved #12 blade was used for ease of handling and ready visualization of the blade tip in the oral cavity.

Animals were sacrificed at 3, 6, 9, 12, 24, 48 and 72 hours after wounding. These time intervals were determined by preliminary experiments to be most representative of the sequential events which occur in the wound healing process in albino rat gingiva.

Preparation of Wounded Tissues for Light and Electron Microscopy

Male albino rats weighing approximately 150 Gm. were anesthetized with chloral hydrate and by means of an intracardiac cannula they were perfused with a fixative consisting of 2% formaldehyde and 2% glutaraldehyde in a $0.15M$ cacodylate buffered at pH 7.3. Simultaneously, fixative was instilled into the oral cavity. The animals were then put into plastic bags filled with fixative and stored in the refrigerator overnight. The following morning the wounded incisor gingiva was removed as a block and trimmed of excess tissue. Next, the tissues were rinsed in cacodylate buffer for one hour, and subsequently postfixed for two hours in 1% osmium tetroxide buffered with $0.15M$ cacodylate at pH 7.3. After this post-fixation the tissues were again rinsed in buffer, then dehydrated and imbedded in Araldite. One micron sections were stained with methylene blue-azure II and examined with a light microscope. Thin sections were cut with a diamond knife on a Porter-Blum MT-2 microtome and mounted on uncoated grids. Most sections were double stained with alcoholic uranyl acetate and lead citrate, some tissues having been previously stained *en bloc* in 2% uranyl acetate in 50% ethyl alcohol during dehydration. Other sections were stained with 1% potassium permanganate solution [25]. The sections were examined with either an RCA EMU-3F or an AEI EM 6B electron microscope.

RESULTS

Three hours after wounding a zone of necrosis extends laterally from the incision and involves both the epithelium and connective tissue. The necrotic debris is intermixed with the fibrin and inflammatory exudate. There is a sharp demarcation between necrotic epithelial cells and those which appear to have survived the wounding procedure (Fig. 19-1). Necrotic cells and cells with intact plasma membranes and organelles are adjacent to one another. Some desmosomal connections are still present between the plasma membranes of viable and necrotic cells (Fig. 19-1). At the wound tip, only basal and lower spinous cells remain viable, the upper spinous, granular and horny cells having undergone necrosis (Fig. 19-2). Between viable cells at the wound edge, the intercellular spaces are wider, and compared to normal epithelium, microvilli are more numerous and desmosomes are less numerous. Filaments have detached from desmosomes and are aggregating into bundles and whorls; some have mitochondria entrapped between them. Lipid droplets are numerous in the cytoplasm. Smooth and rough endoplasmic reticulum and Golgi complexes are also present (Fig. 19-1). The basal lamina persists in contact with the connective tissue at the wound edge, even though the epithelial cells above it have died. However, the basal lamina is

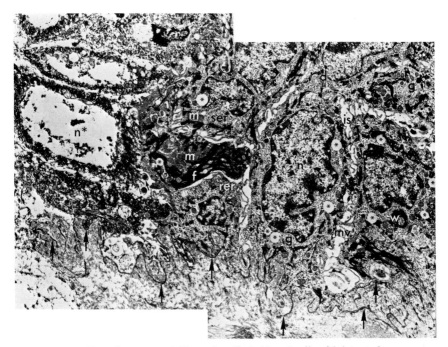

Fig. 19–1.—Three-hour wound. Necrotic cells (*n**) and cells with intact plasma membranes and organelles are adjacent to one another. Some desmosomal connections (*small arrows*) are still present between the plasma membranes of viable and necrotic cells. Between viable cells at the wound edge, the intercellular spaces (*is*) are wide, microvilli (*mv*) are numerous and desmosomes (*d*) are few in number. Filaments are arranged into bundles (*f*) and whorls (*w*). Mitochondria (*m*), lipid droplets (*), smooth endoplasmic reticulum (*ser*), rough endoplasmic reticulum (*rer*), Golgi complexes (g) are also present. The basal lamina (*large arrows*) persists in contact with the connective tissue at the wound edge, even though the epithelial cells above it have died. The basal lamina (*large arrows*) is discontinuous as well as displaying foldings and projections into the edematous connective tissue below. (montage) × 8,850.

discontinuous, as well as displaying foldings and projections into the edematous connective tissue below (Fig. 19-1).

Migration of epithelial cells begins between 3 and 6 hours after wounding. At 6 hours several cells have migrated past the cut edge of the basal lamina and protrude into the clot and exudate (Fig. 19-3). The free edge of the leading cells exhibits pseudopodial and microvillous projections. No pale club shaped cortical projections of the migrating cells were observed [12].

Filaments which have detached from desmosomes form whorls or bundles and these are mainly perinuclear in disposition (Figs. 19-3 and 19-4). Mitochondria and ribosomes become enmeshed within these whorls of tonofilaments. Interestingly, the whorls or bundles are located mainly in that part of the cytoplasm opposite to the leading edge (Figs. 19-4 and 19-5). Lipid droplets and mitochondria are also more numerous in this trailing cytoplasm of the migrating cells. Compared to the upper cells of the wound edge and to normal basal cells, the

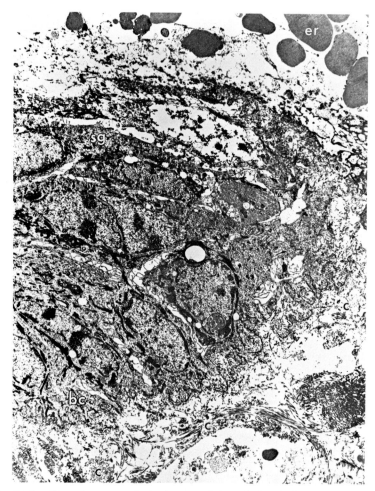

Fig. 19–2.—Three-hour wound. At the wound tip, only basal (*bc*) and lower spinous cells (*sc*) remain viable following wounding, the upper spinous, granular and horny cells having undergone necrosis. Erythrocytes (*er*) are present in the exudate near the epithelial tip. Collagen (*c*) fibrils are separated by edema fluid. × 4,725.

cytoplasm of the basal and suprabasal cells contains few filaments (Figs. 19-3 and 19-4). On the other hand, the profiles of Golgi complexes, smooth and rough endoplasmic reticulum show an increase in number, and the free ribosomes remain plentiful. Lysosomes are present in the cytoplasm of cells of the wound edge (Fig. 19-6).

Intercellular spaces are wide and microvilli are numerous and well developed between basal and suprabasalar cells and less so between upper cells of the wound edge (Figs. 19-3 and 19-4). Desmosomes are fewer in number than in the 3-hour wound, and filaments inserting into them are shorter and finer than in

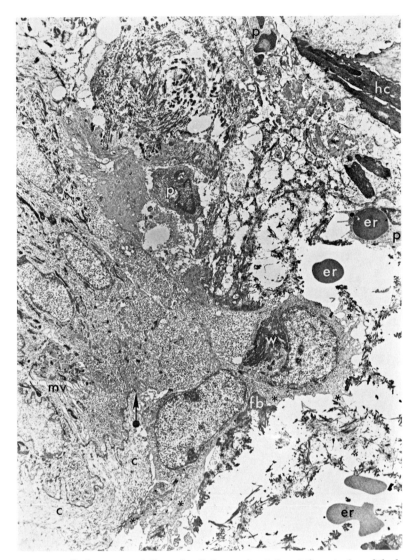

Fig. 19–3.—Six-hour wound. Several cells have migrated past the cut edge of the basal lamina (●→) and protrude into the fibrin (*fb*) clot and exudate. The free edge of the leading cells exhibit pseudopodial and microvillous projections (*). Collagen (*c*), microvilli (*mv*), whorl of filaments (*w*), erythrocyte (*er*), polymorphonuclear leuko-cyte (*p*), horny cells (*hc*). × 4,725.

control incisor gingiva (Figs. 19-3 and 19-6B). They resemble those of normal molar gingiva. Spaces are present between basal cells and the basal lamina, and these appear to be produced by the detachment of these cells from the basal lamina (Fig. 19-4).

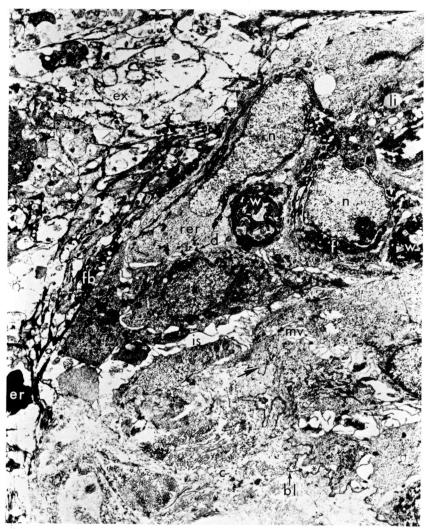

Fig. 19–4.—Six-hour wound. The migrating cells of the wound tip protrude past the cut edge of the basal lamina (*bl*) and collagen (*c*) into the wound exudate (*ex*) which contains some erythrocytes (*er*). The intercellular spaces (*is*) between the lower cells are wide and microvilli (*mv*) are numerous and well developed. Some microvilli (*mv*) are joined by small, infrequently occurring desmosomes (*d*). Spaces (*), present between the basal cells and the basal lamina (*bl*), are apparently produced by the detachment of these cells from the basal lamina. The cells contain whorls (*w*) of filaments and these are usually located near the nucleus (*n*) in the cytoplasm opposite the leading edge. Rough endoplasmic reticulum (*rer*) and lipid droplets (*li*) are also present in these cells. (montage) × 7,480.

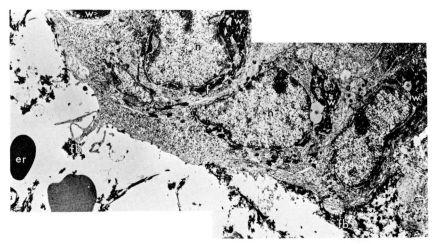

Fig. 19–5.—Six-hour wound. Epithelial cells extend into the wound exudate past the cut edge of the collagen (*c*) and make contact with fibrin (*fb*). Note that the whorls (*w*) and bundles of filaments (*f*), lipid droplets (***) and mitochondria (*m*) are located mainly in the trailing cytoplasm of the migrating cells. Erythrocytes (*er*) are present in the wound exudate. (montage) × 8,670.

Migration of epithelial cells across the wound is well advanced 9 hours after wounding, as is detachment of basal cells from the basal lamina (Fig. 19-7A). Migrating cells move along the fibrin strands and through the inflammatory exudate (Fig. 19-7B). A "poly-band" [10] is not present, however, both neutrophils and monocytes are usually present near the free borders of the migrating cells and microvilli projecting from these cells frequently make contact with the leukocytes (Fig. 19-7B).

The cells appear to migrate by means of pseudopods and long microvillous projections. The leading cells are frequently elongate with the plane of the long axis parallel to the fibrin strand (Fig. 19-7B and 19-8A). The cells migrate as a group connected by small, infrequently occurring desmosomes. Some cells at the leading edge are connected to adjacent cells only by a few desmosomes joining the long microvilli (Fig. 19-7). Intercellular spaces are especially wide between these cells at the leading edge. Cells at the edge fan out in all directions apparently using the fibrin net as a guide.

Some of the migrating cells appear to engulf fibrin and cellular debris (Figs. 19-7B and 19-8B) and contain inclusions which are considered to be phagolysosomes (Fig. 19-8B). There is some variation in cell contents in the migrating cells. Some cells contain only few filaments (Figs. 19-7B and 19-8A), while others contain whorls or dense bundles of filaments (Figs. 19-7A and 19-9A). Most migrating cells contain lipid droplets, lysosomes and inclusions of material ingested from the wound exudate (Figs. 19-8B, and 19-9B and C); rough endoplasmic reticulum is present and smooth endoplasmic reticulum and the Golgi complex are well developed.

In some sections of the 9-hour wounds, leading epithelial cells from opposing

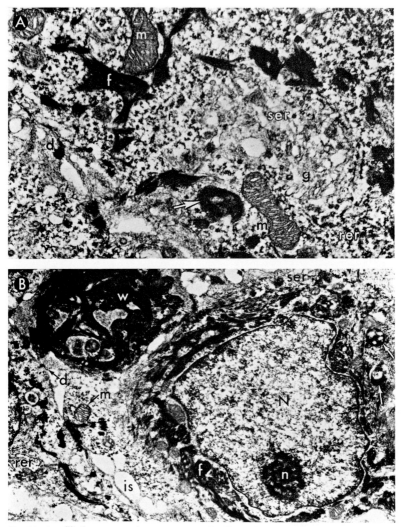

Fig. 19–6.—Six-hour wound. A, contents of cells at the wound edge include lysosomes (*arrow*), Golgi complex (*g*), smooth (*ser*) and rough (*rer*) endoplasmic reticulum, mitochondria, filaments (*f*) and ribosomes (*r*). The cells are joined by small, infrequently occurring desmosomes (*d*). × 31,350. B, the cells at the wound edge exhibit whorls (*w*) and bundles of filaments (*f*), lysosomes (*arrows*), rough (*rer*) and smooth (*ser*) endoplasmic reticulum and mitochondria (*m*). The cells are connected by small desmosomes (*d*). Intercellular space (*is*), nucleus (*N*), nucleolus (*n*). × 17,405.

Fig. 19–7.—Nine-hour wound. A, migrating cells at the wound tip appear to be moving along the fibrin (*fb*) strands by means of pseudopods (■→) and microvillous projections (*mv*). Some cells are connected to adjacent cells only by a few desmosomes (✳→) joining the long microvilli. Whorls (*w*) of filaments and lipid droplets (*li*) are present in these migrating cells. Spaces (✳) are present where basal cells have detached from the

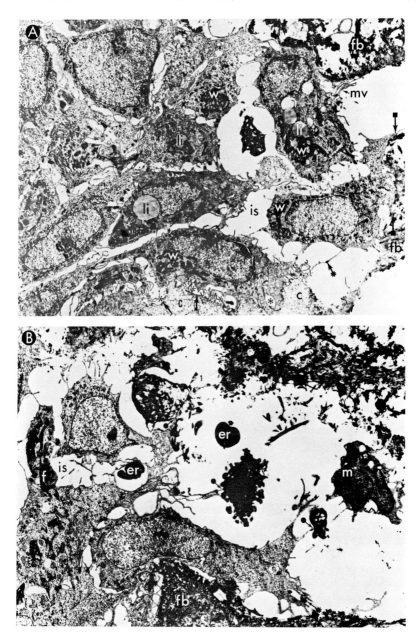

basal lamina (*arrows*) which remains in contact with the collagen (*c*). Intercellular spaces (*is*) are wide between cells at the leading edge. × 6,090. **B**, cells are migrating over the fibrin (*fb*) through the wound exudate by means of pseudopodia and microvillous projections. Some of the microvillous projections are making contact (•→) with macrophages (*m*) in the wound exudate. Erythrocytes (*er*) are also present. Intercellular spaces (*is*) are wide between cells at the wound edge. × 5,762.

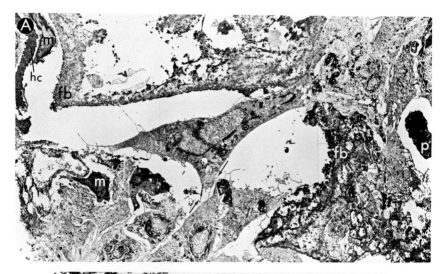

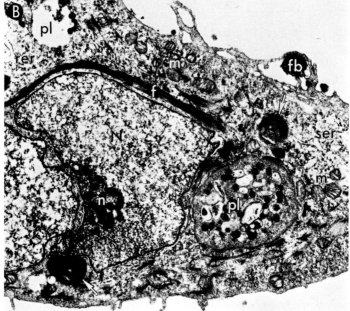

Fig. 19–8.—Nine-hour wound. A, leading epithelial cells from opposing sides (*arrows*) have touched and formed a desmosome (✳→) which joins the two edges. The migrating cells appear to be using the fibrin (*fb*) net as a guide. Polymorphonuclear leukocytes (*p*), monocytes (*m*) and horny cells (*hc*) are present in the wound exudate. (montage) × 2,940. B, this is a higher magnification of a part of the leading migrating cell on the right in A. Fibrin (*fb*) in the process of being phagocytized. Phagolysosome (*pl*), lysosomes (*arrows*), filaments (*f*), smooth (*ser*) and rough (*rer*) endoplasmic reticulum, mitochondria (*m*), filaments (*f*), nucleus (*N*), nucleolus (*n*). × 25,665.

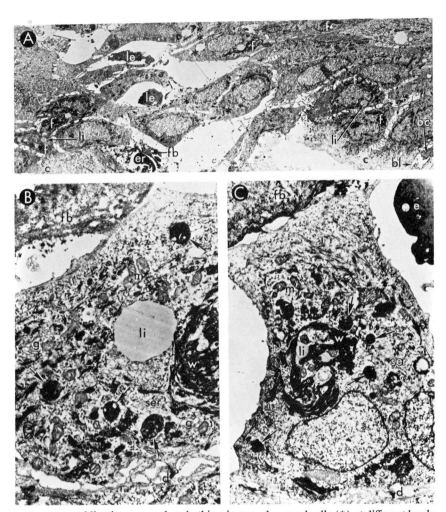

Fig. 19–9.—Nine-hour wound. **A,** in this micrograph several cells (*) at different levels have made contact. They form desmosomes with opposing and neighboring cells resulting in several layers across the wound. Fibrin (*fb*), erythrocytes (*er*) and leukocytes (*le*) are present in the wound area between the cut edges of collagen (*c*). Filaments (*f*) and lipid droplets (*li*) are conspicuous in many of these migrating cells. On the right, note the spaces between the basal cells (*bc*) and the basal lamina (*bl*) due to the detachment of the basal cells from the basal lamina (montage) × 2,100. **B,** part of a migrating cell in contact with fibrin (*fb*). Cell contents include lysosomes (*arrows*), lipid droplets (*li*), whorls (*w*) of filaments, smooth (*ser*) and rough (*) endoplasmic reticulum, Golgi complexes (*g*) and mitochondria (*m*). Desmosomes (*d*) joining the cells are small and sparse. × 18,480. **C,** this is another example of a migrating cell at the wound edge. Cellular contents are similar to those in B. An erythrocyte (*e*) is also present near the epithelial cell. × 13,865.

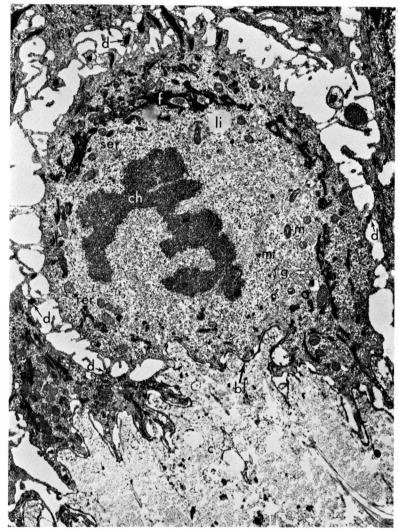

Fig. 19–10.—Nine-hour wound. This is a mitotic cell located near the original wound edge. It is attached to the basal lamina (*bl*) by hemidesmosomes and to adjacent cells by desmosomes (*d*). The chromosomes (*ch*) are placed centrally, as are the microtubules (*mt*) which radiate from them toward the opposite poles of the cell where the centrioles are. Filaments (*f*), smooth (*ser*) and rough (*rer*) endoplasmic reticulum, Golgi complexes (*g*), lipid droplets (*li*) and mitochondria (*m*) are dispersed toward the periphery of the cell. × 12,980.

sides can be seen to have touched (Figs. 19-8A and 19-9A). The microvillous projections come into contact with one another and when this happens desmosomes are formed between them. In some sections just individual cells from each side have met (Fig. 19-8A), while in others several cells at different levels have made contact (Fig. 19-9A). In this latter instance desmosomes are formed not only with opposing cells, but with neighboring ones. This results in the formation of several layers of cells across the wound and cessation of migration.

Occasionally, a mitotic cell is observed near the original wound edge (Fig. 19-10). Such cells are usually basalar or suprabasalar in location, and they are either attached to surrounding cells by desmosomes (which are few in number) or to the basal lamina by hemidesmosomes. Filaments, mitochondria, rough endoplasmic reticulum, Golgi complexes and lipid droplets are disposed toward the periphery of the cell. The chromosomes are placed centrally, as are the microtubules which radiate from them toward the opposite poles of the cell, where the centrioles are located.

DISCUSSION

Epithelialization of Incisions

The healing of incisions in the incisor gingiva of the albino rat progresses much more rapidly than those in human gingiva [26], human epidermis [12], mouse epidermis [13] and rabbit epidermis [10].

In our studies epithelialization is accomplished by 12 hours. Remodeling of the epithelium and connective tissue repair are completed in 72 hours. By comparison, epithelialization of incisions in human gingiva [26] took 28 hours for completion. Interestingly, remodeling of the epithelium takes the same length of time as in our studies, 72 hours, although connective tissue repair is not complete at this time. By comparison, epithelialization of gingivectomy wounds in man [27] and in rats [28] occurred in about 6 days.

Epithelialization of incision wounds in the epidermis of rabbits [10], man [12] and mice [13] was completed by 72 hours, although it took 2 to 7 additional days for the epithelium to return to normal.

Tissue Necrosis

As in incisions of the skin [6, 10, 13], we observe a zone of necrosis extending laterally from the line of the incision in response to the trauma of wounding. In the 3-hour wounds, we are able to demonstrate a sharp delineation between the necrotic cells and those which survived the wounding procedure. At this stage the basal lamina beneath the necrotic cells still persists on a base of edematous and degenerating collagen.

Epithelial Migration

There is usually no evidence of migratory activity in the epithelial cells at the wound margin until approximately 24 hours after wounding in epidermis [10, 12, 13], 18 hours after wounding in human gingival epithelium [26] and 6 hours after wounding in our experience. Therefore, initiation of migratory activity following incision wounds in rat gingival epithelium occurs 3 to 4 times faster than in rabbit [10], mouse [13] and human [12] epidermis and in human gingival epithelium [26].

Method of Migration

Recent ultrastructural studies of healing incision wounds in man [12] and mouse [13] have interpreted movement of epithelial cells to be associated with pseudopodial projections. Odland and Ross [12] described the pseudopodial projections as varying from ordinary microvilli to large, blunt, pale projections of the cytoplasm which contain no organelles, except for ribosomes and a few tonofilaments, while those observed by Croft and Tarin [13] were simply described as small. Pseudopodia in our study vary in form from ordinary microvilli to very long thin microvillous projections extending from larger cytoplasmic processes. We do not observe the large, blunt, pale cortical projections described by Odland and Ross [12].

We agree with previous investigators [4, 8, 29–32], who considered migration of epithelial cells to be a combined ameboid and mass movement. Recent studies [10, 12, 13] have reinforced the concept of mass movement of migrating epithelial cells. The migrating epithelial cells are joined together by desmosomes which are fewer in number and smaller than those in resting epithelium. The cells, therefore, appear to move forward as a column [5, 13]. We find no evidence to support the theory that cells roll over one another to become implanted on the wound surface, as in the movement of a caterpillar track [11].

Cell Types Involved in Migration

Views have varied as to which epithelial cell types are involved in migration across the wound surface. Eycleshymer [14] and Hartwell [18] felt that basal, spinous and granular cells took part in the migration. Bishop [16] felt only upper Malpighian cells migrate across the wound, while Uhlenhuth [15], Matoltsy [17] and Viziam *et al.* [10] concluded only basal cells migrate to cover the wound surface. We note basal and suprabasalar cells exhibiting migratory activity. It was hoped that membrane-coating granules would serve as a marker for spinous cells. However, no membrane-coating granules are noted in the suprabasalar cells of the migrating epithelial tip, even in cells 4 to 5 layers above the basal cells. Two possibilities exist to account for the absence of membrane-coating granules in these cells. Either the cells have not yet differentiated into spinous cells, and hence, no membrane-coating granules have been formed, or membrane-coating granules disappeared from preexisting spinous cells in response to the trauma of wounding. The latter possibility may be comparable to the disappearance of membrane-coating granules following ultraviolet injury [33].

Many of the upper cells of the migrating tip contain numerous filaments arranged to form bundles and whorls. Also, Golgi vesicles, rough endoplasmic reticulum and filaments are more evident than in the basal cells. This suggests that the cells have an increased metabolic activity and that differentiation has begun [34]. This may indicate that, in addition to basal cells, spinous cells participate in the migratory activity. However, the absence of membrane-coating granules prohibits positive identification of these suprabasalar cells as spinous cells.

The Plane of Migration of the Epithelial Cells

Opinions have varied as to the plane of migration of the epithelial cells. The cells have been recorded as traveling through the wound clot [19], through a layer of fresh exudate under the scab [20], and through the connective tissue [6, 11]. In skin wounds of rabbits [10] and mice [13] the plane of invasion was between healthy and necrotic tissue delineated by a band of polymorphonuclear leukocytes ("poly-band"). Our observations are similar to those of Odland and Ross [12], who did not observe the formation of a poly-band [10]. They noted that the advancing epithelium appeared to follow a plane defined by the fibrin net, which in turn was enclosed by a serous exudate which contained inflammatory cells. This plane lies deep to the wound scab.

The Mechanism by Which Epithelial Cells Invade Along the Plane of Migration

Gillman and Penn [19] proposed that epithelial cells invade along the plane of migration by the production of proteolytic enzymes, and this concept received some apparent support when Grillo and Gross [21] demonstrated high collagenolytic activity in migrating epithelium at the wound margin. Phagocytic activity in regenerating salamander epidermis was noted by Taban [35] and Weber and Köln [36]. At the ultrastructural level, Odland and Ross [12] demonstrated apparent phagocytic inclusions in migrating epithelial cells in human skin wounds. Croft and Tarin [13] made similar observations in the skin wounds of mice and proposed intracellular digestion of ingested particles to be a part of the mechanism of epithelial invasion. In our material we observed migrating cells which appeared to be engulfing fibrin and cellular debris and contained membrane bound inclusions which we interpret as phagolysosomes. Our findings agreed with the above proposals that epithelial cells are capable of phagocytosis and we demonstrated for the first time migrating epithelial cells which appeared to be engulfing particulate matter. We also feel that phagocytic leukocytes play some role in assisting the epithelial invasion along the plane of migration.

The Role of Mitosis in Epithelialization

We did not study mitotic activity in the present investigation, except to describe the mitotic cells found at the wound edge during ultrastructural studies. There has been a diversity of opinion as to the role of mitosis in epithelialization.

Hartwell [18] stated that mitotic activity increases at the wound edge only after migratory activity has ceased. Several workers [27, 38] noted fluctuating peaks and lows of mitotic activity following wounding. Marchand [39], Werner [40] and Bullough and Laurence [41] observed relatively low mitotic activity at the wound edge during the initial stages of epithelialization. Some studies [18, 32, 42, 43] reported the absence of dividing cells in the migrating tip, while Holmes [3] related thickening of the migrating tip to increased mitotic activity. Further, Viziam *et al.* [10] and Matoltsy and Viziam [44] stated that epithelial cells in the migrating tip divide and differentiate while they move over the wound surface.

The Fine Structure of Migrating Cells

The fine structure of migrating epithelial cells has been described in skin wounds in man [12] and mouse [13]. Intracellular filaments were sparse, but ribosomes were relatively prominent. Migrating cells contained inclusions which the above authors interpreted as phagocytosed material and structures morphologically similar to lysosomes. Endoplasmic material was more prominent and desmosomes were fewer than in resting epidermis. The pseudopodial projections described above were also noted.

In our material we note a variation in the contents of migrating epithelial cells. Some cells have only few filaments, while others contain whorls or dense bundles of filaments. These whorls and bundles were not described in previous studies [12, 13]. In addition to lysosomes, phagocytic inclusions and rough endoplasmic reticulum were reported by previous investigators [12, 13], whereas in our study most migrating cells contain lipid droplets, and the Golgi complexes and smooth endoplasmic reticulum are well developed. These latter findings cor relate with the presence of lysosomes and phagocytic inclusions in the migrating cells. Gordon *et al.* [45] believed that the Golgi complex plays a major role in supplying hydrolytic enzymes to the phagocytic vacuole. Also, studies of various cell types [46–49] including epidermis [50] proposed the possible role of the Golgi complex in the production of primary lysosomes. Novikoff *et al.* [47] demonstrated the presence of acid phosphatase activity within the rough endoplasmic reticulum and suggested that the hydrolytic enzymes are produced there. The conspicuous rough endoplasmic reticulum (resting cells contain only small amounts) in these phagocytic cells would seem to corroborate this possibility.

Cessation of Cell Migration

We were fortunate to observe the meeting of cells from opposite sides of the repairing epithelium and noted the presence of desmosomes joining projections from opposing cells. In tissue culture studies, Vaughn and Trinkhaus [51] found ruffled membranes of migrating epithelial cells to be particularly adhesive parts of the cell, and that stable adhesions tended to be formed rapidly between contacting cells of epithelial cell masses. In our studies desmosome formation appears to be a rapid process once the microvillous projections from opposing cells touched. In some sections we found cells at several different levels contacting cells from the opposing migrating epithelial mass, and these are joined by desmosomes. Further, as cells from opposite sides interdigitate, desmosomal junctions are also formed between neighboring cells, and this results in the formation of several layers of cells across the wound surface. The formation of desmosomes between microvillous projections of homologous cells of opposing epithelial tips appears to be an important factor in cessation of migration. These findings satisfy the requirements for "contact inhibition" [52] and are adaptable to the "coaptation theory" [53]. Weiss [53] stated that cells have specific stereochemical bonds (templates) which can be saturated only by contact with homologous cells. An equilibrium exists when these templates are safurated, but when a wound is created, the defect disturbs this equilibrium and permits cells to resume their inherent propensity of movement [53]. One could propose that the desmosomal junctions between homologous cells correspond to the saturated templates of Weiss [53] which are responsible for the equilibrium in resting epithelium. When a wound is created, desmosomal connections are broken and the free edge of the wound is lined by epithelial cells lacking desmosomal contact with homologous cells. The cells then migrate until they meet cells from the opposite epithelial edge and form desmosomes. This results in cessation of migration and equilibrium returns. Similarly, desmosomes may be responsible for "contact inhibition" [52] between epithelial cells. When a wound is produced, the deficit of cells interrupts these junctions, and there is a loss of contact inhibition. When epithelial cells from opposite edges meet and form desmosomes between them, contact inhibition is restored and migration ceases.

These proposals are in concurrence with the findings of Chiakulas [23] who noted cessation of migration of epithelium in amphibians only when homologous cell contact occurred. He observed the failure of epithelium from the intestinal tract to fuse with that of the skin—there was either a piling up of cells at this junction, or they migrated past one another. The inability of heterologous epithelial cells to form desmosomal junctions between them would correlate with his findings.

Croft and Tarin [13] stated that contact inhibition might play a part, but it can be considered only as one of many factors. We agree that many factors are probably involved in bringing about cessation of migration. But we feel that the establishment of desmosomal connections between homologous cells of opposing epithelial edges and the attachment of basal cells to the fibrin base by the formation of hemidesmosomes play a significant role.

Dyskeratotic Cells

In the early stages after wounding many epithelial cells resemble dyskeratotic (abnormally keratinizing) cells seen in various skin diseases [54–56], and ultraviolet light injury [33]. These dyskeratotic cells contain dense bundles or whorls of filaments, none of which appear to be attached to desmosomes. We found mitochondria, lipid droplets and ribosomes entwined within the whorls of filaments. Interestingly, there is a polarity in the location of the filament masses. They are usually located in the trailing cytoplasm of the migrating cells, and there is a relatively filament free cytoplasm in the leading portion of the migrating cells. There is also a reduction in the number of desmosomes and an increase in the intercellular space. Microvilli are numerous and well developed.

In a recent ultrastructural study of Hailey-Hailey disease (benign familial chronic pemphigus), Gottlieb and Lutzner [56] noted microvillar changes and abnormal filament configurations which closely resemble those we observed. They proposed that the combination of these two findings in the same lesion was a pathognomonic sign of Hailey-Hailey disease. We feel that these changes in the microvilli and filaments represent a response to injury (whether by physical trauma or disease process) by the epithelial cell and are not pathognomonic of any specific disease process.

ACKNOWLEDGMENTS

The author wishes to express his sincere appreciation to Dr. Alan Peters, Waterhouse Professor and Chairman of Anatomy, Boston University School of Medicine, for his critical evaluation and valuable suggestions during the preparation of this paper.

This work is part of a study submitted in partial fulfillment of the requirements for the degree of Doctor of Philosophy in the Division of Medical Sciences, Boston University School of Medicine where the author was a postdoctoral trainee in dermatology and supported by training grant 5-T-01-AM05295 from the National Institute of Arthritis and Metabolic Diseases.

REFERENCES

1. Greulich, R. C.: Aspects of Cell Individuality in the Renewal of Stratified Squamous Epithelia, in Montagna, W., and Lobitz, W. C. (eds.): *The Epidermis* (New York: Academic Press, Inc., 1964).
2. Peters, C.: Über die Regeneration des Epithels der Cornea, Inaug. Diss., Bonn., 1891.
3. Holmes, S. J.: The behavior of epidermis of amphibians when cultivated outside the body. J. Exper. Zool. 128:13, 1914.
4. Herrick, E. H.: Mechanism of movement of epidermis, especially its melanophores, in wound healing, and behavior of skin grafts in frog tadpoles, Biol. Bull. 63:271, 1932.
5. Lash, J. W.: Studies on wound closure in urodeles, J. Exper. Zool. 128:13, 1955.
6. Ordmann, L. J., and Gillman, T.: Studies in the healing of cutaneous wounds. I. The healing of incisions through the skin of pigs, Arch. Surg. (London) 93:857, 1966.
7. Fraisse, P. H.: Die Regeneration von Geweben und Organen bei den Wirbeltieren, besonders, Amphibien und Reptilien, Cassel und Berlin, 1885.
8. Barfurth, D.: Zur Regeneration der Gewebe, Anat. u. Entwicklungsmech. 37:406, 1891.
9. Rand, H. W.: The behavior of the epidermis of the earthworm in regeneration, Arch. Entwicklungsmech. Organ. 19:16, 1905.
10. Viziam, C. B., Matoltsy, A. G., and Mescon, H.: Epithelialization of small wounds, J. Invest. Dermat. 43:499, 1964.
11. Winter, G. D.: Movement of Epidermal Cells over the Wound Surface, in Montagna, W., and Billingham, R. E. (eds.): *Advances in Biology of Skin (Wound Healing)* (New York: Pergamon Press, 1964).
12. Odland, G., and Ross, R.: Human wound repair. I. Epidermal regeneration, J. Cell Biol. 39:135, 1968.
13. Croft, C. B., and Tarin, D.: Ultrastructural studies of wound healing in mouse skin. I. Epithelial behavior, J. Anat. 106:63, 1970.
14. Eycleshymer, A. C.: The closing of wounds in larval Necturus, Am. J. Anat. 7:317, 1907.
15. Uhlenhuth, E.: Cultivation of the skin epithelium of the adult frog, *Rana pipiens,* J. Exper. Med. 20:614, 1914.
16. Bishop, G. H.: Regeneration after experimental removal of skin in man, Am. J. Anat. 76:153, 1945.
17. Matoltsy, A. G.: In vitro wound repair of adult human skin, Anat. Rec. 122:581, 1955.
18. Hartwell, S. W.: *The Mechanism of Healing in Human Wounds* (Springfield, Ill.: Charles C Thomas, 1955).
19. Gillman, T., and Penn, J.: Studies on repair of cutaneous wounds, Med. Proc. 2 (Suppl. 3):121, 1956.
20. Zahir, M.: Effect of scabs on the rate of epidermal regeneration in the skin wounds of guinea pigs, Nature 199:1013, 1963.
21. Grillo, H. C., and Gross, J.: Collagenolytic activity during mammalian wound repair, Developmental Biol. 15:300, 1967.
22. Weisman, G.: The role of lysosomes in inflammation and disease, Ann. Rev. Med. 18:97, 1967.
23. Chiakulas, J. J.: Cell movement in amphibian epithelia, J. Exper. Zool. 121:383, 1952.
24. Abercrombie, M., and Middleton, C. A.: Epithelial-Mesenchymal Interactions Affecting Locomotion of Cells in Culture, in Fleischmajer, R., and Billingham, R. E.

(eds.): *Epithelial-Mesenchymal Interactions* (Baltimore: Williams & Wilkins Company, 1968).

25. Martinez, I. R., Jr.: Ultrastructural studies of wound healing in albino rat gingiva. I. Inflammatory response, mesenchymal-epithelial cell contacts and connective tissue repair (In preparation).

26. Mittelman, H. R., Toto, P. D., Sicher, H., and Wentz, F. M.: Healing in the human attached gingiva, Periodontics 2:106, 1964.

27. Ramfjord, S. P., and Costich, E. R.: Healing after simple gingivectomy, J. Periodont. 34:401, 1963.

28. Stahl, S. S.: Healing of gingival tissues following various therapeutic regimens— A review of histologic studies, J. Oral Thera. & Pharm. 2:145, 1965.

29. Born, G.: Über Verwachsungversuche mit Amphibien Larven, Arch. Entwicklungsmech. Organ. 4:517, 1897.

30. Oppel, A.: Causal-morphologische zellenstudien, Arch. Entwicklungsmech. Organ. 36:371, 1912.

31. Poynter, C. W. M.: Some observations on wound healing in the early embryo, Anat. Rec. 16:1, 1919.

32. Arey, L. B.: Wound healing, Physiol. Rev. 16:327, 1936.

33. Wilgram, G. F., *et al.*: Sunburn effect on keratinosomes, Arch. Dermat. 101:505, 1970.

34. Matoltsy, A. G., and Parakkal, P. F.: Keratinization, in Zelickson, A. S. (ed.): *Ultrastructure of Normal and Pathologic Skin* (Philadelphia: Lea & Febiger, 1967).

35. Taban, C.: Quelques problemes de regeneration chez les urodeles, Rev. Suisse Zool. 62:387, 1955.

36. Weber, W., and Köln, V.: Experimentelle untersuchungen uber das problem der wundheilung bei *Salamandra maculosa* Saur, Roux Arch Entwicklungsmech. Organ. 149:528, 1957.

37. Sullivan, D. J., and Epstein, W. L.: Mitotic activity of wounded human epidermis, J. Invest. Dermat. 41:39, 1963.

38. Hell, E. A., and Cruickshank, C. N. D.: The effect of injury upon the uptake of 3H-thymidine by guinea pig epidermis, Exper. Cell Res. 31:128, 1963.

39. Marchand, F. J.: Der Process der Wundheilung mit Einschluss der Transplantation, XVI, Stuttgart, Germany, F. Enke. 528, 1901.

40. Werner, R.: Experimentelle Epithelstudien. Ueber Wachstun Regeneration, Amitosenund Riesenzellen-Bildung des Epithels, Bruns' Beitr. Klin. Chir. 34:1, 1902.

41. Bullough, W. S., and Laurence, E. B.: Technique for the study of small epidermal wounds, Brit. J. Exper. Path. 38:273, 1957.

42. Howes, E. L.: The rate and nature of epithelialization in wounds with loss of substance, Surg. Gynec. & Obst. 76:738, 1943.

43. Washburn, W. W., Jr.: Wound Healing as a Problem of Growth, in Nowinski, W. W. (ed.): *Fundamental Aspects of Normal and Malignant Growth* (New York: Elsevier Press Inc., 1960).

44. Matoltsy, A. G., and Viziam, C. B.: Further observations on epithelialization of small wounds. An autoradiographic study of incorporation and distribution of 3H-Thymidine in the epithelium covering skin wounds, J. Invest. Dermat. 55:20, 1970.

45. Gordon, G. B., Miller, L. R., and Bensch, K. G.: Studies on the intracellular digestion process in mammalian tissue culture cells, J. Cell Biol. 25:41, 1965.

46. Essner, E., and Novikoff, A. B.: Cytological studies on two functional hepatomas: Interrelations of endoplasmic reticulum, Golgi apparatus and lysosomes, J. Cell Biol. 15:289, 1962.

47. Novikoff, A. B., Essner, E., and Quintana, N.: Golgi apparatus and lysosomes, Fed. Proc. 23:1010, 1964.

48. Smith, R. E., and Farquhar, M. G.: Lysosome function in the regulation of the anterior pituitary gland, J. Cell Biol. 31:319, 1966.

49. Friend, D. S., and Farquhar, M. G.: Functions of coated vesicles during protein absorption in the rat vas deferens, J. Cell Biol. 35:357, 1967.

50. Wolff, K., and Schreiner, E.: Epidermal lysosomes. Arch. Dermat. 101:276, 1970.

51. Vaughn, R. B., and Trinkaus, J. P.: Movements of epithelial sheets in vitro, J. Cell Sci. 1:407, 1966.
52. Abercrombie, M., and Heaysman, J. E. H.: Observations on the social behavior of cells in tissue culture. II. "Monolayering" of fibroblasts, Exper. Cell Res. 6:293, 1954.
53. Weiss, P.: Specificity in Growth Control, in Butler, E. (ed.): *Biological Specificity and Growth* (Princeton: Princeton Univ. Press, 1955).
54. Charles, A.: An electron microscope study of Darier's disease, Dermatologica 122: 107, 1961.
55. Caulfield, J. B., and Wilgram, G. F.: An electron-microscope study of dyskeratosis and acantholysis in Darier's disease, J. Invest. Dermat. 41:57, 1963.
56. Gottlieb, S. K., and Lutzner, M. A.: Hailey-Hailey disease—an electron microscopic study, J. Invest. Dermat. 54:368, 1970.

This work was performed while Dr. Martinez was a Public Health postdoctoral trainee in dermatology, Boston University Medical Center, and was supported by U.S. Public Health Training Grant No. 5-T-01-AM05295 from the National Institute of Arthritis and Metabolic Diseases.

20

Evaluating the Effects of Hemostatic Agents
on the Healing of Superficial Wounds

David R. Harris, Maj. MC,* and Jerry R. Youkey, Lt. MSC

Superficial surgical wounds are treated with numerous and varied modalities to control blood flow. The more conventional approaches to hemostasis include the application of direct pressure or Gelfoam® to promote clot formation, cauterizing chemicals (silver nitrate, phenol or ferric subsulfate) and the use of electrodesiccation. Recently, two new hemostatic agents, the alkyl-2-cyanoacrylates and topical thrombin, were evaluated as hemostatic superficial wound dressings with favorable results [1–4]. Neither of these modalities has been compared in controlled studies to the more conventional hemostatic methods enumerated above. In such a comparison, one is aware that ferric subsulfate NF (Monsel's solution and electrodesiccation stop bleeding by traumatizing the viable wound bed. However, the mechanisms by which the cyanoacrylates [1, 2], topical thrombin [5], direct pressure or Gelfoam® [6] control bleeding do not rely on tissue injury. We anticipated that this fundamental difference would affect both the rate and quality of wound healing.

The present communication compares the effects of each of these agents on early superficial wound repair.

METHODS AND MATERIALS

Preparation of the Experimental Animal. The domestic pig was selected as the experimental animal because his epidermal architecture and rate of healing closely resemble that of man. The back of a 50-pound animal was shaved with an Oster® heavy duty electric animal clipper. Loose hair was removed and the skin was cleaned with a germicidal soap (pHisoHex®), rinsed with tap water and dried with toweling. General anesthesia was induced with intravenous pentobarbitol and maintained by penthrane® gas (methoxy flurane).

Preparation of Experimental Sites. Thirty-five separate 2.6 × 2 cm. wound sites,

---

*Division of Dermatology, Letterman Army Institute of Research, Presidio of San Francisco, California.

2 cm. equidistant from one another, were mapped symmetrically over the mid-portion of the pig's back and a 0.3 mm. defect was created at each site with a Castroviejo dermatome (Storz Instrument Co.). Each hemostatic agent was applied to five separate wounds in a predetermined random pattern (random numbers table).

Immediately after wounding, the bleeding base was blotted once with coarse mesh gauze and the hemostatic agent was applied. Isobutyl 2-cyanoacrylate (Johnson & Johnson) was sprayed in a thin film for approximately one second. Topical thrombin solution (Parke, Davis and Company) was applied with a syringe at a concentration of 1000 units per ml. by flooding the bleeding site, waiting 10 seconds, and blotting the wound surface dry with coarse mesh gauze. Ferric subsulfate solution NF (Merck and Co.) was swabbed over each wound base with a cotton-tipped applicator. Powdered Gelfoam® (The Upjohn Company) was sprinkled from its container in quantities sufficient to cover the entire wound base. Electrodesiccation was effected by using a "Hyfrecator" (The Birtcher Corporation) on the white outlet at a setting of 50; gently running the needle tip over the entire wound base. Direct pressure was applied by hand for 2 minutes with coarse mesh gauze. Bleeding from the 5 control wounds was allowed to stop spontaneously.

Evaluation. On days 0, 3, 7, 10 and 14 respectively, each wound was photographed and wedge-shaped excisions, approximately 5 × 10 mm., were then obtained using the sharp scalpel technique. Excisions within a single wound site were at least 3 mm. from one another. All specimens were fixed in 10% formalin and processed for light microscopy in the conventional manner. Eight representative, 6 μ thick histological sections from the central portion of each specimen were stained routinely with hematoxylin and eosin and examined for the rate of epidermal migration and degree of maturation, granulation tissue proliferation and for the presence of implants (incorporation of fragments of the hemostatic agent into granulation tissue).

RESULTS

Ferric Subsulfate (Monsel's) Solution

Day 0. Application caused immediate hemostasis by chemical cautery of the wound surface to a depth of 125 μ. This initial injury was clearly identified as a more darkly stained magenta band through the dermis at the wound base.

Day 3. A band of dried collagen underlying the initially cauterized dermis was incorporated into and doubled the thickness of the eschar. Degenerating inflammatory cells were seen to infiltrate the base of this eschar. Epidermis, migrating primarily from wound edges through a cleavage plane below the inflammatory infiltrate, covered less than 20% of the wound base (Fig. 20-1A).

Day 7. Eschar remained unchanged. Epidermal regeneration, now primarily from appendages, was essentially complete. However, the epidermis remained largely undifferentiated, a few layers in thickness with no stratum corneum and few pseudo-rete pegs. Granulation tissue was evident to a depth of 200 μ below the epidermis.

Day 10. Maturation of epidermis with the production of stratum corneum, as well as slight thickening of the dermal scar, had occurred (Fig. 20-1B).

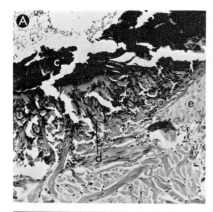

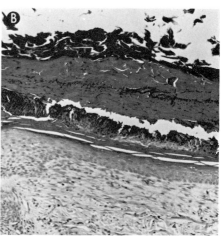

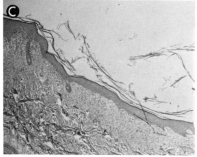

Fig. 20–1.—Ferric subsulfate (Monsel's solution. A, Day 3. A band of dried collagen (*d*) underlies the initially cauterized, densely stained, dermis (*c*). Epidermis is migrating through a cleavage plane below these dermal elements (*e*). × 100. B, Day 10. Epidermal regeneration and differentiation is complete. Note that twice the normal amount of dermal collagen is incorporated into the eschar (approximately 250μ). × 100. C, Day 14. Pseudo-rete-pegs are diminished with granulation tissue proliferation noted to the midreticular dermis. × 35.

Day 14. With desquamation of stratum corneum, the eschar had been shed. Pseudo-rete-pegs were diminished with granulation tissue proliferating to the midreticular dermis (Fig. 20-1C).

Gelfoam® Powder

Day 0. Two or three generous applications of Gelfoam® were necessary at times to stop blood flow. This resulted in an initial coagulum of Gelfoam® powder, serous exudate and masses of red blood cells at the wound surface which appeared on subsequent biopsies as a 300 μ thick surface crust.

Day 3. The original crust had thickened by incorporation of a 200 μ wide band of dermal collagen and masses of inflammatory cells. Early migration, both from wound edges and appendages, was evident, but epithelial tongues remained thin and undifferentiated (Fig. 20-2A).

Day 7. Eschar had thickened slightly, indicating more dermal drying. Epidermis covered 90% of the wound bed and stratum corneum was evident. Granulation tissue proliferated to a depth of 200 μ in the reepithelized zones, but was absent at those points which remained denuded (Fig. 20-2B).

Day 10. Migration was complete, although the epidermis remained thin and fragile. With the first desquamation of stratum corneum, eschar was beginning to lift (Fig. 20-2C).

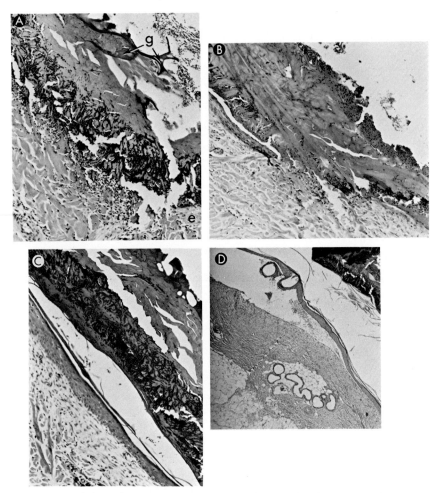

Fig. 20–2.—Gelfoam® powder. **A,** Day 3. Early migration is evident (*e*). Gelfoam fragments are incorporated into dermal eschar (*g*). × 100. **B,** Day 7. Epidermis is covering over 90% of the wound bed. Slight eschar thickening indicates more dermal drying. × 100. **C,** Day 10. Migration is complete, but epidermis remains thin and immature in zones. × 100. **D,** Day 14. Thin sheets of fragile, immature cells are easily separated from underlying granulation tissue. × 35.

Day 14. Zones of hyperplastic epidermis alternated with thin sheets of fragile, immature cells which separated easily from underlying granulation tissue (Fig. 20-2D).

Thrombin Solution

Day 0. A solution of 1000 units/ml. stored at 4°C provided effective hemostasis even after 2 weeks of daily use. After wounding, 2 or 3 applications were necessary in each case to control hemorrhage. No immediate crust formation or damage to the wound base was associated with hemostasis.

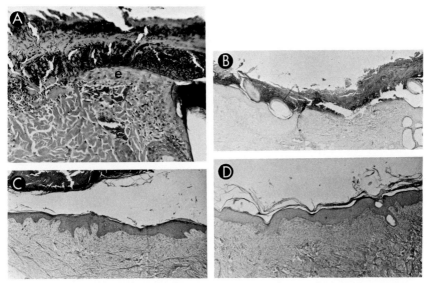

Fig. 20–3.—Topical thrombin solution. **A,** Day 3. A 225μ eschar contains a band of dried collagen and a dense inflammatory infiltrate. Epidermal migration (*e*) covers less than 15% of the base. × 100. **B,** Day 7. Thin, undifferentiated epidermis, migrating primarily from appendages covers 70% of the wound bed. × 35. **C,** Day 10. Hyperplastic epidermis with numerous pseudo-rete-pegs, has migrated completely, covering the defect. × 35. **D,** Day 14. Epidermis remains hyperplastic with zones of fibrosis evident to the midreticular dermis. × 35.

Day 3. A 225 μ eschar had formed containing a band of dried dermis and a dense inflammatory infiltrate. Initial epidermal migration, both from appendageal remnants and from wound edges, covered less than 15% of the base (Fig. 20-3A).

Day 7. Eschar had begun to separate with a strip of thin undifferentiated epidermis, migrating primarily from appendages, covering over 70% of the wound bed (Fig. 20-3B).

Day 10. A hyperplastic epidermis with numerous pseudo-rete-pegs now completely covered the defect. Rather sparse granulations were evidenced from 125 μ to 175 μ below the epidermis (Fig. 20-3C).

Day 14. Eschar was lifting with adequate horny layer formation. The epidermis remained hyperplastic in zones and fibrosis now was evident to the midreticular dermis (Fig. 20-3D).

Electrodesiccation

Day 0. The wound base was desiccated to a depth of 175 μ instantaneously effecting hemostasis.

Day 3. As was seen with Monsel's solution, eschar contained a double layer of dried collagen. Epidermis, migrating both from the wound edges and from avulsed appendages, covered approximately 10% of the wound surface (Fig. 20-4A).

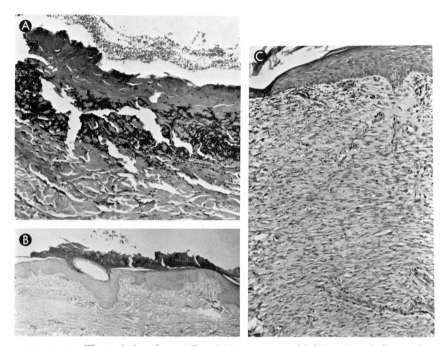

Fig. 20–4.—Electrodesiccation. **A,** Day 3. As was seen with Monsel's solution, eschar contains twice the normal amount of dried collagen. × 100. **B,** Day 7. Epidermis now covers 90% of the defect and shows zones of hyperplasia. × 35. **C,** Day 14. Migration is complete, with maturation of the epidermis continuing. A dense fibrosis is shown completely replacing normal connective tissue to a depth of 275–400μ. × 100.

Day 7. Eschar remained unchanged, while epidermis now covering 90% of the defect showed zones of hyperplasia and a generous stratum corneum (Fig. 20-4B).

Day 10. Migration was now completed, and maturation of the epidermis continued. Underlying granulation tissue was dense in some zones.

Day 14. Sloughed eschar contained appendageal and dermal remnants. A dense fibrosis completely replaced normal connective tissue in most specimens at a depth of 275–400 μ (Fig. 20-4C).

Isobutyl 2-Cyanoacrylate Spray

Day 0. Polymerization of the monomer upon contact with the moist dermal wound base brought immediate hemostasis. The bond between cyanoacrylate and the wound base was so complete that the polymer filled each dermal irregularity. No tissue injury was observed (Fig. 20-5A).

Day 3. Some eschar formed in zones between the wound base and the cyanoacrylate, indicating spotty drying of the wound surface. In these areas, a relatively thin, immature epidermis was estimated to cover 10% of the wound surface. However, in zones devoid of crust where cyanoacrylate remained bonded to the wound bed, no migration was evident. This histologic picture

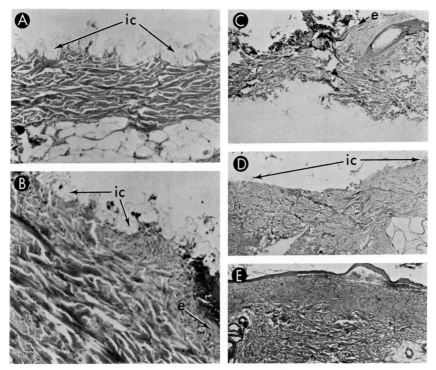

Fig. 20–5.—Butyl 2-cyanoacrylate spray. **A,** Day 0. The monomer (*ic*) polymerizes upon contact, forming a tenacious bond with the wound bed. No dermal injury is noted. × 100. **B,** Day 3. Thin epidermal tongues (*e*) are seen below those areas where eschar had formed between the wound base and the cyanoacrylate. Where the polymer (*ic*) remained bonded, no migration is evident. × 100. **C,** Day 7. In broad zones where cyanoacrylate remains bonded to the wound bed, only spotty migration of epidermis (*e*) is seen. There is no dermal injury or inflammation in these zones. × 35. **D,** Day 10. Re-epithelization is still variable (60–100%). Denuded wound bed is often covered with fragments of firmly adhering cyanoacrylate (*ic*). × 35. **E,** Day 14. Migration is complete. The epidermis remains thin, fragile, and is easily lifted from underlying granulations. × 35.

suggested an association between shedding of the cyanoacrylate, crust formation and epithelial migration (Fig. 20-5B).

Day 7. Spotty eschar formation remained. Extent of reepithelization was variable, from less than 20% to approximately 80% of the wound bed. The association between overlying eschar and underlying epithelial migration remained evident. In zones where the bond between cyanoacrylate and the wound bed remained tenacious, no migration of epidermis was seen, either from the edges or from appendages. Nor was there dermal injury or inflammation in these zones (Fig. 20-5C).

Day 10. Eschar became more confluent as migration proceeded. However, reepithelization was still somewhat variable (60–100%). Denuded wound bed often still had fragments of cyanoacrylate firmly adhering with no inflammatory infiltrate evident at the base (Fig. 20-5D).

Day 14. Migration was complete, but like the Gelfoam® treated wounds, immature epidermis remained so tenuous that it was lifted free from the underlying granulations in every section. Fibrosis was evident to a depth of 200 μ (Fig. 20-5E).

Pressure

Day 0. Welling of blood stopped after applying pressure for 2 minutes, but serous oozing continued for an undetermined time.

Day 3. A 200 μ thick eschar had formed and contained a wide, dense band of inflammatory cells at its base. Immediately beneath this band, migration of epithelium from appendageal remnants was well established (Fig. 20-6A).

Day 7. The scab had thickened and was beginning to lift. It consisted primarily of dried collagen and pyknotic inflammatory cells. Hyperplastic epidermis covered the entire wound surface. A thin band of granulations was seen in the papillary dermis between extensive pseudo-rete-pegs (Fig. 20-6B).

Day 10. Eschar was sloughed. Epidermis showed a well defined granular layer and normal stratum corneum, but remained hypertrophic in most areas. Fibrosis was evident to a depth of 200 μ (Fig. 20-6C).

Fig. 20–6.—Pressure. A, Day 3. Beneath the eschar, migration of epithelium (*e*) from appendageal remnants is well established. × 100. B, Day 7. Hyperplastic epidermis covers the entire wound surface. × 35. C, Day 10. Epidermis shows a well defined granular layer and normal stratum corneum, but remains hypertrophic with many pseudo-rete-pegs evident. × 35. D, Day 14. Scar, evident to a depth of 200μ, remains unchanged, and underlies a well formed but still hyperplastic epidermis. × 35.

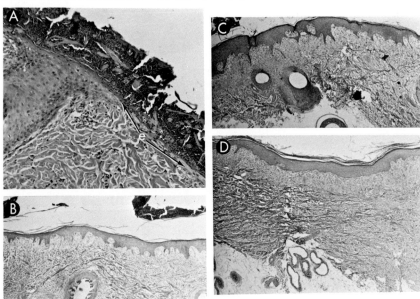

Day 14. Cellular scar remained unchanged and underlies a well formed, but still slightly hyperplastic epidermis (Fig. 20-6D).

Control Wounds

There were no histological differences observed between control wounds and wounds treated with direct pressure.

DISCUSSION

Winter has observed that crust formation at the base of air exposed superficial wounds results in desiccation of a thin layer of dermal tissue at the surface of the wound bed [7]. A band of inflammatory cells migrates into the base of this dried collagen forming a "leukocytic" layer through which migrating epidermis will pass. This dried connective tissue, having been cleaved by the advancing epidermis, becomes incorporated into the overlying eschar. In the present study this sequence of healing did not change regardless of the method of hemostasis used. However, variation was evident in the amount of connective tissue incorporated into eschar, in the rate of migration and maturation of the epidermis, and in the depth of fibrosis over the 14-day trial.

Both the control untreated sites and those wounds treated by application of pressure were completely covered by hyperplastic epidermis by the seventh day. At day 10, as a measure of epidermal differentiation, stratum corneum had been produced and shed in quantities sufficient to cast off eschar. By 14 days, underlying fibrosis, replacing the dermal defect, averaged 200 μ in depth (Figs. 20-6B, C and D).

Although complete migration lagged a day or two, wounds dressed with topical thrombin showed as much epidermal maturation and no more scar at 10 to 14 days than the control and pressure treated sites (Figs. 20-3C and D). This was not surprising. Topical thrombin (bovine origin) causes no tissue injury or does it interfere in any way known with normal reepithelization. It clots the fibrinogen of the blood directly. A concentration of 1000 units/ml. is capable of clotting an equal volume of blood in less than one second [5]. Stallings and Wilson [3] carefully removed this clot by gentle blotting after applying topical thrombin to split-thickness skin donor sites in humans. These authors were impressed by the virtual absence of pain after 24 hours and noted repair rates comparable to those observed in the present study.

Gelfoam® is a partially denatured skin gelatin and its hemostatic action is achieved through the release of thromboplastin within the sponge (or powder) to produce a blood clot [6]. In the present study, Gelfoam® treated sites showed a rate of epithelization comparable to wounds treated by pressure and with thrombin. However, with Gelfoam® the epidermis still remained thin, immature and fragile at 14 days and showed little of the hyperplasia seen with pressure and thrombin (Fig. 20-2D). Clinically, this observation may be irrelevant. Hagstrom *et al.* [6] sprinkled a 5 to 10 mm. layer of Gelfoam® over human donor sites observing, as Stallings did with thrombin [3], that patients were relatively pain free. Both these authors noted also that neither thrombin nor Gelfoam® impeded or accelerated the rate of superficial wound healing in man. Nor were resulting scars judged to differ cosmetically from those of untreated donor sites.

Nonetheless, in the present study thrombin offered two clear advantages—hemostatic action was consistently superior to Gelfoam® while migration and the maturation of the epidermis approximated that of the control and pressure treated sites.

Surprisingly, we found that wounds treated with either electrodesiccation or with ferric subsulfate (Monsel's) solution NF showed no more lag in reepithelization than the control or the thrombin and pressure treated sites. When the wound bed was initially cauterized by ferric subsulfate solution NF or dehydrated with the desiccating current, approximately 225 μ to 400 μ of dried connective tissue was eventually incorporated into eschars. This net loss in dermal wound bed averaged twice that identified in the scabs at either the control sites or in the wounds of all the other modalities evaluated, including cyanoacrylate (Figs. 20-1A and 20-4A). The finding of a deeper dermal injury in ferric subsulfate treated and electrodesiccated wounds suggests that a longer period would be necessary for complete reepithelization. Previously, Winter [8] had pointed out that with forced air drying of the wound surface, a much deeper layer of dermal tissue is dehydrated. This injury forces epidermal cells to migrate vertically down the wound edge before moving horizontally through the dermal tissue below the artificially created dry layer. While forced air drying may be directly analogous to pretreatment with chemical cautery or electrodesiccation, we found that the bulk of our regenerated epithelium was contributed, not from wound edges, but from appendages. Thus, when we consider migratory rate, it appears to matter little whether 150 or 400 μ of connective tissue bed is incorporated into the crust of a superficial wound, as long as viable appendageal remnants remain below. This view is consistent with the observations of Sawhney et al. [9] who found epithelization time consistent irrespective of the thickness of the split graft removed.

However, the cosmetic appearance of wounds treated with these destructive modalities has not been compared clinically with the other hemostatic methods evaluated here. We did note that the granulation tissue replacing the dermal defect in wounds treated either by cautery or by desiccation averaged 120–130 μ in depth greater than those treated with non-destructive modalities (Fig. 20-4C). Since normal dermis does not regenerate, this deeper level of fibrosis probably reflects nothing more than the net loss of connective tissue. Resulting scars either should be clinically less pleasing than those treated with nondestructive modalities or should take a longer period of time to remodel. This point needs clarification with controlled observations.

The higher homologues of the alkyl 2-cyanoacrylates polymerize rapidly, forming adherent films when applied to moist living tissue [1]. With the application of isobutyl 2-cyanoacrylate in the present study, polymerization resulted in instantaneous hemostasis, as well as the most clinically pleasing wounds which showed little crust formation over the first 10 days. However, biopsies revealed a lag in epithelization averaging 3 to 7 days wherever the cyanoacrylate remained in close adherence to the underlying wound bed (Figs. 20-5B, C and D). This finding confirmed the previous observations of Ousterhout et al. [2], who applied higher homologues of alkyl 2-cyanoacrylate to split-thickness wounds in minipigs. These authors found a similar lag, with control wounds epithelizing in 6 to

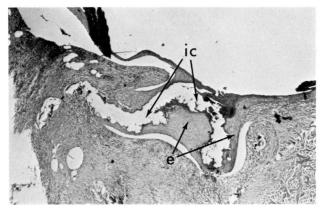

Fig. 20–7.—In cyanoacrylate covered, deep punch biopsy wounds, epidermis (*e*) migrating from the wound edges is diverted to form a new cleavage plane around cyanoacrylate (*ic*) fragments at the wound base. × 35.

12 days vs. 15 to 21 days for the cyanoacrylate treated sites. In the present study, isobutyl cyanoacrylate treated wounds closed by 14 days, but the regenerated epidermis remained poorly differentiated and fragile in comparison to other wounds. Ousterhout suggested that the intimate bond to underlying structures formed by the cyanoacrylate might have mechanically retarded epithelization. Our finding, associating migrating epithelium with overlying scab, which presumably formed where the cyanoacrylate cracked or flaked off, supports this concept. Moreover, we recently evaluated this material in deep dermal punch wounds [10]. Biopsies here showed epidermis migrating from wound edges, and then being diverted to form a cleavage plane around the closely adhering fragments of cyanoacrylate at the wound base (Fig. 20-7).

Certainly, cyanoacrylate must offer a mechanical impediment when it forms such a tenacious, flexible band that no dermal drying is seen for over one week, as was the case in some of our wounds. However, we are not suggesting that dermal drying serves to stimulate migration. This concept is contrary to findings from the domestic pig studies of Winter [8] and Harris and Keefe [11] and the work in humans of Hinman and Maibach [12]. These authors showed that occlusive membranes prevent drying and improve the rate of reepithelization in both superficial and deep dermal wounds. All of these observations merely demonstrate the necessity for a moist plane of migration, whether it be at the base of dried and separating connective tissue or on the surface of an occluded wound bed.

While Ousterhout *et al.* [1] noted cyanoacrylate implants in 6 of 20 biopsies during their clinical trials, we found no dermal implants in our split-thickness domestic pig wounds. Ousterhout's group applied cyanoacrylate with a modified Paasche spray gun using ultra-high purity nitrogen as the propellent. It is possible that this system provided too much pressure and acted as a dermojet, imparting some cyanoacrylate fragments into the mid-dermis. In the present study, cyanoacrylate was deposited only at the surface of the superficial wound bed and was shed completely with the scab. Our propellent was in standard pressurized spray cans of the type used in most commercially available cosmetics.

It is possible also that the domestic pig possesses a dermal bed which is more resistant to surface implantation than the human. This possibility needs investigation.

The future of the higher alkyl 2-cyanoacrylate homologues in the treatment of superficial wounds remains undetermined. On the one hand, clinical trials have shown only minor differences between cyanoacrylate treated and control donor sites both in the healing time necessary for separation of eschar and in the long term cosmetic appearance of the wound site [1]. At the same time, this material, in spray form, offers convenient and extraordinary effective hemostasis and patients experience much greater comfort throughout the period of healing. Furthermore, numerous investigators have offered no evidence of systemic toxicity from cyanoacrylate implants [1, 2, 4, 13].

On the other hand, the higher cyanoacrylate homologues are slowly absorbed, degraded and metabolized [14, 15]. Does 1 or 2 weeks of discomfort during healing or convenience to the surgeon justify possible long term implantations? Until a standard system of delivery causing no dermal implantation is developed and validated, routine use of cyanoacrylates in the treatment of superficial wounds cannot be justified.

Our observations suggest that topical thrombin solution provides the most acceptable hemostatic dressing of any we evaluated. With this material, early reepithelization and epidermal maturation were not impaired, nor was there injury to the wound bed. Moreover, a solution, once mixed, remains active for at least two weeks when stored at 4°C. Thus, in a concentration of 1000 units/ml., topical thrombin provides a consistently effective and inexpensive hemostatic agent.

The effects of this preparation and other hemostatic modalities on deep dermal wounds will be the subject of a future communication.

SUMMARY

Superficial cutaneous wounds were created in a young domestic pig with a dermatome. Hemostasis was effected in individual groups of wounds by electrodesiccation and by applying ferric subsulfate (Monsel's) solution NF, powdered Gelfoam®, topical thrombin solution, isobutyl 2-cyanoacrylate spray and direct pressure. Biopsies taken at days 0, 3, 7, 10 and 14 following application were evaluated histologically for the rate of epidermal migration and the degree of maturation, granulation tissue proliferation and for the presence of implants.

Wounds showing most rapid reepithelization and epidermal differentiation with the least underlying fibrosis were treated either with topical thrombin, or by applying direct pressure. Rate and quality of healing in these wounds approximated that seen in control wounds, where bleeding was allowed to stop spontaneously. Gelfoam® treated sites healed as quickly as controls but displayed a less mature, more fragile epidermis.

On contact, electrodesiccation immediately dehydrated and Monsel's solution chemically cauterized connective tissue at the base of wounds. These injuries, not seen on application of other hemostatic agents, resulted in a net loss of dermal wound bed averaging twice that of all the other modalities evaluated. While there was no lag in epidermal migration, these deeper dermal injuries were associated with more prominent fibrosis at 14 days.

Wounds sprayed with isobutyl 2-cyanoacrylate showed the tenacious polymerized film bonded to broad sections of undamaged dermal bed for the first 7 days after wounding. These zones were crust free, showed no inflammatory reaction and were associated with both delayed epithelial migration for the first 10 days, and a thinner, more fragile epidermis at 14 days. No cyanoacrylate implants were seen.

These histological findings, coupled with the efficient hemostatic action of thrombin, suggest that topical thrombin solution would provide the most effective dressing of any evaluated in this study.

REFERENCES

1. Ousterhout, D. K., Tumbusch, W. T., Margetis, P. M., and Leonard, F.: The treatment of split-thickness skin graft donor sites using n-butyl and n-heptyl 2-cyanoacrylate, Brit. J. Plastic Surg. 24:23, 1971.
2. Ousterhout, D. K., Johnson, E. H., and Leonard, F.: Topical treatment of minipig split-thickness skin graft donor sites using 2-cyanoacrylate homologues, J. S. Res. 10:213, 1970.
3. Stallings, J. O., and Wilson, M. H.: Another way to manage the split-thickness skin donor site, J. Trauma 53A:185, 1971.
4. Bhaskar, S. N., and Cutright, D. E.: Healing of skin wounds with butyl cyanoacrylate, J. Dent. Res. 48:294, 1969.
5. Miller, A. B.: Topical Thrombin (bovine origin), in *Physicians Desk Reference* (Oradell, N.J.: Medical Economic, Inc.).
6. Hagstrom, W. J., Landa, S. J., Elstrom, J. A., Stuteville, O. H., and Beers, M. D.: The use of a hemostatic agent as a definitive dressing in the management of the donor site in partial thickness skin grafting, Plast. & Reconstruct. Surg. 39:628, 1967.
7. Winter, G. D.: Formation of the scab and the rate of epithelization of superficial wounds in the skin of the young domestic pig, Nature 193:293, 1962.
8. Winter, G. D.: Effect of air drying and dressings on the surface of a wound, Nature 197:91, 1963.
9. Sawhney, C. P., Subbarajir, G. V., and Chakravarte, R. N.: Healing of donor sites of split skin grafts. An experimental study in pigs, Brit. J. Plast. Surg. 22:359, 1969.
10. Harris, D. R., and Youkey, J. R.: Evaluating the effects of hemostatic agents in wound healing. II. Deep wounds (In preparation).
11. Harris, D. R., and Keefe, R. L.: A histologic study of gold leaf treated experimental wounds, J. Invest. Dermat. 52:487, 1969.
12. Hinman, C. D., and Maibach, H. I.: Effect of air exposure and occlusion on experimental human skin wounds, Nature 200:377, 1963.
13. Woodward, S. C., Hermann, J. B., Cameron, J. L., Brandes, G., Pulaski, E. J., and Leonard, F.: Histotoxicity of cyanoacrylate tissue adhesive in the rat, Ann. Surg. 162:113, 1965.
14. Reynolds, R. C., Fassett, D. W., Astill, B. D., and Casarett, L. J.: Absorption of methyl-2-cyanoacrylate-2-HC from full-thickness skin incisions in the guinea pig and its fate in vivo, J. S. Res. 6:132, 1966.
15. Ousterhout, D. K., and Gladieux, G. V.: Cutaneous absorption of n-alkyl alpha-cyanoacrylate, J. Biomed. Mater. Res. 2:157, 1968.

21

Wound Healing in a Patient with Darier's Disease: Preliminary Observations

Gary L. Peck, M.D.* and Peter M. Elias, M.D.*

Keratosis Follicularis (Darier's disease) is an uncommon, chronic genodermatosis of unknown etiology beginning in childhood with predilection for intertriginous areas. The primary lesion is a brownish-red keratotic follicular papule. Multiple lesions may form with involvement of the interfollicular epidermis. The clinical course is variable with seasonal exacerbations making therapy difficult to evaluate. Vitamin A in large doses however is reportedly effective in some patients [1]. The characteristic histology includes suprabasalar lacunae, acantholysis, and premature individual cell keratinization ("corps rounds"). Other frequently encountered changes include acanthosis, basal proliferation of rete ridges, and papillomatosis [2].

During studies in which dermatome strips were taken from a patient with Darier's disease, it was found that sites involved with active disease appeared to heal faster than uninvolved skin. Experiments were then undertaken to determine whether the more rapid healing might be due to accelerated epidermal migration following injury and to study the effect of experimental wounding on the clinical course of both involved and uninvolved skin.

METHODS

Dermatome Stripping. Strips of skin were taken from a 62-year-old female patient with Darier's disease using a Castroviejo ophthalmologic keratotome (Storz Instrument Co.). Strips were approximately 2 cm. in width, 5 cm. in length and 0.2 mm. thick, determined by using a 0.2 mm. spacer in the shaving head. Sites included several areas of the back, upper abdomen and hips. Bleeding was controlled with pressure only. Telfa gauze dressings were used for one to two days, and no other topical therapy was applied. The wounds were then left open, measured and photographed daily.

Incisional Wound Healing. Multiple linear incisions, approximately one cm. in

---

*Department of Dermatology, National Institutes of Health, Bethesda, Maryland.

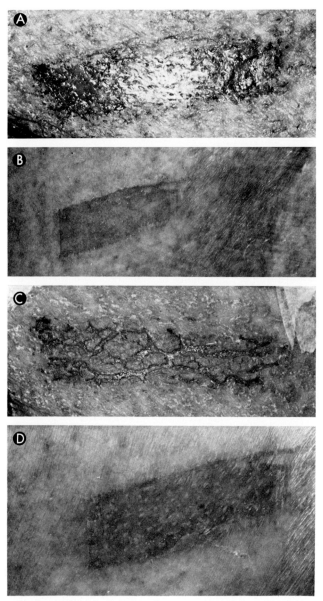

Fig. 21–1.—A, dermatome stripped site from involved skin on left hip, one day after stripping. Epithelial migration has begun from the wound margins and results in an irregular border. B, dermatome stripped site from uninvolved skin one day after stripping. Signs of epithelial migration are not visible. C, dermatome stripped, involved skin, 3 days after stripping. Thick epithelium, derived from both the wound margins and wound bed, has almost completely covered the wound site. D, dermatome stripped, uninvolved skin, 3 days after stripping. A very thin translucent layer of epithelium covers this site. Several islands of follicular epithelium are clearly visible.

length, were made in diseased skin areas of the right anterior forearm and in clinically uninvolved skin of the left anterior forearm. Because the involved skin surface is more irregular than uninvolved skin, and because the epidermis is variably thickened in dermatoses such as Darier's disease, the standard blade guard device can not be used to ensure equal depth of incisions [3]. We, therefore, chose minimal capillary bleeding as a measure of comparability of incision depth. Telfa gauze was the only dressing employed. Four mm. punch biopsies were taken at zero time, and 3, 6, 12, 18, 24, 48 and 72 hours after wounding. Each biopsy was divided transversely to the wound into two approximately equal pieces. One piece was fixed in cold phosphate-buffered glutaraldehyde, post-fixed in osmium tetroxide, imbedded in Epon 812, and 1–2 μ thick sections were stained with Azure II-methylene blue. The other half was routinely fixed in formaldehyde and imbedded in paraffin prior to sectioning and staining. Sections were cut coronally to the incision.

RESULTS

Dermatome Stripping. Involved sites healed more rapidly than uninvolved skin following dermatome stripping (Fig. 21-1). Two weeks after stripping, the uninvolved site remained larger and more erythematous than the involved site. Furthermore, a zone approximately 10 cm. wide of previously diseased skin around stripped sites on the left hip was observed to have clinically regressed by this time. Clinical regression of involved skin surrounding dermatome stripped sites was repeatedly observed (Fig. 21-2).

Five months after the initial stripping experiment, the patient had a generalized exacerbation of her disease, which spared previously dermatomed sites of *uninvolved* skin (Fig. 21-3). Clinically, the uninvolved stripped sites are now hypopigmented and slightly atrophic. Histologically, the epidermis and pilosebaceous apparatus appear normal except for diminution of the rete ridge pattern and flattening of the papillary dermis.

Incisional Wound Healing. The sequential histologic changes of involved and uninvolved skin following incisional wounds are illustrated in Figure 21-4. Wounds in involved sites healed faster than those in uninvolved skin.

DISCUSSION

Our observations indicate that the accelerated wound healing in involved skin of Darier's disease may be related to rapid epidermal migration. In fact, the whole process of epidermal repair including epidermal cell migration, mitosis and transit time [4] and differentiation, may be accelerated in Darier's disease. Since the results reported here represent preliminary work on a single patient with Darier's disease, interpretations must be made with appropriate caution. Future efforts should be directed toward confirming these data in other patients with Darier's disease. In addition, more information about the events occurring during early wound healing probably could be obtained by more frequent biopsies between the sixth and twelfth hours after incision. Psoriasis and lamellar ichthyosis, other diseases characterized by increased rates of epidermal DNA synthesis,

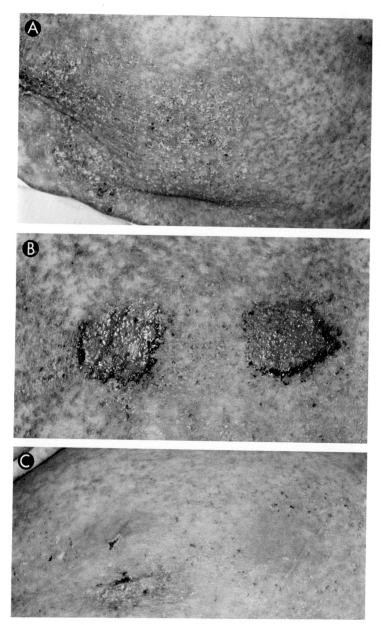

Fig. 21–2.—A, Darier's disease of upper abdomen prior to dermatome stripping. B, upper abdomen one day after dermatome stripping. C, upper abdomen three weeks after dermatome stripping. The diseased skin surrounding the stripped sites has healed.

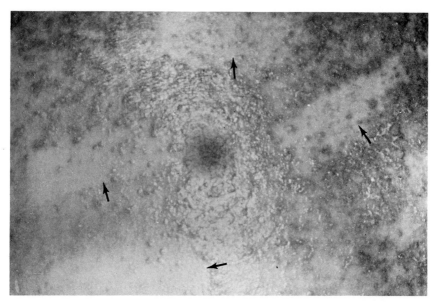

Fig. 21–3.—Upper back, five months after dermatome stripping of uninvolved skin. Recurrent Darier's disease almost completely spares dermatome stripped sites (*arrows*).

might be similarly examined for accelerated rates of wound healing in involved skin.

The mechanism whereby dermatome stripping is followed by a prolonged clinical remission in our patient with Darier's disease is unknown, especially since trauma is usually regarded as an aggravating factor in exacerbating dermatologic diseases, such as psoriasis and lichen planus. This discrepancy may be due to the fact that our work describes trauma to *involved* skin in Darier's disease, and the isomorphic response describes the appearance of a lesion following trauma to *uninvolved* skin [5]. This phenomenon along with our final observation that the dermatome stripped sites of *uninvolved* skin remained disease free during a generalized exacerbation are in accord with the finding that electrodesiccation and curettage are effective as a treatment for Darier's disease [6].

SUMMARY

Dermatome strips were taken from a patient with Darier's disease at involved and uninvolved sites. Involved sites healed considerably faster than uninvolved sites. Accelerated healing could be due to a more rapid epidermal migration because superficial linear incisions healed more quickly in involved sites (12 hours) than in uninvolved sites (48 hours). Additional findings included: (1) disease-free dermatome stripped sites remained free of disease when a generalized flare surrounded these sites five months later and (2) on five occasions Darier's disease surrounding dermatome stripped diseased sites clinically regressed within two to three weeks of stripping.

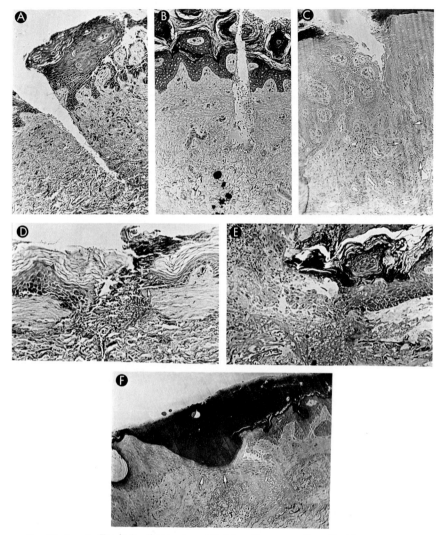

Fig. 21–4.—A, Darier's disease immediately after wounding. Incision extends into papillary dermis. Azure II. × 25. **B,** uninvolved skin immediately after wounding. Incision extends into papillary dermis. PAS. × 25. **C,** Darier's disease 12 hours after wounding. Epithelialization is complete (*arrows*). No migration was seen prior to 12 hours. Azure II. × 25. **D,** uninvolved skin 12 hours after wounding. No epithelial migration is seen (*arrows*). Azure II. × 25. **E,** uninvolved skin 24 hours after wounding. A wedge of epidermal cells has begun to migrate beneath the overlying crust. Azure II. × 100. **F,** uninvolved skin 48 hours after wounding. Epithelialization is complete (*arrows*). Azure II. × 100.

REFERENCES

1. Burgoon, C. F., Graham, J. H., Urbach, F., *et al.*: Effects of Vitamin A on epithelial cells of skin, Arch Derm. 87:63, 1963.
2. Pinkus, H., and Mehregan, A. H.: *A Guide to Dermato-Histopathology* (New York: Appleton-Century-Crofts, 1969).
3. Viziam, C. B., Matoltsy, A. G., and Mescon, H.: Epithelialization of small wounds, J. Invest. Dermat. 43:499, 1964.
4. Frost, Phillip: Unpublished data.
5. Farber, E. M., Roth, R. J., Aschheim, E., *et al.*: Role of trauma in isomorphic response in psoriasis, Arch. Dermat. 91:246, 1965.
6. Shelley, W. B., Arthur, R. P., and Pillsbury, D. M.: A view of keratosis follicularis (Darier's Disease) as a neoplastic process, Arch. Derm. 80:332, 1959.

Index